Becoming a CBT Therapist

Whilst there are many texts that introduce trainees to the overarching theory, formulations, and interventions used in Cognitive Behavioural Therapy (CBT), few describe the lived experience of being a CBT therapist and of making it through training. *Becoming a CBT Therapist* takes prospective trainees on a journey from applying for a place on a training course through to navigating the challenges of CBT training and developing in their career once qualified.

Featuring contributions from experienced CBT tutors, supervisors, and practicing therapists, this book is the first to detail the practical, emotional, and psychological challenges of embarking upon and sustaining a career in this field. From adjustment to learning new skills, to the role transition from their existing role and identity, through to the practicalities of how to demonstrate competence during their training, the book covers an array of topics which are a must-read for aspiring CBT therapists. The chapters offer practical advice for developing a range of key skills, such as how to succeed at interviews, maintain a work–study–life balance, and deal with imposter syndrome.

Packed full of vignettes and reflective exercises, this book is a must-read for those looking to apply for CBT training, currently undertaking training, or involved in supporting trainees through the various challenges they will encounter.

Jason Roscoe is Course Director for the CBT training programmes at Bangor University. He has previously worked as a senior lecturer in CBT at the University of Cumbria and as course accreditation manager for the British Association for Behavioural and Cognitive Psychotherapies (BABCP). He has published research on CBT training and supervision and also operates a small private practice.

'Training in CBT can be rewarding yet daunting. The pressures on novice therapists to demonstrate competence with standard protocols while delivering good outcomes is considerable. This new volume will be a valuable vade mecum for therapists in training. Written in an accessible style with useful tips and clinical illustrations, I predict it will become essential reading for all those setting out on their path as cognitive behaviour therapists.'

Dr Stirling Moorey, *BABCP President Elect, CBT therapist, trainer and supervisor*

'A personal, honest and reflective account of the pathway to becoming a CBT therapist, which encompasses the broad scope and landscape of current CBT practice. Full of practical, encouraging guidance, with clear illustrative examples to prepare and engage trainees – a must read for any aspiring CBT Therapists!'

Katy Emerson, *Lecturer in Cognitive Behavioural Therapy, Cardiff University*

'This book is a must for everyone considering a career in CBT. Providing a clear and helpful insight into the journey that one must follow to become a therapist, from contemplating this challenge, including the pathway they have to follow along with the potential pitfalls that they are likely to encounter. The book offers very useful tips on how to survive training and beyond and is an essential companion for anyone embarking on the beautiful journey of training as a CBT therapist.'

Arlinda Hasani, *Clinical Lead, Talking Therapies, Derby*

'This book offers a wealth of highly relevant advice and guidance to accompany the journey from being a trainee through to establishing oneself as a newly qualified CBT Therapist. It offers pragmatic wisdom and guidance, with authors sharing their authentic experiences of CBT training and practice. This book will be an invaluable aid to CBT therapists over the course of their training and subsequent qualified practice. It will also be a key resource qualified therapists can continue to refer to as they grow and develop throughout their career.'

Dr Mathew Horrocks, *Assistant Professor of Mental Health and Psychological Therapies, University of Nottingham*

Becoming a CBT Therapist

Thriving in Training and Beyond

Edited by Jason Roscoe

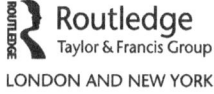
Routledge
Taylor & Francis Group

LONDON AND NEW YORK

First published 2025
by Routledge
4 Park Square, Milton Park, Abingdon, Oxon OX14 4RN

and by Routledge
605 Third Avenue, New York, NY 10158

Routledge is an imprint of the Taylor & Francis Group, an informa business

British Library Cataloguing-in-Publication Data
A catalogue record for this book is available from the British Library

Library of Congress Cataloging-in-Publication Data
Names: Roscoe, Jason, editor.
Title: Becoming a CBT therapist : thriving in training and beyond / edited by Jason Roscoe.
Other titles: Becoming a cognitive behavioral therapy therapist
Description: Abingdon, Oxon ; New York, NY : Routledge, 2025. | Includes bibliographical references and index.
Identifiers: LCCN 2024046034 (print) | LCCN 2024046035 (ebook) | ISBN 9781032550060 (hardback) | ISBN 9781032550053 (paperback) | ISBN 9781003428527 (ebook)
Subjects: MESH: Cognitive Behavioral Therapy—education | Psychotherapists—education | Vocational Guidance
Classification: LCC RC489.C63 (print) | LCC RC489.C63 (ebook) | NLM WM 18 | DDC 616.89/1425—dc23/eng/20241209
LC record available at https://lccn.loc.gov/2024046034
LC ebook record available at https://lccn.loc.gov/2024046035

ISBN: 978-1-032-55006-0 (hbk)
ISBN: 978-1-032-55005-3 (pbk)
ISBN: 978-1-003-42852-7 (ebk)

DOI: 10.4324/9781003428527

Typeset in Times New Roman
by Apex CoVantage, LLC

Contents

24   **From surviving to thriving: going the distance as
     a CBT therapist**   291

JASON ROSCOE

Afterword   295

LUCY HALE

Contributors

Shah Alam is a clinical psychologist, a British Association for Behavioural and Cognitive Psychotherapies (BABCP)-accredited CBT therapist, and a visiting lecturer from East London. He developed the Valued Voices Mentoring scheme, which looks to support racially minoritised aspiring clinical psychologists, and is the co-chair of the BABCP Equality and Culture Special Interest Group (SIG).

Jessica Baines is a high-intensity CBT therapist working for an NHS Talking Therapies Service part-time and has recently set up a private practice. Prior to high-intensity training, Jessica was a senior psychological wellbeing practitioner (PWP) and supervisor.

Natalia Barnes is a lecturer and a self-practice/self-reflection (SP/SR) lead at the University of East Anglia. Her main current focus is on helping other therapists work on their own experiences and use techniques on themselves to help them develop in their personal and professional lives.

Jo Anne Bates is a high-intensity CBT therapist in an NHS Talking Therapies for Anxiety and Depression Service. Jo Anne's clinical and research interests include the impact of the therapist on the effectiveness of therapy and the use of imagery across disorders.

Tobyn Bell is a compassion-focused therapy trainer, supervisor, and psychotherapist and is part of the training committee for the Compassionate Mind Foundation. He is currently employed as a lecturer and operational lead in the School of Health Science at the University of Manchester.

Denika Campbell-Lee is a clinical psychologist who completed her doctorate degree and graduated from Newcastle University in 2023.

Anjali Mehta Chandar is a lecturer at the Charlie Waller Institute, University of Reading, and runs a private practice, Brighter Life Therapy, working with children and adults in both community and school settings. She has a passion for supporting autistic young people with depression and anxiety.

Elaine Davies is a counsellor and CBT therapist. Elaine is also a BABCP Fellow, Chair of the BABCP Supervision SIG, and Secretary for the BABCP EDI Committee.

Ashley Fulwood has been working for the national charity OCD-UK since 2004, which he co-founded. During the last 19 years, he has worked to offer a voice for people affected by OCD and to offer advice, support, and, most importantly, hope through the difficult times. He is also the co-author of the book *FAQs on OCD*, which was published in 2022.

Lucy Hale is a chartered clinical psychologist and a BABCP-accredited practitioner and trainer. Lucy currently works as Academic Director on the Doctorate of Clinical Psychology Training Programme at King's College London. She has been involved in training clinical psychologists for over eight years and developed and led a pathway to BABCP accreditation on a clinical psychology programme for several years.

Andrew Haley is a cognitive behavioural therapist, a cognitive analytic therapy practitioner, and an Eye Movement Desensitisation and Reprocessing (EMDR) practitioner. He works in a Step 3+ NHS Talking Therapies Service.

Laura Hamill currently works as a cognitive behavioural therapist within a Talking Therapies service in Lancashire. Laura has a particular interest in trauma, perinatal mental health, and the use of compassion-focused chair work.

Taf Kunorubwe is a BABCP-accredited CBT therapist, supervisor, and trainer. He has also led Low-Intensity CBT (LICBT) and CBT training courses in Wales. Currently, he works part-time in private practice with a special interest in enhancing access and outcomes for clients from diverse backgrounds.

Allán Laville is Professor of Equity in Psychology and teaches clinical psychology at the School of Psychology and Clinical Language Sciences (SPCLS), University of Reading. Allán is a National Teaching Fellow and Senior Fellow of the Higher Education Academy, an Associate Fellow of the British Psychological Society (BPS), Co-Chair of the Equity, Equality, Diversity and Inclusion Committee, and a member of the Scientific Programme Advisory Group for the BABCP. He is also a member of the BPS Equality, Diversity, and Inclusion Strategic Board.

Gavin Lawton is a BABCP-accredited cognitive behavioural therapist. Gavin has worked across community psychosis services and between 2017 and 2023 worked at the University of Hull as Programme Director for the CBT portfolio before returning to Rotherham Doncaster and South Humber NHS Trust in 2023 as Lead Psychological Professional for the Acute Care Service.

Rebecca Light is a BABCP-accredited cognitive behavioural therapist and EMDR therapist and has worked in a range of child and youth mental health services within the NHS for the past 22 years, offering CBT for Children and Young People and supervision.

Julia Limper-Menapace is a cognitive behavioural therapist in private practice and a lecturer and programme director on the Postgraduate Diploma in high-intensity CBT course at the University of Reading. Her passion lies in destigmatising practitioner lived experience of mental health difficulties and implementing SP/SR techniques to improve practitioner wellbeing and promote more effective practice.

Jim Lucas is a BABCP-accredited cognitive behavioural therapist, supervisor, and teaching fellow on the CBT Postgraduate Programme at the University of Birmingham. He is an association for contextual behavioral science (ACBS) peer-reviewed acceptance and commitment therapy trainer and founder of Openforwards CBT & Counselling, a Birmingham-based psychology practice offering evidence-based psychotherapies.

Natalie Meek is Lecturer in Clinical Psychology at the University of Reading in the Charlie Waller Institute and has a private practice working as a cognitive behavioural psychotherapist with a special interest in supporting clients living with long-term physical health conditions. Natalie is bisexual and disabled and passionate about ensuring that training and therapy are accessible to all.

Helen Moya is a chartered psychologist and an accredited cognitive behavioural therapist. She was Course Director of a CBT training programme for six years and has practised CBT in different services and independently. Helen runs a private practice, Moya CBT, where she offers CBT treatment for clients, clinical supervision, and career advice for those interested in becoming or developing as a CBT therapist.

Joanne Myers is a CBT therapist with over a decade of experience using guided self-help and CBT to help people with common mental health difficulties. She offers freelance clinical training and recently started conducting group supervision.

Cheryl Nicholls is a cognitive behavioural therapist and the deputy service manager for the NHS Blackpool Talking Therapies Service. Cheryl was a PWP and a senior PWP prior to undertaking her CBT training.

Sam Palin is a cognitive behavioural therapist working for impact on Teesside. Sam studied at Northumbria University and obtained a BSc in psychology and an MSc in health psychology. Sam has a keen clinical interest in Post-Traumatic Stress Disorder (PTSD)/Trauma and in particular childhood emotional neglect.

Jessica Palmer is a BABCP-accredited cognitive behavioural therapist working at Think Wellbeing Wigan, part of Greater Manchester Mental Health NHS Trust.

Vickie Presley is a BABCP-accredited CBT therapist and supervisor and Course Director for the Postgraduate Diploma in Cognitive Behavioural Therapy at Coventry University. Vickie's research activities to date have focused on therapist factors, including the relationship between therapist schemas, professional development, and therapeutic outcomes in CBT.

Alex Preston is Course Lead for the high-intensity CBT programmes at Keele and Staffordshire Universities. He is also a fully accredited therapist and supervisor, working clinically within a Talking Therapies service. He specialises in the treatment of obsessive-compulsive disorder and has a keen interest in aspects that improve the tolerability of treatment.

Sarah Priestley is a cognitive behavioural psychotherapist and Programme Lead on the Postgraduate Diploma in High Intensity Psychological Interventions (HIPI) at the University of Lincoln. Sarah has worked in various Improving Access to Psychological Therapies (IAPT) services and within non-traditional IAPT settings and has a particular interest in the delivery of clinical supervision within CBT.

Mathew Pugh is a clinical psychologist, cognitive behavioural psychotherapist, advanced schema therapist, and voice dialogue facilitator. He is a teaching fellow and research supervisor at University College London and Lead Resource Developer for Psychology Tools. He also co-directs www.chairwork.co.uk: an international provider of chairwork-related training, supervision, and research.

Jason Roscoe is Course Director for the CBT training programmes at Bangor University. He has previously worked as a senior lecturer in CBT at the University of Cumbria and as course accreditation manager for the British Association for Behavioural and Cognitive Psychotherapies (BABCP). He has published research on CBT training and supervision and also operates a small private practice.

Sarah D. Rees brings over 20 years of experience to the field of mental health and has spent more than a decade successfully running a busy private practice in Cheshire. Founder of the popular Substack community, 'Therapists Corner', Sarah has supported thousands of therapists in establishing and expanding their private therapy practices.

Natasha Scullane is a BABCP-accredited cognitive behavioural therapy (CBT) therapist and supervisor. Natasha has over 15 years' experience working in primary care mental health services in the NHS and has recently started in private practice.

Cassie-Ann Simmonds has worked within secondary care services as a registered mental health nurse and a CBT therapist and has a clinical interest in working with individuals with severe and enduring mental illness.

Heather Howard Thompson is a cognitive behavioural psychotherapist in full-time private practice, and her company Yorkshire Psychotherapy Ltd was established in 2015. She has a particular interest in working with complex trauma and emotional dysregulation, including working with neurodivergent clients.

Sam Thompson is a mental health nurse and BABCP-accredited cognitive behavioural therapist. He has also undertaken a PGDip in clinical supervision. Sam has supervised clinicians with both low- and high-intensity CBT experience and is passionate about improving accessibility to high-quality supervision and training.

Eleanor Vialls is Lecturer in Clinical Psychology at Reading University, delivering training on the PWP, and MSci Applied Psychology courses. Eleanor is a qualified PWP, having completed her training in 2016 and then qualifying as a supervisor in 2018.

Mathew Wilcockson is a CBT therapist, supervisor, trainer, and EMDR consultant of 20 years' experience, currently working in secondary care, specialising in foreign language speakers and somatic presentations. He is also a lecturer on the University of Coventry Postgraduate Diploma in CBT.

Jo Williams is a BABCP-accredited CBT therapist and senior lecturer at Cardiff University. Jo is Programmes Director of both the Postgraduate Certificate and Diploma in CBT and has spearheaded the development of the first Level 2-BABCP-accredited training in Wales.

Acknowledgements

There are many people who have made this book possible, and possibly too many to list here! To Karen Taylor, everything that has taken place in my career would not be possible had you not seen something in me that day! To Rufus Harrington, thanks for your passion and creativity as a tutor and supervisor. To Julie Taylor, Liz Bates, Sue Wilbraham, and Peter Elliot, who have all played a part in giving me the confidence to write. To Will Curvis, who kindly shared his experience of putting together an edited book, and to Grace at Routledge, thank you for believing in the book. To my wife Fran, who has been my number one cheerleader from the beginning, and my dad, who has always encouraged me to give things a go and never be afraid of failing. Finally, to my mum – I know you would have been so proud of me.

Foreword

Sir Isaac Newton is credited with having said, 'If I have seen further, it is by standing on the shoulders of Giants'. The next generation of scientists advances by building on the findings of their predecessors. In the world of therapy, this phrase has been used to describe our indebtedness to those from whom we have learned (both directly and indirectly).

Whilst cognitive behavioural therapy (CBT) is one of the most popular therapies, it is unfortunately difficult to find someone who is a true expert in it. There is a lot to know and a lot to learn, and it can be hard to know where to start. Many CBT trainers, such as myself, look back at our own training and wonder if we could do it all over again, how would we do it differently? We wonder how we could have been more efficient and effective in our training. We wonder about opportunities we took advantage of and those we let slip away. Furthermore, we wonder if we would have made the same career choices had we understood how these systems worked before we entered into them.

Often clinicians who are new to CBT are eager to get more tools for their toolbox, whilst the experienced CBT practitioner recognises that CBT is more than a bag of tricks, but rather a way of thinking. In some ways, CBT is a victim of its own success. Oversimplified and misconstrued ideas such as positive thinking have spread faster and further than the actual therapy. Learning to do CBT well now involves learning the therapy and unlearning some misconceptions. CBT can at times be made into a strawman argument where the theory is misrepresented as being entirely based on distorted cognitions. A good CBT therapist knows that many of our clients' thoughts are at least partially true and that many of the folks we work with are in extremely challenging situations. Similarly, complaints about CBT within what was the Improving Access to Psychological Therapies (IAPT) initiative are often actually indicative of challenges in the NHS in general.

Back when I worked for Dr Aaron T Beck, as one of his CBT trainers, I was lucky enough to watch him demonstrate his skills. It was one of the greatest pleasures of my life. I was always struck by how seamlessly he applied both relationship skills (e.g. empathy, genuineness, humour) and change strategies (e.g. Socratic questioning and problem-solving). Learning to do CBT with both the head and heart is a skill that needs to be cultivated.

I still vividly remember my first time getting high-quality supervision in CBT. It was a wonderful and challenging experience. I remember carefully reviewing my recorded sessions with my supervisor. I remember the amount of vulnerability it required, and I also remember that as I leaned into that discomfort, my skills improved immensely. The people I was working with started getting better at a more rapid rate. It started to click. I started to enjoy it more. I learned how to both make it my own and do it well.

Now, when I work with supervisees, what I often tell them is you get out what you put in. If you are someone who wants to get the most out of your life and experience as a clinician, this book will help you learn how and where to invest your time and effort so that you get the largest return on your investment. The skills it takes to be a CBT practitioner extend beyond the therapy room. There are skills related to understanding the occupational and business side of the practice. There are skills related to managing stress and vicarious trauma. Finally, there are skills related to managing and addressing our own assumptions and expectations. Self-practice and self-reflection are also important parts of this process.

This book is geared towards teaching clinicians who are learning CBT how to think and approach training like a pro. The wisdom in this book can act as a mentor from trainers and clinicians who have been down this path before you. There is an emphasis on practical and experiential methods. The writers are focused on walking you through their own thought process and helping you explore your own. Highly nuanced topics like experiential learning, culturally responsive care, and navigating hiring systems are explored. There is much to learn, and you do not have to reinvent the wheel. Read this book and learn from the collective experiences of other clinicians. If you stand on the shoulders of these giants, you too will see further.

Scott Waltman, PsyD, ABPP
Clinical Psychologist
Author, *Socratic Questioning for Therapists and Counselors: Learn to Think and Intervene like a Cognitive Behavioral Therapist*
President-Elect, Academy of Cognitive & Behavioral Therapies

Preface

Jason Roscoe

What does it mean to be a cognitive behavioural therapist (CBT), and what is it like to work as one? Not only that, how does one survive the training experience and thrive post-qualification? These are questions that have rarely been answered in existing textbooks or research. The key aim of this book is to help you gain a deeper understanding of what it *means* and *takes* to be a CBT therapist.

The concept of this book came to my mind a few years ago, when I was working as a course tutor on what was referred to then as an IAPT course (now Talking Therapies for Anxiety and Depression [TTAD]). For those unsuccessful at interview, I had wanted to point them in the direction of a book that would give them some useful, practical information that they can use to inform their answers to interview questions next time round. I was often surprised about how little trainees knew what they were signing up for when they chose CBT as a career pathway. It also struck me that many of the challenges that came up for trainees in supervision or during lectures were not always addressed by the CBT books that describe the 'how to' aspects of the job.

Written from a UK perspective by an ensemble of highly experienced CBT practitioners, trainers, and researchers, each chapter will describe one of these challenges, offering insight into the lived experience of those who have been there, done it, and got the T-shirt. The wisdom that is contained within this book reaches beyond the confines of TTAD training. As the foreword alludes to, there are universal challenges for those undertaking CBT training that transcend the context of where therapy is delivered.

How to make the best use of this book?

The book is intended to be interactive, encouraging you to make notes as you go along, and uses a combination of personal experiences, case illustrations, tips, and reflective exercises to deepen your understanding of each step towards becoming a CBT therapist. Hopefully, the book takes you on a journey that illustrates what it is like not just to train and work as a CBT therapist across a range of contexts but also to thrive as one despite these challenges.

Book structure

When considering the content and flow of the book, I asked myself one key question, and that was, 'If I was considering a career as a CBT therapist, what things would I want to know up front?' Firstly, I would want to know the environments in which I might gain employment and how I could get there. I would want to know of key literature to read before I attended an interview, and I would want an idea of some of the challenges that lay ahead. These questions informed the first two parts of the book, and the final part answered a second question, 'How might I enhance my skills and progress in my CBT career once qualified?'

The book has therefore been structured in a chronological order, starting with what you need to know before commencing CBT training, through to what it is typically like being on a training course, and concluding with ideas about how one might begin to shape their own identity and career as a CBT therapist.

Some chapters are deliberately longer than others as they address pivotal issues such as readiness for training, quality of supervision, and practising CBT with flexibility and fidelity. Whilst it might be tempting to skip to specific chapters which sound most appealing, I would advise against this. Immerse yourself in the journey that this book will take you on – all that remains for me to say now is, good luck!

Introduction

Jason Roscoe

Getting a place on a cognitive behavioural therapy (CBT) training course can be extremely challenging – preparing for interviews, participating in role-plays, and, in some cases, moving to another part of the UK. Then comes the challenge of letting go of your old ways of working and experiencing the sense of 'conscious incompetence' that comes with learning any new skill. With all this in mind, it is important to spend some time considering, 'is this the right job for me?' This book will help you to answer this and other pertinent questions related to becoming a CBT therapist.

The rise of CBT

Where, at one time, the practice of CBT and the dissemination of its research were dominated by psychologists, it has now become (almost) a profession in its own right. Training to be a CBT therapist is now a popular career choice amongst psychology graduates and those in health and social care roles (many of which are referred to as 'core professions'; BABCP, 2023). In England, this largely relates to the rollout of the adult Improving Access to Psychological Therapies (IAPT) programme in 2008 (Clark, 2011). Across other parts of the UK, CBT is also recommended as one of the first-line treatments for a range of mental health problems (e.g. National Health Service Education for Scotland, NES, 2011; National Psychological Therapies Management Group and Public Health Wales, 2016).

There are now training pathways for applying CBT with children and young people, serious mental health conditions such as eating disorders, and more recently, accreditation pathways within Clinical Psychology Programmes (Daley et al., 2022; HEE, 2019). The demographic of CBT trainees is very broad, and the skills that they start their training with vary considerably (e.g. Liness et al., 2019; Waltman et al., 2017). There are also different motivations for undertaking training, for example, gaining a place on a CBT training course can be a long-held ambition that fits well with how one thinks and how they like to work. For others, the decision to undertake this career pathway might be strongly influenced by the incentive of a higher salary, more favourable shift patterns, or long-term employment prospects (Ball & Corrie, 2024; Roscoe & Wilbraham, 2024).

DOI: 10.4324/9781003428527-1

The absence of statutory regulation

A challenge for those of us concerned with benchmarking the standard of clinical practice is that 'CBT therapist' is not a protected title (Moorey, 2022). In theory, anyone can call themselves one. The absence of statutory regulation of all psychotherapies means that there is no objective definition of the skills and knowledge that are required to be competent in this role. At present, organisations such as the British Association for Behavioural and Cognitive Psychotherapies (BABCP) offer several frameworks (e.g. their minimum training standards and Core Curriculum) for ensuring high standards based on expert consensus and the best available evidence on CBT training (BABCP, 2021, 2023; Muse et al., 2022). Whilst accreditation does not always guarantee therapist competence or fidelity to the evidence base, in this book, we view BABCP accreditation as part of the process of becoming an accountable and credible CBT therapist.

Learning to think and act like a CBT therapist

Whilst there are age-old debates about what is and is not CBT, this book adopts the viewpoint that CBT is both a way of *doing* things and a way of *seeing* things. This transcends specific techniques and models and is governed by a set of shared principles and processes (see Hayes & Hofmann, 2018). In the first edition of her book 'Cognitive Therapy: Basics and Beyond', Judith Beck (1995) outlined ten principles which underpin good practice and might be considered the 'hallmarks' of CBT (e.g. formulation-driven, problem-focused, and structured).

I propose that these principles can be subsumed under three S's that encapsulate how to think and act like a CBT therapist:

- *Style* (how we interact with clients)
- *Stance* (how we view the onset and resolution of mental health problems)
- *Skills* (the techniques and formulations that we apply in clinical practice)

The transition from a previous professional role to that of a competent CBT therapist often involves a change in our *style* of interaction with clients, shifting from advising to eliciting information through guided discovery (Roscoe et al., 2022). In training, we learn theories and methods that help us to make sense of our client's problems in a particular way. For some trainees, this requires a change in how they conceptualise distress and bring about meaningful change – in other words, altering their *stance*. Finally, we learn new *skills* for bringing about symptom amelioration through focused and structured interventions, some of which are transdiagnostic and some which are disorder specific. Some individuals and professional backgrounds appear to influence the speed at which this alteration of style, stance, and skills occurs (Roscoe et al., 2022; Wilcockson, 2020). This book is concerned with helping you, as the reader, to understand the psychological as well as practical processes involved in becoming a CBT therapist.

Overview of Parts I–III

The book starts by helping you to understand the various myths that exist about CBT. People hold all kinds of misconceptions about CBT, and these may influence their decision to train in this modality. For example, some people think that CBT is simple to master because aspects of it are easy to grasp and disseminate (e.g. many mental health professionals use CBT methods such as activity scheduling or thought challenging and will draw out five areas maintenance diagrams). This can lead some to believe that there is little more to learn, and the training experience can be a huge shock to the system! Other chapters in Part I offer practical suggestions on the existing skills and qualifications that are needed to access CBT training, the implications of undertaking this training in various parts of the UK, and tips on how to excel at interviews. Finally, some of the psychological and emotional challenges of training are addressed. Aside from the expected stress that comes with learning a new skill, completing essays, and building a caseload, for those with existing mental health problems, there is the additional consideration of how this will be impacted by the training experience. Training requires us to practise CBT techniques on ourselves or to hear about other life stories that may echo our own painful experiences. It is hoped that by the end of this part, potential applicants can make an informed decision about choosing CBT as a career path.

In Part II, the focus is on how to make the most of your training experience. The chapters in this part will provide the reader with insights from those who have taught or supervised on CBT training courses as well as those who have survived the training. Topics such as how to maximise use of supervision through to the importance of getting out of the clinic room with clients to undertake behavioural experiments are covered. The value of 'shadowing' qualified peers in learning how to convert theory into practice is also discussed. There is also consideration as to the ways in which CBT has historically under-emphasised important aspects of a client's identity and the inherent challenges of belonging to a minority group.

Finally, Part III looks at how novice CBT therapists can begin to expand their toolkit by developing 'meta-competencies' (Roth & Pilling, 2007). During CBT training, there is often considerable focus on the disorder-specific models; however, the capacity to adapt treatment protocols to the individual client is imperative given that many clients present with one of more challenges to treatment. Extensive comorbidity, chronicity, socio-economic disadvantage, multiple relapses, alcohol and substance abuse, and relational difficulties all have the potential to disrupt the implementation of short-term therapy as they are laid out in the manuals (Moloney & Kelly, 2004). This can lead CBT therapists, especially novices, to assume that if therapy is not proceeding as they expect, it is somehow their fault or that CBT is unsuitable for specific populations. This book aims to show that CBT can be adapted in many ways whilst recognising it is not a fix-all approach.

Part III introduces ideas about how to make sessions more experiential, moving away from a reliance upon pen and paper exercises to more emotive and energetic in-session activities such as chair work. There are examples of what it is like to practise CBT in various settings, including specialist services and an invitation for the reader to reflect on how their own beliefs and behaviours can 'get in the way' of providing effective therapy. The book concludes with both a summary of what it takes to thrive as a CBT therapist and a consideration of how the field of clinical psychology training is changing to incorporate a CBT pathway with its associated benefits and challenges.

References

Ball, C., & Corrie, S. (2024). "Bridging the gap": A reflexive thematic analysis of the experiences of therapy trainees transitioning from psychodynamic counselling to cognitive behavioural therapy. *Counselling and Psychotherapy Research, 24*(2), 631–641.

Beck, J. S. (1995). *Cognitive therapy: Basics and beyond.* Guilford press.

British Association for Behavioural and Cognitive Psychotherapies. (2021). *Core curriculum reference document.* https://babcp.com/Core-Curriculum

British Association for Behavioural and Cognitive Psychotherapies. (2023). *BABCP minimum training standards for the practice of cognitive behavioural therapy.* https://babcp.com/Minimum-Training-Standards

Clark, D. M. (2011). Implementing NICE guidelines for the psychological treatment of depression and anxiety disorders: The IAPT experience. *International Review of Psychiatry, 23,* 318–327. https://doi.org/10.3109/09540261.2011.606803

Daley, J., Hale, L., & Patton, B. (2022). Clinical psychology trainees' experiences of following a specialised cognitive behavioural therapy (CBT) pathway accredited by the British association of behavioural and cognitive psychotherapies (BABCP): A pilot evaluation. *Clinical Psychology Forum, 349,* 28–34.

Hayes, S. C., & Hofmann, S. G. (Eds.). (2018). *Process-based CBT: The science and core clinical competencies of cognitive behavioral therapy.* New Harbinger Publications.

Health Education England. (2019). *National curriculum for cognitive behavioural therapy for severe mental health problems.*

Liness, S., Beale, S., Lea, S., Byrne, S., Hirsch, C. R., & Clark, D. M. (2019). The sustained effects of CBT training on therapist competence and patient outcomes. *Cognitive Therapy and Research, 43,* 631–641.

Moloney, P., & Kelly, P. (2004). Beck never lived in Birmingham: Why CBT may be a less useful treatment for psychological distress than is often supposed. *Clinical Psychology,* 4–10.

Moorey, S. (2022). Cognitive behavioral therapy in the United Kingdom. In M. D. Terjesen & K. A. Doyle (Eds.), *CBT in a global context.* Springer.

Muse, K., Kennerley, H., & McManus, F. (2022). The why, what, when, who and how of assessing CBT competence to support lifelong learning. *The Cognitive Behaviour Therapist.* https://doi.org/10.1017/S1754470X22000502

National Health Service Education for Scotland, NES. (2011). *The matrix. Mental health in Scotland: A guide to delivering evidence-based psychological therapies in Scotland.* Retrieved April 15, 2017, from www.nes.scot.nhs.uk/media/20137/Psychology%20Matrix%202013.pdf

National Psychological Therapies Management Group and Public Health Wales. (2016). *Matrics Cymru: The Welsh matrix. A guide to delivering evidence-based psychological therapy in Wales.* Retrieved February 15, 2017, from www.1000livesplus.wales.nhs.uk/matrics-cymru-draft-consultation

Roscoe, J., Bates, E. A., & Blackley, R. (2022). 'It was like the unicorn of the therapeutic world': CBT trainee experiences of acquiring skills in guided discovery. *The Cognitive Behaviour Therapist, 15,* E32. https://doi.org/10.1017/S1754470X22000277

Roscoe, J., & Wilbraham, S. (2024). 'When it goes well, it works fantastically': Motivations to train and their impact on the practice of CBT. *The Cognitive Behaviour Therapist.* https://doi.org/10.1017/S1754470X24000060

Roth, A. D., & Pilling, S. (2007). *The competences required to deliver effective cognitive and behavioural therapy for people with depression and with anxiety disorders.* HMSO, Department of Health.

Waltman, S., Hall, B. C., McFarr, L. M., Beck, A. T., & Creed, T. A. (2017). In-session stuck points and pitfalls of community clinicians learning CBT: Qualitative investigation. *Cognitive and Behavioral Practice, 24*, 256–267.

Wilcockson, M. D. (2020). Transition to cognitive behavioural therapy from different core professional backgrounds: Three grounded theory studies. *The Cognitive Behaviour Therapist, 13*, E35. https://doi.org/10.1017/S1754470X20000331

Part I

Making the switch

Chapter 1

What is a CBT therapist?

Jo Williams

Introduction

What do you think of when someone says they are a cognitive behavioural (CBT) therapist? Do you have an image of Freud sitting near a couch or the look of a stern therapist sitting across a desk from a client, or do you think of a warm, supportive person smiling encouragingly at them?

> ### Reflective exercise
>
> Write down the first three words that come to mind when you think about a CBT therapist.
>   Keep this list to reflect upon at the end of this chapter.

Now let's compare your thoughts to those of some practicing CBT therapists. I asked some colleagues for a definition of what a CBT therapist is. Do these explanations fit with your thoughts?

> '*I help people become more aware of the psychological aspects of their mental health issues, using formulation and monitoring to improve this awareness. I then apply both cognitive and behavioural change methods to work on maintenance factors and more deeply held beliefs to achieve an outcome*'.
>   '*I think there are a lot of misconceptions about what we do: being rigid, modular, disorder led, technique focused. However, principally we help people to understand and modify meaning in relation to their lives. We use psychological theory (behavioural and cognitive) to inform how we make change, but ultimately working with meaning is central to our work*'.
>   '*My primary focus is on helping individuals identify and understand the connections between their thoughts, feelings, and behaviour. I work collaboratively*

DOI: 10.4324/9781003428527-3

with clients to explore and challenge unhelpful thought patterns and beliefs that may contribute to emotional distress or behavioural challenges'. (In addition, this therapist also referred to the 'misconceptions' related to CBT being 'impersonal or uncaring' and that it is considered a 'superficial intervention'.)

Interestingly, the misconceptions of CBT were a theme across most of the responses received, as well as the importance of conceptualisation. A conceptualisation (or formulation) is a technique that CBT therapists use with clients to piece together the puzzle related to the maintenance factors linked to the client's mood. It is a highly beneficial tool (Redhead et al., 2015). The misconceptions of CBT will be brought into this chapter to further explore what a CBT therapist really is. The chapter will achieve this by debunking some of the main myths surrounding CBT for you to receive an honest interpretation of what we do.

What is CBT?

There is so much that we could talk about here; this could be a chapter itself; however, various theorists and researchers have covered these topics in detail. To explore the historical underpinnings of CBT, I'd recommend Rachman (2009) on the evolution of CBT in the book *Science and Practice of Cognitive Behaviour Therapy* (Clark & Fairburn, 2009). Whilst the development of CBT is key to your learning, the aim of this chapter is to give a more personal and experiential feel.

CBT is a talking therapy which is generally a time limited/short-term psychotherapy that typically focuses on current difficulties. Each treatment session is structured to help a client get the most out of it. Within a session, the therapist and client will collaboratively explore and understand the client's difficulties and then use this understanding to work towards the clients' goals using an evidenced-based approach.

CBT proposes that emotions and the resulting physiological sensations are a result of maladaptive beliefs and unhelpful patterns of behaviour. These behaviours keep us safe in the short term but will maintain the difficulties in the long term. See the vignette of Kelly for an example of this practice.

Case vignette: Kelly (Social anxiety)

Kelly is at a busy restaurant for a family birthday. Kelly has thoughts that she is weird/different, that people will not like her, or that she will offend them. Kelly's anxiety rises and she becomes increasingly worried about people being able to notice her anxiety. Kelly thinks she is becoming red, obviously sweating, and starting to shake. Kelly thinks that she will be rejected if people notice how anxious she is or if they realise how weird she is. To stop people noticing, Kelly is sat in a darker corner of the room and the end of the table, playing a game on her phone, avoiding making eye contact or looking at anyone else. Kelly is trying to avoid people speaking to her, but the more she keeps away, the more Kelly's beliefs about being weird are reinforced, because no one is speaking to her. Kelly's anxiety would rise if someone came and spoke to her so avoiding people keeps Kelly's anxiety manageable in the short term. However, in the long term this maintains Kelly's anxiety because she doesn't have the opportunity to disconfirm her unhelpful thoughts and test out what would happen if she was to speak to someone.

Formulation is key

A CBT therapist would often start by putting this information that Kelly has provided into a 'hot cross bun' model (Padesky & Greenberger, 1995) or might opt to go straight into disorder-specific formulation (e.g. Clark & Wells, 1995). By being able to learn ways to better manage the unhelpful thoughts and behaviours, people can reduce the intensity/duration or frequency of their mood difficulties and thus reduce the distressing physiological sensations that accompany these. Ultimately, CBT encourages clients to become their own therapists, considering skills and tools to be used for years to come. This is the basis of CBT. Formulation and treatment are more nuanced than this but understanding the basics can help us to consider what we do.

Key Point: Hold the importance of working collaboratively and using conceptualisation in your mind as your read through some of the misconceptions.

Common myths about CBT

There are many statements made about CBT and CBT therapists that aren't based on truth and misinformation about CBT can influence how people perceive CBT therapists. These myths exist within our clients as well as other mental health professionals. Many trainee clinicians come into the role holding beliefs that these myths are true (Dobson & Dobson, 2018). In this section, I will look to dispel eight of the most common myths.

CBT is about thinking positively

I have repeatedly heard people say that CBT is just about positive thinking. Let's start by saying that positivity and optimism have their place. However, health is more closely related to the absence of pessimism rather than the presence of optimism (Scheier et al., 2021).

CBT is more complex than just thinking positively. Within CBT, a client works with a therapist to develop the skills needed to better manage unhelpful thinking habits. Change happens in relation to maladaptive cognitions (Beck, 1970) and aims to realign thinking with reality. By helping us to explore illogical thought patterns and framing them in a more realistic way, CBT aims to alleviate distress (Beck et al., 1979). This includes testing out the validity of maladaptive beliefs (Clark & Wells, 1995). Challenging maladaptive beliefs requires a range of skills and techniques. Simply focusing on positive thinking undermines the complex work that we do. It also undermines the tough situations our clients are facing. Imagine telling a depressed client to think positive thoughts, I would be surprised if that client came back to the next session!

It is also worthy of note that being overly positive can be as problematic as negative thinking. Positive thoughts aren't always appropriate to the current situation and can lead someone to taking the wrong or no action. Think about someone who lives their life with one rule: good vibes only! Now this person is in a house that was on fire, all the fire alarms are sounding, and their thoughts were, '*well isn't this warm and cosy*'. The person isn't going to go anywhere, this action is unhelpful. More recently people refer to 'toxic positivity', which is the use of encouraging statements to minimise painful emotions. CBT does not, in any way, play into the minimisation of emotions.

CBT is rigid, manualised, and therefore the same for everyone

CBT is not a one-size-fits-all approach. A therapist will collaborate with a client to develop a shared description and understanding of the difficulty as well as what maintains it (Beck, 1995). A case conceptualisation is fundamental to better understand each person's experience of a presenting problem (Dobson & Dobson, 2018). A conceptualisation is a layer-by-layer exploration (Kinderman & Lobban, 2000) of the client's experience of that presenting problem and is therefore unique to an individual and their experiences. A CBT therapist will consider the individual they are working with and is responsive to the needs, problems, and diagnoses of a client, as well as considering different interpersonal aspects (Norcross & Wampold, 2011).

Understanding our clients and what maintains their difficulties is the foundation for all other work carried out. The conceptualisation is like the foundation of a house; the client's and therapists understanding of the difficulty needs to be clear for any effective interventions to take place. Our work is always collaborative, and a conceptualisation will allow a client to decide how best to apply the evidence-based techniques to their individual situation.

CBT only focuses on the 'here and now'

CBT is a treatment that has many layers. CBT starts by addressing factors that are currently maintaining a client's difficulties. What starts the problem off may not be what is maintaining it. The advantage of focusing on the present time is that we have the power to control/change certain aspects. It is an empowering concept to know that we can change things.

However, this does not mean that CBT doesn't explore the past. Kuyken et al. (2009) argue that when a problem is chronic, a longitudinal conceptualisation is necessary. A longitudinal conceptualisation links current difficulties with a number of other factors, including core beliefs, developmental factors, predisposing factors, and significant past experiences. However, it is important to add that historical factors that the client considers to be important to understanding the present difficulties can be included within a cross-sectional or descriptive case conceptualisation (Padesky, 2020). Therefore, historical experiences can be discussed in developing the client's and therapist's understanding of the current problem.

Understanding historical contexts can help therapists to consider potential therapeutic relationship difficulties that may arise. For example, if I know someone has been rejected by a number of important people in their lives, then I will prepare for the ending of therapy carefully so that this is not considered another rejection. Similarly, if I know someone has beliefs about the importance of pleasing other people then I need to ensure that the client isn't doing or saying things just to please me.

CBT ignores emotion

CBT therapists are interested in emotions! Cross-sectional and descriptive conceptualisations demonstrate that CBT sees that thoughts, behaviours, moods, physiological sensations, and environmental factors are all interlinked (Padesky, 2020). CBT considers that we can better understand emotional experiences and reduce the intensity/duration/frequency of them by reflecting upon unhelpful cognitive and behavioural habits that maintain them in the present. Emotions form part of the fundamental concept of CBT. Often, asking about mood helps the client to consider other elements of the cross-sectional conceptualisation. The emotion is usually the first thing the client notices because the accompanying physiological sensations are distressing. Using the emotions to help the client to break down their experience is pivotal.

CBT does not acknowledge the importance of a therapeutic relationship

This is a myth I have encountered on more than a few occasions. It is a big misconception about CBT stemming from its early behavioural roots. CBT prioritises the collaboration of client and therapist in working together with a common goal in mind (Beck et al., 1979). The therapeutic relationship interlinked with the therapy techniques (Dobson, 2022) is considered imperative and that a strong, constructive relationship is essential in achieving positive outcomes within CBT (Okamoto et al., 2019).

I can't begin to imagine why someone would continue to attend therapy if they didn't feel comfortable, valued, safe, and respected. How would our clients even fathom engaging in work, such as reliving, or behavioural experiments if the therapeutic relationship wasn't strong. This is a fundamental concept; it is the grounding of all we do. Now, I am not saying we are all perfect at it, after all, therapists are human too. Therefore, we need to know how to recognise and repair ruptures within a relationship. Feedback is used to 'check in' with a client to help us identify any problems at the end of a session; however, we are also skilled at paying attention to the implicit as well as the explicit meanings within a session. My role is not to tell someone what to do but to use guided discovery and Socratic questioning to help a client explore potential solutions for themselves (Wells, 1997).

Exposure techniques are cruel

Exposure techniques, in principle, sound like they are a very difficult and distressing technique for a client to engage with. However, they are underpinned by research; we understand the rationale behind them, and this psychoeducation is worked through with the client following a descriptive case conceptualisation. This is not a technique that is forced on anyone and can only be conducted with a strong therapeutic relationship. Exposure-based approaches are carried out collaboratively, with the client choosing what they want to work on. The client can gauge the level of emotional intensity to pitch their exposure so that it is manageable and achievable. In addition, at the start of exposure, when anxiety is likely to be high, safety behaviours can be planned (Dessert et al., 2023). A client will be supported to carry out the goals they set in relation to the exposure task, in line with the case conceptualisation and evidence base.

Exposure techniques are so powerful, they work. Until you see the shifts people can make, it is hard to grasp. Exposure is a scary concept for many trainee therapists; it isn't until you see how it works in action that you can develop your confidence.

Personal reflection

I remember being petrified of working with PTSD, the concept of re-living seemed so far from what I wanted to do. I wanted to protect and rescue the client, to stop them from feeling the distressing emotions. But that would mean colluding with the client and helping to maintain their distress long term.

Exposure works, but we need to learn to tolerate our own distress with these techniques as much as our client's need to learn to tolerate theirs.

CBT is a sticking plaster providing only temporary relief

Some view CBT as a 'sticking plaster', a temporary relief that often leaves clients feeling better for only a short period of time. This is a controversial topic and is sometimes less about CBT generally and more about the way it is delivered within services. The National Institute for Health and Care Excellence (NICE) guidelines make evidence-based recommendations related to session numbers. Due to a variety of reasons, services may offer fewer sessions than recommended. Some clients have reported that the sessions offered within what was formerly known as Improving Access to Psychological Therapies (IAPT) weren't sufficient (MIND, 2010, 2013), despite their being guidance emerging to emphasise the need for an adequate number of sessions (Clark, 2019; NCCMH, 2024.). It is worth noting that there isn't as robust reporting of CBT in primary care in the other nations of the UK. However, there are anecdotal reports of fewer sessions being offered across the nations and sectors.

Similarly, services may offer CBT with a therapist who has received minimal training and who has minimal supervision or continued professional development opportunities. Judgements are made about CBT as a whole at this point, rather than understanding the delivery contexts. These contexts will impact upon how effective CBT is for a client.

When delivered within the guidance of the evidence base, CBT has been shown to be an effective therapy. Research has demonstrated that CBT has continued to be effective in one- to three-year follow-up studies (DiMauro et al., 2013; Dugas et al., 2003; Paykel et al., 2005; Von Brachel et al., 2019; Watanabe et al., 2010; Wiles et al., 2016). Several meta-analyses of Randomised control trials have also demonstrated the long-term effectiveness of CBT (Chambles & Ollendick, 2001; Norton & Price, 2007). In summary, it is not a sticking plaster when delivered within the recommended guidelines, within the evidence base.

CBT does not meet the needs of minoritised ethnicities

Admittedly most of the development and research into CBT has historically focused on English-speaking, secular (sometimes Christian) populations in Western countries. As a result, a common myth is that CBT is only for people raised in Western societies, living by Western values, and speaking English.

However, let's be frank: CBT is just as effective when delivered in a culturally responsive way to meet the needs of the client. Whether in the form of Culturally

Sensitive CBT, which retains the core components of CBT with smaller adjustments on an individual basis, or in the form of culturally adapted CBT, which maintains the core components of CBT but involves more substantial modifications to better suit a specific ethnic group (Beck, 2016).

Personal reflection

I try to be open and honest with a client if I have not had any experience of their culture or background, I strive to remain curious and keen to learn. As a White therapist, I also must sit with the discomfort of knowing that I am incredibly privileged to have not had some of the experiences my clients' have had (such as racism). It is a very humbling experience that they have shared with me but it also raises some feelings of sadness and guilt. Equally, I have learnt about positive experiences and the pride that my clients have being a part of their community and how integral it is to them. Being privy to this information makes me feel incredibly fortunate, enriching my clinical work.

The emerging evidence base shows that CBT can be effective, acceptable, and feasibly delivered for clients from diverse backgrounds in western countries (Huey et al., 2023), those in non-Western countries (Latif et al., 2021), with clients from religious backgrounds (Golker & Cioffi, 2021; Mir et al., 2015), and with the assistance of interpreters (d'Ardenne et al., 2007). Moreover, there is a recognition that what may get in the way of this is a therapist's avoidance or lack of confidence in asking the client about their cultural experiences and experiences of racism (Naz et al., 2019).

Ultimately, therapists need to guard against their own biases to avoid generalisations about differences between groups (Carter, 1991), self-reflect on their own cultural contribution (Richardson & Molinaro, 1996), acknowledge the implicit cultural assumptions inherent within CBT (Kunorubwe, 2023), utilise theoretical frameworks to guide the modification (Naeem et al., 2023), and collaboratively agree to work with the client/s as to what degree to integrate their background into therapy.

Reflective exercise

Have you heard any of these myths? Did you believe any of them? If so, where did you develop that understanding?

Key points

To summarise, let's think about the role in line with the quotes in the introduction. CBT therapists are

- collaborative;
- use formulation to elicit change;
- support clients to challenge unhelpful thoughts and maintaining behaviours;
- consider the therapeutic relationship as pivotal to their role;
- skilled in exploring both the past and present;
- scientist-practitioners, we use evidence base to inform our therapy. We do what research tells us works;
- efficient in using Socratic questioning and guided discovery;
- self-reflective;
- open to working with the client and their individual experiences.

Reflective exercise

Revisit the three words you noted at the start of the chapter and consider whether any of them have changed after reading about what we actually do.

Conclusion

What is a CBT therapist?

This question, in theory, should be easy to answer having reviewed what CBT is and is not. There are a range of practitioners that deliver CBT interventions, and this can muddy the waters somewhat. Mental health nurses, occupational therapists, and psychological wellbeing practitioners use elements of CBT within their role; however, they may not be considered CBT therapists. CBT is a complex treatment; it is perhaps far more complicated than many assume when they are starting out. The role requires the completion of very intense and demanding training programmes with stringent quality checks upon your practice.

When we are talking about what a CBT therapist is, we are referring to someone who is trained to work with CBT in line with NICE guidelines. A CBT therapist will be delivering CBT in a way that is collaborative, skilfully underpinned by Socratic questioning and informed by a personal formulation whilst still working in line with the evidence base. CBT therapists come from a variety of careers and professions, including psychologists, mental health nurses, social workers, counsellors, and many others.

A frustration working as an accredited CBT therapist is that it is not a protected title. This means that unlike a doctor, nurse, or psychologist, anyone can call themselves a CBT therapist. Gaining accreditation with The British Association of

Behavioural and Cognitive Psychotherapies (BABCP), a CBT therapist commits to continued professional development in order to maintain their standards of practice, as well as committing to receiving supervision for their practice. In addition, a BABCP-registered CBT therapist will commit to adhering to the standards of conduct, performance, and ethics.

Key Point: BABCP registration allows a client to have the peace of mind that their therapist is well trained and experienced; this is so incredibly important given that many of our clients will be vulnerable.

Being a CBT therapist is a varied job with no one day being the same. It is a job that allows you to sit with people talking about their most difficult experiences, to listen when people share their most shameful secrets, to me this is the biggest honour. To think that I can create an environment that enables someone to be truly open and honest, a space where someone can feel safe and feel they can trust me. Being a CBT therapist plays on every emotion that can be experienced and at times is the best job in the world, sometimes it's one of the toughest.

Ultimately, our clients are our main focus. Therefore, it makes sense that this chapter concludes with a perspective from someone who has experienced CBT:

My CBT therapist had a significant impact on my treatment when I was suffering with OCD; he taught me to use cognitive behavioural techniques to deal with the symptoms. He had a way of making me feel like I was doing it myself, but now, looking back, I can see that there was a distinct process and he was guiding me through it. I gained so much insight and confidence through my sessions with a CBT therapist.

Beth Evans

Acknowledgements

I would like to say a very heartfelt thank you to several people who have contributed to this chapter. Katy Emerson and Dave Hitt and Taf Kunorubwe at Cardiff University, thank you for proof reading and offering your expert opinions on what a CBT therapist is as well as contributing to discussion related to the myths surrounding CBT. Furthermore, I would like to extend my appreciation to Beth Evans for her overview of her experience working with a CBT therapist.

Further reading

For further details of what CBT is, please visit: https://babcp.com/what-is-cbt.

Mueller, M., Kennerley, H., McManus, F., & Westbrook, D. (2010). *Oxford guide to surviving as a CBT therapist.* Oxford University Press.

Whittington, A., & Grey, N. (2014). *How to become a more effective CBT therapist. Mastering metacompetence in clinical practice.* Wiley Blackwell.

References

Beck, A. T. (1970). Cognitive therapy: Nature and relation to behaviour therapy. *Behaviour Therapy*, *1*(2), 184–200. https://doi.org/doi.org/10.1016/S0005–7894(70)80030–2

Beck, J. S. (1995). *Cognitive therapy: Basics and beyond.* Guilford Press.

Beck, A. (2016). *Transcultural cognitive behavioural therapy for anxiety and depression: A practical guide.* Routledge.

Beck, A. T., Rush, A. J., Shaw, B. F., & Emery, G. (1979). *Cognitive therapy of depression.* Guilford Press.

Carter, R. T. (1991). Cultural values: A review of empirical research and implications for counselling. *Journal of Counselling & Development*, *70*(1), 164–173. https://doi.org/10.10002/j.1556-6676.1991.tb01579

Chambles, D. L., & Ollendick, T. H. (2001). Empirically supported psychology interventions: Controversies and evidence. *Annual Review of Psychology*, *52*, 685–716. https://doi.org/10.1146/annurev.psych.52.1.685

Clark, D. M. (2019). *IAPT at 10: Achievements and challenges.* www.england.nhs.uk/blog/iapt-at-10-achievements-and-challenges/

Clark, D. M., & Fairburn, C. G. (Eds.). (2009). *Science and practice of cognitive behaviour therapy.* Oxford University Press.

Clark, D. M., & Wells, A. (1995). A cognitive model of social phobia. In R. Heimberg, M. Liebowitz, D. A. Hope, & F. R. Schneier (Eds.), *Social phobia: Diagnosis, assessment and treatment* (pp. 69–93). Guilford Press.

d'Ardenne, P., Ruaro, L., Cestari, L., Fakhoury, W., & Priebe, S. (2007). Does interpreter-mwediated CBT with traumatized refugee people work? A comparison of patient outcomes in East London. *Behavioural and Cognitive Psychotherapy*, *35*(3), 293–301. https://doi.org/10.1017/S1352465807003645

Dessert, A., Lynch, A., McMillon, A., Terrill, M., & MacNeil, B. (2023). Doctoral clinical psychology student commentary on common myths about CBT: Lessons learned for competency-based training. *The Cognitive Behaviour Therapist*, *16*, e7. https://doi.org/1017/S1754470X23000016

DiMauro, J., Domingues, J., Fernandez, G., & Tolin, D. F. (2013). Long term effectiveness of CBT for anxiety disorders in an adult out patient clinic sample: A follow-up study. *Behaviour Research and Therapy*, *51*(2), 82–86. https://doi.org/10.1016/j.brat.2012.10.003

Dobson, K. S. (2022). Therapeutic relationship. *Cognitive and Behavioural Practice*, *29*, 541–544. https://doi.org/10.1016/j.cbpra.2022.02.006

Dobson, D., & Dobson, K. S. (2018). *Evidence-based practice of cognitive-behavioural therapy.* Guilford Press.

Dugas, M. J., Ladoucer, R., Leger, E., Freeston, M. H., Langlois, F., Provencher, M. D., & Boisvert, J. M. (2003). Group cognitive behavioural therapy for generalised anxiety disorder: Treatment outcome and long term follow up. *Journal of Consulting and Clinical Psychology*, *71*(4), 821–825. https://doi.org/10.1037/0022-006x.71.4.821

Golker, C., & Cioffi, M. C. (2021). Cultural adaptations of cognitive behaviour therapy for the Orthodox Jewish community: A qualitative study of therapists' perspectives. *The Cognitive Behaviour Therapist*, *14*, e3. https://doi.org/10.1017/S1754470X20000616

Huey, S. J., Park, A. L., Galan, C. A., & Wang, C. X. (2023). Culturally responsive cognitive behavioural therapy for ethnically diverse populations. *Annual Review of Clinical Psychology*, *19*, 51–78. https://doi.org/10.1146/annurev-clinpsy-080921-072750

Kinderman, P., & Lobban, F. (2000). Evolving formulations: Sharing complex information with clients. *Behavioural and Cognitive Psychotherapy*, *28*, 307–310. https://doi.org/10.1017/S1352465800003118

Kunorubwe, T. (2023). Cultural adaptations of group CBT for depressed clients from diverse backgrounds: A systematic review. *The Cognitive Behaviour Therapist*, *16*, e35. https://doi.org/10.1017/S1754470X23000302

Kuyken, W., Padesky, C. A., & Dudley, R. (2009). *Collaborative case conceptualisation.* Guilford Press.

Latif, M., Awan, F., Gul, M., Husain, M. O., Husain, M. I., Sayyed, K., Magsi, T., Naz, S., Aylem, O., Phiri, P., Irfan, M., Ayub, M., & Naeem, F. (2021). Preliminary evaluation of a culturally adapted CBT-based online programme for depression and anxiety from a lower middle-income country. *The Cognitive Behaviour Therapist, 14,* e36. https://doi.org/10.1017/S1754470X21000313

MIND. (2010). *We need to talk, getting the right therapy at the right time.* www.mind.org.uk/media-a/4428/we-need-to-talk-getting-the-right-therapy-at-the-right-time.pdf

MIND. (2013). *We still need to talk, a report on access to talking therapies.* www.mind.org.uk/media-a/4426/we-still-need-to-talk_reports.pdf

Mir, G., Meer, S., Cottrell, D., McMillan, D., House, A., & Kanter, J. W. (2015). Adapted behavioural activation for the treatment of depression in Muslims. *Journal of Affective Disorders, 180,* 190–199. https://doi.org/10.1016/j.jad.2015.03.060

Naeem, F., Sajid, S., Naz, S., & Phiri, P. (2023). Culturally adapted CBT – the evolution of psychotherapy adaptation frameworks and evidence. *The Cognitive Behaviour Therapist, 16,* e10. https://doi.org/10.1017/S1754470X2300003X

National Collaborating Centre for Mental Health. (2024). *The improving access to psychological therapies manual.* www.england.nhs.uk/publication/the-improving-access-to-psychological-therapies-manual/

Naz, S., Romilly, G., & Bahu, M. (2019). Addressing issues of race, ethnicity and culture in CBT to support therapists and service managers to deliver culturally competent therapy and reduce inequalities in mental health provision for BAME service users. *The Cognitive Behaviour Therapist, 12,* e22. https://doi.org/10.1017/S1754470X19000060

Norcross, J. C., & Wampold, B. E. (2011). Evidence-based therapy relationships: Research conclusions and clinical practices. In J. C. Norcross (Ed.), *Psychotherapy relationships that work: Evidence-based responsiveness* (pp. 423–430). Oxford University Press.

Norton, P. J., & Price, E. C. (2007). A meta-analytic review of adult cognitive-behavioural treatment outcome across the anxiety disorders. *The Journal of Nervous and Mental Disease, 195*(6), 521–531. https://doi.org/10.1097/01.nmd.0000253843.70149.9a

Okamoto, A., Dattilio, F. M., Dobson, K. S., & Kazantzis, N. (2019). The therapeutic relationship in cognitive-behavioural therapy: Essential features and common challenges. *Practice Innovations, 4*(2), 112–123. https://doi.org/10.1037/pri0000088

Padesky, C. A. (2020). Collaborative case conceptualisation: Client knows best. *Cognitive and Behavioural Practice, 27*(4), 392–404. https://doi.org/10.1016/j.cbpra.2020.06.003

Padesky, C., & Greenberger, D. (1995). *Clinicians guide to mind over mood.* Guilford Press.

Paykel, E. S., Scott, J., Cornwall, P. L., Abbott, R., crane, C., Pope, M., & Johnson, A. L. (2005). Duration of relapse prevention after cognitive therapy in residual depression: Follow-up of controlled trial. *Psychological Medicine, 35*(1), 59–68. https://doi.org/10.1017/s003329170400282x

Rachman, S. (2009). The evolution of cognitive behaviour therapy. In D. M. Clark & C. G. Fairburn (Eds.), *Science and practice of cognitive behaviour therapy* (pp. 3–26). Oxford University Press.

Redhead, S., Johnstone, L., & Nightingale, J. (2015). Clients' experiences of formulation in cognitive behaviour therapy. *Psychology and Psychotherapy: Theory, Research and Practice, 88*(4), 453–467. https://doi.org/10.1111/papt.12054

Richardson, T. Q., & Molinaro, K. L. (1996). White counsellor self-awareness: A prerequisite for developing multicultural competence. *Journal of Counselling & Development, 74*(3), 238–242. https://doi.org/10.1002/j.1556–6676.1996.tb01859.x

Scheier, M. F., Swanson, J. D., Barlow, M. A., Greenhouse, J. B., Wrosch, C., & Tindle, H. A. (2021). Optimism versus pessimism as predictors of physical health: A comprehensive reanalysis of dispositional optimism research. *American Psychologist, 76*(3), 529–548. https://doi.org/10.1037/amp0000666

Von Brachel, R., Hirschfeld, G., Berner, A., Willutzki, U., Teisman, T., Cwik, J. C., Velten, J., Schulte, D., & Margraf, J. (2019). Long-term effectiveness of cognitive behavioural therapy in routine outpatient care: A 5 to 20 year follow up study. *Psychotherapy and Psychosomatics*, *88*(4), 225–235. https://doi.org/10.1159/000500188

Watanabe, N., Furukawa, T. A., Chen, J., Kinoshita, Y., Nakano, Y., Ogawa, S., Funayama, T., Ietsugu, T., & Noda, Y. (2010). Change in quality of life and their predictors in the long term follow-up after group cognitive behavioural therapy for social anxiety disorder: A prospective cohort study. *BMC Psychiatry*, *10*, 81–91. https://doi.org/10.1186/1471-244X-10-81

Wells, A. (1997). *Cognitive therapy for anxiety disorders: A practice manual and conceptual guide*. Wiley.

Wiles, N. J., Thomas, L., Turner, N., Garfield, K., Kaunali, D., Campbell, J., Kessler, D., Kuyken, W., Lewis, G., Morrison, J., Williams, C., Peters, T. J., & Hollinghurst, S. (2016). Long-term effectiveness and cost effectiveness of cognitive behavioural therapy as an adjunct to pharmacotherapy for treatment-resistant depression in primary care: Follow-up of the CoBalT randomised controlled trial. *Lancet Psychiatry*, *3*(2), 137–144. https://doi.org/10.1016/S2215-0366(15)00495-2

Chapter 2

Pathways to becoming a cognitive behavioural therapist

Helen Moya

Introduction

On average, the journey to become a CBT therapist can take around eight years, so understanding the different routes, and which one best fits your background, qualifications, and experience, is essential to navigate through the process. In this chapter, we will consider the different pathways to becoming an accredited CBT therapist in the UK. There are stages to this journey, and we will discuss each stage and option in turn, using a pathway map. This will help you to identify which pathway best suits you. Information on the essential knowledge and clinical experience required to access CBT training is presented and the various ways you can meet them. Storied accounts by people from different clinical backgrounds bring this information to life by describing their CBT career journey with tips relating to the specific pathway followed.

Understanding the CBT therapist role

Before embarking on this career path, make sure you fully understand the role of a CBT therapist. Sometimes we pursue a career choice and spend many years preparing for it only to find that it does not live up to expectations.

> **Top tips: learning about the CBT role**
>
> - If you are not already working in a psychological therapy service, speak to CBT therapists and learn about the day-to-day tasks and demands of the role.
> - If you do currently work in a service such as Talking Therapies (e.g. as a low-intensity therapist), make sure you are fully aware of the differences between low and high-intensity CBT. Along with working with more complex presentations, there is a difference in recovery rates. This is often overlooked when applying for high-intensity training.

DOI: 10.4324/9781003428527-4

The current landscape of public sector psychological therapy services is very fraught and under-resourced. There is pressure to deliver therapy in very challenging circumstances, and there are high rates of CBT therapists leaving the NHS due to burnout. Although this is being addressed at an organisational and political level, it is important to have realistic expectations. This will enable you to prepare fully for the journey ahead, paying attention to your own wellbeing to build and maintain resilience.

Figure 2.1 provides a CBT career roadmap that outlines the most common pathways to becoming a CBT therapist. It should be noted that there are always some anomalies to the journey, but the road map provides an overview to help you assess the options. The road map has been reproduced from Moya (2024) with permission from the publishers.

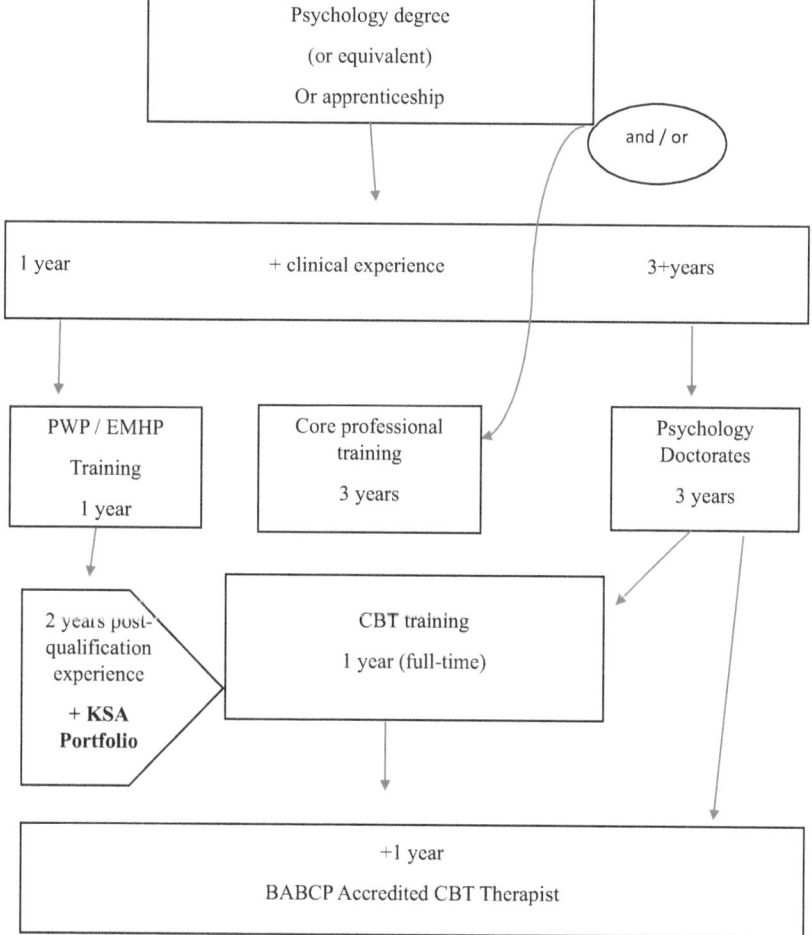

Figure 2.1 CBT career roadmap

Source: Moya, 2024. Reproduced with permission from Pavillion Publishing

Psychology knowledge

It is worth noting that CBT is a specialist approach that was originally aimed at mental health professionals from different core professional backgrounds who want to use CBT in their clinical role. Since the introduction of the Improving Access to Psychological Therapies (IAPT) initiative in 2008, alternative pathways to becoming a CBT therapist have become more common. Most of these will begin with a psychology degree.

CBT is a psychological therapy which is based on theory from various branches of psychology, including clinical, developmental, social, and cognitive psychology. For this reason, it is advantageous to have a psychology-related degree. This does not have to be a pure psychology degree, but having a substantive amount of psychology theory included in the curriculum helps to evidence certain knowledge, skills, and attitudes.

As stated above, the psychology knowledge can be gained through core professional training. The British Association for Behavioural and Cognitive Psychotherapies (BABCP) website provides an up-to-date details of what roles are considered core professions:

- see https://babcp.com/Core-Professions

Core professional training applies psychology knowledge through clinical skills, which makes it more suited to moving directly into CBT training following a 12-month period of consolidation. It is possible to proceed into a CBT career without a psychology undergraduate degree or core profession. This is achieved by completing an apprenticeship into a psychological wellbeing practitioner (PWP) training role. These are designed to encourage people without a formal university degree to access psychological therapy training and supported by NHS England. More details can be found at the end of this chapter.

Clinical experience

Without a core profession, you will need substantive clinical experience of a minimum of four years before starting CBT training. The pathway map shows the different routes to gaining this experience.

Psychological wellbeing practitioner/educational mental health practitioner route

For these roles, you are normally required to have at least six months to a year of relevant mental health clinical experience following the completion of a psychology related degree. See the work experience options table for examples of clinical roles. Training for PWP and EMHP roles is one year at the postgraduate level and is combined with a full-time paid post in a service. Part-time options may be available.

Following training, you are required to complete two further years of clinical practice before starting CBT training, which makes up the four years of equivalent clinical experience to that of a core professional. You will also need to complete a Knowledge, Skills, and Attitudes (KSA) portfolio either before applying for CBT training (if a Level 2-accredited course with BABCP) or following training to apply for practitioner accreditation. There is a section on completing a KSA later in the chapter.

Psychology doctorate route

Following the completion of a psychology degree, a popular career choice is clinical or counselling psychology. Both courses include CBT theory and practice as part of the curricula. However, access to the training is challenging due to the level of competition. This means that most courses will not consider you without a substantive amount of postgraduate clinical experience. On average, this is three years.

Most candidates pursuing this pathway will apply for Assistant Psychologist (AP) roles within a range of services within the NHS. Whilst this will allow access to the doctoral programmes, they do not have the same currency for CBT training access. If you decide to apply for CBT training as a stepping-stone to the clinical or counselling courses, then you would need more than AP experience alone. This will depend on the specific AP post, but many are supportive roles that do not include delivery of clinical skills.

One advantage of the doctoral route, if you want to practise CBT in the role, is that many of the programmes now have course accreditation status from the BABCP. This means that the programme covers all the minimum training standards (MTS) set by the BABCP for individual practitioner accreditation. Once you pass the course, you can apply for practitioner accreditation in the same way as any other Level 2 course graduates (BABCP, 2023).

If you are completing a non-accredited course, then you can either do the high-intensity training after the doctorate or make up the gaps of the MTS in practice and apply directly to the BABCP for individual practitioner accreditation. In recent years, in England and Wales, there has been some funding made available for clinical psychologists to undertake 'top-up' training in CBT (see Lack et al., 2024).

Alternative route – apprenticeships

The main pathways have been presented; however, in some cases, it is possible to advance to CBT training without a psychology degree or core profession. One such route is via an apprenticeship scheme. Access and availability of these vary around the UK, and funding can change from year to year. This option allows people without the traditional requirements to build knowledge and skills on the job. Suited particularly to people who may not have gained academic credentials in a school or college setting but have the potential to achieve the standard required to successfully complete CBT training at a low-intensity level.

Apprenticeships provide a pathway into the PWP role. They are government funded and place emphasis on lived experience in addition to academic ability. There is a minimum requirement to have Level 2 English and maths, and in line with all government-funded schemes, applicants need to have lived in the UK for a minimum of three years. Training as a PWP is comparable to the standard route, but assessments may be marked at a graduate level instead of postgraduate level. These adjustments allow for parity in assessment.

Key Point: Apprentices fulfil the same requirements following training in terms of a minimum of four years mental health clinical experience before entering a high-intensity CBT training programme.

There is a new apprenticeship being offered in the UK which has a wider reach than the PWP role. This is called the clinical associate in psychology (CAP) which is a postgraduate-level post. It is aimed predominantly at psychology graduates who have an interest in applying psychology to common mental health problems. It is a distinct career option aimed at closing the gap between the AP role and the qualified clinical or counselling psychologist role. It provides access to a range of psychological therapies, with psychological formulation and evidence-based psychological interventions guiding practice. It is an 18-month programme which is awarded at master's level.

Top tip: accessing apprenticeships

PWP apprenticeships – more information can be found on the NHS England website.

Suitable work experience options

To gain the required clinical experience, you will need to consider the relevance of each role. For example, a role where you are providing physical care alone will demonstrate compassion and empathy but will not demonstrate skills relating to delivery of psychological support. In these circumstances, you can turn to the therapists and other members of the multidisciplinary team to discuss potential options for developing clinical skills. A good question to ask yourself in any role is 'how is this experience going to prepare me for CBT practice?' You could also list the specific skills and see how they relate to the role of the CBT therapist. This may be listening skills or making sense of someone's distress from a CBT perspective.

Top tips: relevant work experience

- Healthcare assistant role in any NHS mental health or learning disability setting
- Assistant Psychologist (psychology graduate)
- Open door charity – www.opendoorcharity.com/volunteer/
- MIND www.mind.org.uk/get-involved/volunteering- participating/
- Scope – www.scope.org.uk/volunteering/
- Mencap – www.mencap.org.uk/get-involved/work-with-feeling
- Childline – www.childline.org.uk/get-involved/
- Samaritans – www.samaritans.org/support-us/volunteer/
- International medical corps – https://internationalmedicalcorps.org.uk/volunteer
- National Citizens Service (NCS) – https://wearencs.com

This list provides some ideas and suggestions for work experience prior to clinical training. It is not exhaustive, and you should always check your local area for any services or projects providing psychological support. A more detailed guide is linked in the resources section at the end of the chapter. The more diverse your experience, the better placed you will be to access training later. The most important thing is that you enjoy the experience and be prepared to learn. Approaching any position as a tick-box exercise will minimise its potential value and will not instil the professional attitude required to be a mental health professional.

KSA portfolio

As stated above, if you do not have a core profession, then you will be required to provide evidence of equivalence in the form of the KSA portfolio (BABCP, 2020). This is a framework divided into criteria across knowledge, skills, and attitudes expected of a mental health professional. A complete portfolio consists of 14 criteria, and details can be obtained on the BABCP website under the Accreditation tab.

The BABCP has recently changed the requirements for submission of a KSA based on individual background. Shortened versions of the portfolio are allowed under certain circumstances. The most common condensed KSA is for registered PWPs with the BABCP. This is a relatively new professional standing offered by the BABCP to recognise a standard of clinical practice of a minimum of 12 months following qualification as a PWP or EMHP. Meeting the requirements of registration acknowledges that many of the KSA criteria have also been met. As such, the shortened version only requires evidence of criteria 4, 13, and 14 if you have a psychology degree with developmental psychology content. For those without this content then the addition of criterion 1 is required.

Other allied professions without substantive mental health content in their training may also qualify for a condensed version of the KSA.

Pathway stories

Table 2.1 includes the individual accounts of people from different backgrounds who have all successfully completed their training and are now qualified CBT therapists. Each story includes a personal tip on how to get the most out of the journey.

Table 2.1 Example Pathways to CBT Training

PWP	Core professional
After completing my psychology degree I knew I wanted to work in mental health but didn't want to be a clinical psychologist. I had CBT and really found it helpful so knew this was what I wanted to do. I did some work experience for a mental health charity for 6 months then worked in a hospital alongside a multidisciplinary team. I was successful at interview for PWP training and stayed in the role for five years before doing the high-intensity training via the KSA route. I still use both approaches in practice. **Tip** – speak to lots of people but don't compare your journey to theirs. Everyone approaches things differently and brings different strengths to the table.	*I trained as a Learning Disability Nurse many years ago. At the time I didn't know I would become a CBT therapist one day. It was working in academia as a mental health nurse educator when I was introduced to the IAPT (NHS Talking Therapies) initiative which really excited me. I found a placement and did the training alongside my academic role, then combined clinical practice as a CBT therapist with becoming a trainer on the CBT programme at my university.* **Tip** – it is never too late to change career path. If you have a core profession but want to specialise in CBT do some research and speak to people and go for it.
Clinical psychologist	*Apprentice*
When doing my psychology degree I loved the modules on mental health and did some voluntary work alongside my studies. After graduation I did two Assistant Psychologist (AP) roles for a year each with very different client groups. One was in a dementia service, and one was a hospital-based role where I performed clinical assessments and practised producing psychological formulations. CBT was my favourite model. I tried for two years before getting on the clinical psychology doctorate programme but was lucky that it was BABCP accredited so I graduated as both a clinical psychologist and an accredited CBT therapist. **Tip** – this pathway is extremely competitive and takes many years. You need to remain confident and have belief in yourself and try and enjoy every step of the process.	*When I finished sixth form, I didn't know what I wanted to do so decided not to go to university. I became a healthcare assistant in a mental health service. I became interested in psychological interventions that the mental health nurses and psychologists were using. I was able to access PWP training as a graduate certificate through an apprenticeship programme. I went onto to do my CBT training three years later. I have now been qualified for three years and love it.* **Tip** – don't feel inferior for not having a psychology degree. You will learn what you need on the apprenticeship, and no-one will judge you as we all are following the same goal.

Conclusion

This chapter has provided an overview of the different pathways to become a CBT therapist. Although there are specific requirements in terms of knowledge and clinical experience to access CBT training, there is flexibility in how you can acquire them. Storied accounts from individuals with different clinical backgrounds bring the journey to life. There is no short cut to become a CBT therapist, so enjoying each stage of the process is essential. Finally, always check the BABCP website as guidelines can change periodically.

Further reading

Moya, H. (2021). Work experience for psychology students in IAPT. *CBT Today, 48*(2), 32–33.
Moya, H. (2022). CBT career development: Introducing a conceptual model. *CBT Today, 50*(4), 28–30.

A brief guide on becoming a CBT therapist can be found on the Moya CBT website:

www.moyacbt.co.uk/wp-content/uploads/2020/07/CBT-Career.pdf
CBT work experience tips: www.moyacbt.co.uk/wp-content/uploads/2021/02/ Work-experience-guide.pdf

References

British Association for Behavioural and Cognitive Psychotherapies. (2020). *Guidelines for assembling and assessing KSA portfolios or evidence for course assessment.* https:// babcp.com/Knowledge-Skills-Attitudes
British Association for Behavioural and Cognitive Psychotherapies. (2023). *BABCP minimum training standards for the practice of cognitive behavioural therapy.* https://babcp. com/Minimum-Training-Standards
Lack, S., Handley, R., Barr, L., Rivers, M., Patel, A., Coe, M., & Hale, L. (2024). CBT accreditation for clinical psychologists: A limitation or an opportunity to apply and maintain our organisational and systemic influence and leadership? *Clinical Psychology Forum, 375.* https://doi.org/10.53841/bpscpf.2023.1.371.4
Moya, H. (2024). *The CBT career guide: Becoming & developing as a cognitive behavioural therapist.* Pavilion Publishing.

Chapter 3

Charting your path
Navigating the journey to becoming a CBT therapist across the UK

Taf Kunorubwe

Introduction

The journey to becoming an accredited cognitive behavioural (CBT) therapist can be likened to embarking on a challenging yet immensely rewarding voyage – much like trying to travel from the northernmost point of John O'Groats to the southern tip of Land's End, or making your way from the picturesque landscapes of Eryri (Snowdonia) to the famous Clochán an Aifir (Giants Causeway). Much like these, the path is filled with twists and turns, amazing moments, and many long miles and requires some planning.

Across the nations of the United Kingdom (UK), aspiring CBT therapists may follow similar fundamental steps, but regional variations can make the journey distinct. The aim of this chapter is to provide you with some essential context by summarising the difference in the provision and reflecting on the ways in which these may influence your path before, during, and after your CBT training. Note that the Republic of Ireland (ROI) is not considered in this chapter. See Butcher and Chigwedere (2022) for a comprehensive account of CBT in ROI.

Differences in the provision of CBT

Across the nations

The provision of CBT is influenced by the government of each nation, and they are bound by complex historical, political, and societal dynamics. Each government and respective health department implement their own health policies, manage budgets, and structure services and have autonomy in tailoring strategies to meet the specific needs and priorities of their respective regions.

Below are two examples of how the differences play out:

- *Treatment guidelines* – Whilst there are overarching evidence bases, each country has the autonomy to adapt and interpret these recommendations based on their unique healthcare priorities. In England, you will hear about the NICE guidelines; in Scotland, you would refer to the SIGN guidelines and the Scottish

DOI: 10.4324/9781003428527-5

Matrix, or in Wales, you will hear of the Matrics Cymru. These guidelines result in differences in the recommended therapeutic approaches, duration, or frequency of treatment and even whether a specific treatment is available under the National Health Service (NHS).

Key Point: Often, people mistakenly assume that Talking Therapies for Depression and Anxiety (formerly Improving Access to Psychological Therapies or IAPT as it was commonly known) is a UK-wide programme. This is a common misconception, as it is specifically within England and overseen by NHS England (NHS England, 2023). Across the other nations, provision is variable with some offering similar provision and others with no NHS provision.

• *Funding* – NHS provision of CBT varies drastically across the nations. Between 2021 and 2022, funding for all mental health care was £345 million in Northern Ireland (Northern Ireland Audit Office, 2023), £962 million in Wales (Welsh Government, 2023), £1.3 billion in Scotland (Public Health Scotland, 2023), and £12 billion in England (National Audit Office, 2023). Even after accounting for differences in population size, there remains a notable difference in funding. Considering such budgetary constraints, impossible decisions must be made.

Reflective exercise

If you were the decision-maker, what psychological therapies would you fund? What other mental health treatments would you fund? What services would you open or close? How do you ensure access across the nation?

Across the sectors

Provision is also influenced by whether CBT is being provided in the public, private, or third (charity) sector. In the public sector, the NHS provides access to mental health care, including CBT, free of charge to any eligible individual. However, due to limitations in NHS provision and patient choice, CBT may also be accessed outside of the NHS. The private sector provides access to individuals utilising private medical insurance or as 'self-pay' patients (Guy, 2019). The charity sector provides access to CBT at a lower rate or free of charge to supplement formal healthcare systems. This is often with the aim of filling gaps, advocating for healthcare needs, and supporting vulnerable populations with limited access to government-funded healthcare. In this chapter, these sectors are described separately; however, the picture is more complicated, and distinctions are often blurred (Calnan, 2000). Each sector's provision involves trade-offs in terms of accessibility, waiting times, session limits, scope, and cost, influencing individual choices based on preferences, needs, and resources.

Across service types

The provision of CBT is also influenced by service structures, typically organised according to specific issues or the type of support provided. Variation exists in terms of service names, referral routes, entry criteria, therapeutic approaches offered, and even the number of sessions. However, for our purpose, let's broadly describe them as primary care, secondary care, and specialist services.

- Primary care mental health services tend to be the first point of contact for most people accessing psychological therapies. These services typically offer a range of evidence-based psychological therapies (including CBT) for common mental health conditions like depression and anxiety disorders (e.g. Talking Therapies).
- Secondary care mental health services provide more intensive levels of care. These services typically offer a range of evidence-based pharmaceutical, psychological, and social interventions (including CBT) for more complex or severe mental health conditions or when previous treatment hasn't worked (e.g. Community Mental Health Team [CMHT]).
- Specialist services provide a range of highly specialised evidence-based treatments (including CBT and other psychological therapies) for more complex and severe mental health conditions. Treatment often involves a combination of specialist interventions (e.g. Inpatient Eating Disorder Service).

In summary, the provision of CBT across the UK has a complex interplay of factors across multiple domains. Figure 3.1 visualises this interplay (please note, however, that it doesn't cover all possible factors and domains).

- The provision of CBT across the UK will influence your journey to becoming a qualified CBT therapist.
- The country in which you apply will influence the treatment guidelines you follow or even the availability of CBT.
- The sector will influence whether your training post is funded, or if you need to self-fund and even if the clients you see are fee paying.
- The structure of the service will influence whether you are working with mild to moderate or more severe mental health conditions.
- Where you study will influence the extent to which standard training curriculums adequately prepares you for the realities of work.

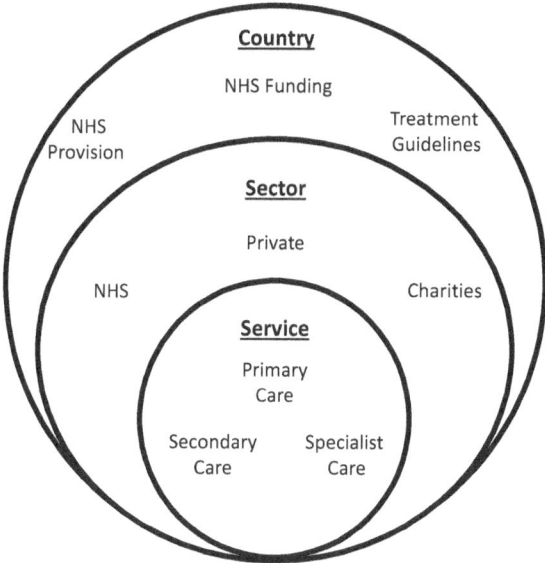

Figure 3.1 Illustrating the factors influencing the provision of CBT across the nations

---

Top tips: course teaching teams

- CBT goes beyond IAPT.
- Explore the diverse applications of CBT and reflect on how you'd like your training to unfold.
- Tailor your path to align with your specific interests and embrace the wealth of opportunities.
- Opportunities exist in the NHS, private companies and in charities. I always suggest potential trainees reflect on the unique dynamics, challenges, and rewards each sector brings.
- Embrace the opportunity to gain varied experiences, broaden your perspective, and contribute positively to your professional growth.

Before starting training

Once you are ready to embark on your journey, it can be helpful to take time to carefully plan the path ahead. Considering how to fund the programme is a critical step in your journey; several funding options are available, depending on the nation, the sector, and your own personal circumstances. Below are some ways in which the provision across the UK will have a direct impact on your experience.

Funding CBT training

You might consider NHS programmes that offer funding, for example a trainee post with the NHS England Talking Therapies. As part of their long-term strategy, significant funding is allocated for CBT training posts (NHS, 2019). Alternatively for NHS staff in Wales, Scotland, or Northern Ireland, there are lesser-known schemes where you apply for funding via the health board. For instance, NHS Education for Scotland (NES) fund places each year for staff across all the health boards in Scotland. In addition, there are occasional opportunities for NHS staff to access funding; these tend to be in response to a service needing therapists or supporting staff progression. Regrettably, levels of funding and opportunities are not uniformly available or accessible.

Another potential pathway to be considered is securing a trainee post within a private or charity organisation that will fund your training. Even though not as prevalent, it is worth knowing about these opportunities. Whilst writing this chapter a search on popular job websites generated a handful of trainee posts with private CBT companies.

The final option is self-funding which can be challenging due to the high costs associated with fees, resources, and living expenses. However, if you are contemplating this route, it is worth exploring if this can be aided through grants, bursaries, and higher education loans. This might be via national, regional, charity or university-based schemes. Please don't feel like you need to go it alone, it's always advisable to discuss finance options with the university's finance department to determine the options best suited to you.

In summary, when seeking funding for CBT training, the availability of financial support can vary depending on your specific circumstances and location within the UK. It's crucial to explore these funding opportunities, engage in discussions with your employer or educational institution, and remain aware of any additional costs to ensure a successful and well-supported CBT training experience.

Securing a trainee opportunity

If you plan to take the path that involves getting a trainee job to gain funding, it is important to familiarise yourself with the positions available. Understanding the terminology used can be an asset during the application process and knowing various job titles within a field broadens the search scope. This increases the chances of finding relevant positions that might be listed under different titles regardless of nations, sectors, and services.

It is also advisable to familiarise yourself with the different requirements and understand the different provisions so you can tailor your application and interview approach to the context. Aligning your skills and experiences with the unique requirements, increases your relevance and competitiveness for the role. For example, when applying to private provider in Wales talking at length about your understanding of NHS Talking Therapies and the evolution of IAPT may be out of context. Or in an interview for a place in Scotland, not referring to the Scottish context and the Scottish Matrix is a missed opportunity.

Finally, recognise that training opportunities in the mental health sector, including CBT, can be in high demand. Stay up to date with the job market by setting reminders or notifications on job listing websites. This proactive approach will enable you to apply promptly when new opportunities become available.

Finding the right CBT training course

Reflecting on whether a particular course is a good fit is a pivotal step. There is an array of courses claiming to equip you to be a CBT therapist, some even using the same language as the accredited training courses, for example, 'Diploma in CBT'. It is essential to check and quality assure the training on offer to ensure it is accredited and meets minimum training standards (see further reading). If your training is funded, there is a good chance the choice of course may not be in your hands. However, make sure you reflect on whether the course is a good fit.

Go beyond the minimum training requirements and investigate the curriculum in depth, aligning it with the specific skills and knowledge areas you aim to develop. For instance, a colleague specifically chose to undertake the PGDip in CBT for Eating Disorders because she is a mental health nurse and would continue working on an inpatient Eating Disorder ward. Also, find out about the areas of specialism or research activity and consider if these align with your areas of interest. Contact the course team or find opportunities to speak to them, for example, course open days. Seek out feedback from previous trainees to gain insight into their experiences and the highs and lows of the course. It's also essential to examine the programme's compatibility with your personal and professional commitments, considering factors like location, schedule, family commitments, carer responsibilities, and workload feasibility. For example, is a full-time course feasible or is a part-time course more compatible? Finally, evaluate how the university and the programme support students with supervision and clinical practice. By thoroughly assessing these aspects, you can ensure that your chosen CBT therapist training programme aligns with your career development and personal goals.

Top tips: course teaching teams

Research the job titles and match your approach accordingly. Do your search for trainee posts with the title of HI, High Intensity, CBT Therapist, Step 3 Therapist, Psychological Therapist, or other variations?

Think pragmatically about the training and where you would realistically be able to commute to/from to maintain a work–life balance that is feasible for the whole period. Be thoughtful about which services/employers you apply to for your training year. Ideally, make applications to those services/ Universities with which you see yourself having an aligned future.

If you do not have a core profession, then familiarise yourself with the Knowledge, Skills, and Attitudes (KSA) process through the resources on the British Association for Behavioural and Cognitive Psychotherapies (BABCP) website. Start your portfolio early, in advance of any future application, to make sure it is complete, see if there is anyone that has been through the process who might be able to mentor or advise.

During training

Detailed accounts of different aspects related to surviving and thriving during your CBT training will be provided within Part II of this book. However, notable considerations are captured below.

Clinical practice and supervision

One aspect that varies is placement and supervision during training. It may be arranged prior to starting the trainee role or the course via service-level agreements involving the university, your employer, and you. For instance, with NHS England Talking Therapies, your clinical practice and supervision will be within the service in which you are employed. In contrast, if you are doing your training via a funded route in Northern Ireland, Wales, or Scotland, clinical practice is often within the health board or service where you work and if possible, your supervisor will be a CBT therapist who also works in the health board.

If you are self-funded, you will probably fulfil your clinical practice in a voluntary placement and may need to source private supervision if there are no CBT therapists within the placement to supervise you. This can incur a significant cost which you will need to consider. Also, bear in mind that due to the scarcity of BABCP-accredited therapists outside of England, it can be challenging to find a supervisor with availability to offer private supervision. Identifying and organising this is your responsibility, but if you're lucky, there may be a placement officer within the university who can assist. Therefore, don't leave it to the last minute, assuming it will be quick to find someone suitable.

Clients and contexts

Variation will also extend to the content of the clinical practice, that is, the level of care and the type of clients. For instance, if your clinical practice is in primary care, you are most likely to see clients presenting with depression and anxiety. In comparison, if your clinical practice is in a CMHT (secondary care), you are more likely to see clients with more severe and enduring difficulties (e.g. bipolar and psychosis).

The context of your clients' lives and their external realities will also influence the type of client you see. For instance, think of the differences for a client who lives in one of the most affluent areas of Berkshire compared to a client in the most deprived areas of the Welsh valleys. Give some thought to the degree to which the demographics of your typical caseload would match the diversity in your area. You can also consider some of the external realities faced by you or the clients. For instance, if you are working in Scotland and treating clients across the 'Highlands and Islands' you may be faced with challenges of being geographically isolated and needing to work (and possibly train) remotely.

Employment status

Another aspect to take into consideration is your employment status and wages. If you are completing your CBT training through a trainee job role, you will typically be employed and, therefore, receive payment for clinical practice and/or attending university. If you have negotiated sponsorship from your employer, you may need to request amendments to your contract to allow you to attend university and engage in clinical practice as part of your existing work, thereby drawing a wage. There isn't standardised pay across nations or contexts, so you may find considerable salary variations.

For those self-funding and completing their clinical practice in voluntary clinical roles, no wage is received. This profoundly impacts a trainee's experience, affecting financial stability and focus on training or clinical practice. Self-funding can be challenging due to the high costs and the loss of income.

Top tips: course teaching teams

Be curious about CBT and its evidence base, theories, and applications, particularly with regards to the experiences of minoritised and marginalised groups and communities – we need more trainees and recent graduates to feel able to ask, 'says who' and 'what about' to support CBT research and application literature to widen and to ensure that services really are actively equitable in their delivery of CBT.

Take the time to think about what support mechanisms you might want to put in place from the outset of the course that are specific to your own individual needs: for example, consideration of childcare needs, access to study skills through the university, referral to the disability team for a dyslexia assessment/support, time for personal care, and opportunity to pursue outside interests.

If you're doing your placement where you already work, make sure to keep the role separate. This separation helps keep your existing position intact and lets you develop CBT therapist, making it easier to learn, minimise the chance to time sinks, and avoid any conflicts of interest.

After training

Detailed accounts of different aspects related to consolidating and expanding your core skills post-training will be provided within Part III of this book. However, notable considerations are captured below.

Job opportunities

The prevalence and spread of job opportunities for qualified CBT therapists vary significantly across nations, sectors, and services. Within the NHS, the devolved management across the nations means that availability of opportunities will vary depending on decisions about funding, priorities, policy, and delivery. Often where NHS provision is limited, the charity sector may attempt to fill gaps; however, job opportunities will be significantly lower due to budgetary constraints of charities. Consequently, where there is limited provision in the public and charity sector, more job opportunities for CBT therapists may arise in the private sector.

Progression opportunities

Progression opportunities after qualifying and consolidating your skills also vary greatly. This may be in relation to supervision, management, training, or even developing specialisms. For instance, due to the smaller number of BABCP-accredited courses in some contexts, the availability of opportunities to lecture may be not as prevalent as on Talking Therapies courses. Another example would be because of the limited number of BABCP-accredited CBT therapists in Wales, there is more demand for therapists offering private supervision.

The evolving landscape of mental health, emerging therapeutic approaches, and the recognition of CBT's efficacy contribute to the avenues available for therapists to advance their careers. The rise of remotely delivered CBT, accelerated by the global pandemic, has not only expanded accessibility but has also opened avenues for therapists to navigate new modes of delivery. The evolving evidence base supporting the effectiveness and adaptability of CBT across a range of disorders, clients, and contexts allows therapists to continually develop.

In summary, the job opportunities for qualified CBT therapists in the UK are influenced by a variety of factors. Understanding the local demand, service delivery landscape, and one's own specialisations is crucial for therapists seeking to establish a successful career in this field.

Top tips: course leads

Apply for your BABCP accreditation as soon as you are ready! Join the BABCP Special Interest Groups (SIGs) or your local branch to promote connection to other CBT therapists. Connect with people when you do training.

Consolidate, consolidate, consolidate. Try to enjoy and be present in your clinical work rather than chasing the next bit of training, the next 'step-up', and the next 'opportunity'. These will all come in due course and sometimes they can come so quickly that the graduate has not had a period of enjoying their own developing competence in CBT.

Consider returning to your institute as a supervisor, lecturer or marker in years to come. Many CBT graduates make great contributions to their programmes after graduating and find it to be a valued adjunct to their clinical work.

Develop your passions and specialist interests! With time, consider developing new competencies like supervision, management, training or research. Nurture specialist interests to broaden your skill set and stay up to date with new and evolving therapeutic approaches.

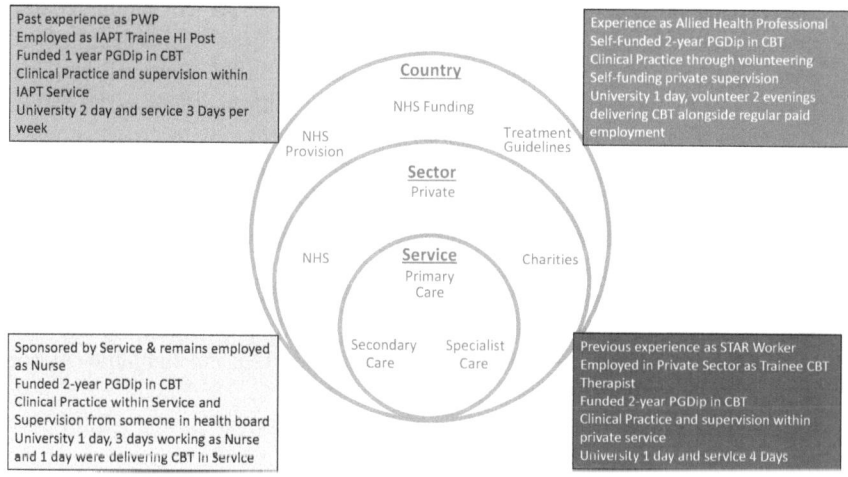

Figure 3.2 Illustrating four different experiences influenced by the provision of CBT across the nations

Conclusion

The journey to becoming a CBT therapist across the UK involves navigating diverse landscapes and unique challenges. Just as traversing from John O'Groats to Land's End or navigating the terrain from Eryri to Clochán an Aifir, each path requires planning, adaptable navigation, and an enduring commitment to the course. Not every journey will be the same, as there may be some similar steps, but each can be radically different. To help illustrate just a few of the pathways, see Figure 3.2.

Regional disparities in healthcare provision, funding, and policy will profoundly impact your path. The choice of an accredited CBT course, funding options, and recruitment processes differ, making it essential for aspiring therapists to adapt their strategies. Meeting the entry requirements and understanding regional variations in placement organisations, paid versus voluntary work, client demographics, and supervision are pivotal during training. Post-training opportunities for CBT therapists vary based on locality, service delivery, and specialisations, with competition and regulatory requirements playing a significant role. In this diverse journey, adaptability and a keen awareness of nuances are crucial for success.

A few words of encouragement regardless of what stage you are at embrace the uniqueness of your journey; if your path looks different, you sometimes feel like you are stuck or it isn't progressing as fast as you would like, remember, that's an integral part of your personal growth and discovery. Not all those who wander are lost.

Key points

- We need to acknowledge that some aspiring CBT therapists will encounter additional barriers due to social, historical, and systemic inequalities (e.g. trainees from the global majority face challenges securing funded positions, and even if successful, they may encounter discrimination, with racism in NHS Talking Therapies an ongoing concern; Kunorubwe et al., 2023).
- Some institutions may prove inhospitable, offer inaccessible support, and display little awareness of the needs of neurodiverse students (Clouder et al., 2020). These and many other examples highlight the additional barriers faced.
- The intention behind sharing these challenges is not to dissuade you from applying but rather to acknowledge the realities. By acknowledging these, we aim to foster a collective understanding and validate your experiences. We can work collectively to address these, fostering a more supportive and equitable environment for all aspiring CBT therapists.
- Finally, this acts as a call to action for those in positions of power, regardless of nation, sector, or service, to take committed actions.

Acknowledgements

I would like to extend my sincere appreciation to all those who graciously contributed their time and shared their invaluable knowledge. This includes Joanne Williams, CBT therapist/Senior Lecturer, at the University of Cardiff. Katy Emerson, CBT therapist/Lecturer, at the University of Cardiff. David Hitt, CBT therapist/Lecturer, at the University of Cardiff. Fiona Switzer, Interim Programme Director/CBT therapist, in South of Scotland Masters Programme in CBT at Queen Margaret University, Edinburgh. Dr Mallika Sharma, Clinical Psychologist/Director of CBT Programmes, at Buckinghamshire New University. Dr Hannah Vickery, Associate Professor/BABCP-accredited clinical psychologist, at University of Reading. Your generosity in sharing your time and wisdom is a testament to the kindness and support that define our CBT community.

Further reading

https://babcp.com/Careers/Accredited-Courses
https://babcp.com/Minimum-Training-Standards
Jenkins, H., Waddington, L., Thomas, N., & Hare, D. J. (2018). Trainees' experience of CBT training: A mixed methods systematic review. *The Cognitive Behaviour Therapist, 11*, e2.
Waddington, L., & Jury, R. (2013). Improving access to psychological therapies: A comparison between two devolved nations. *The Cognitive Behaviour Therapist, 6*, e2.

References

Butcher, G., & Chigwedere, C. (2022). CBT in the Republic of Ireland. In M. D. Terjesen & K. A. Doyle (Eds.), *CBT in a global context*. Springer.
Calnan, M. (2000). The NHS and private health care. *Health Matrix, 10*(3).
Clouder, L., Karakus, M., Cinotti, A., Ferreyra, M. V., Fierros, G. A., & Rojo, P. (2020). Neurodiversity in higher education: A narrative synthesis. *Higher Education, 80*(4), 757–778. https://doi.org/10.1007/s10734-020-00513-6
Guy, M. (2019). Between 'going private' and 'NHS privatisation': Patient choice, competition reforms and the relationship between the NHS and private healthcare in England. *Legal Studies, 39*(3), 479–498.
Kunorubwe, T., Ruth, E., Cantwell, S., Fisher, T., George, I., & Griffiths, R. (2023). *Racism in IAPT is real & anti-racist guidelines are 'great on paper'*. BABCP Conference-2023, Cardiff. https://doi.org/10.13140/RG.2.2.19713.02409
National Audit Office. (2023, February 9). *Progress in improving mental health services in England*. NAO. www.nao.org.uk/wp-content/uploads/2023/02/Progress-in-improving-mental-health-services-CS.pdf
NHS England. (2019, July). *NHS mentalw health implementation plan 2019/20–2023/24*. NHS England. www.longtermplan.nhs.uk/wp-content/uploads/2019/07/nhs-mental-health-implementation-plan-2019-20-2023-24.pdf
NHS England. (2023). *NHS talking therapies, for anxiety and depression*. NHS England. www.england.nhs.uk/mental-health/adults/nhs-talking-therapies/
Public Health Scotland. (2023, April 25). *Quality indicator profile for mental health: An official statistics release for Scotland*. Public Health Scotland. https://publichealthscotland.scot/media/19178/2023-04-25-qipmh-full-report.pdf
Northern Ireland Audit Office. (2023, May 23). *Mental health services in Northern Ireland: Report by the comptroller and auditor general*. Northern Ireland Audit Office. www.niauditoffice.gov.uk/files/niauditoffice/documents/2023-05/00293490%20-%20Mental%20Health%20Report_WEB.pdf
Welsh Government. (2023, April 23). *NHS expenditure programme budgets: April 2021 to March 2022*. Welsh Government. www.gov.wales/sites/default/files/pdf-versions/2023/4/2/1682411438/nhs-expenditure-programme-budgets-april-2021-march-2022.pdf

Chapter 4

Maximising your chances at interview

Cheryl Nicholls and Sarah Priestley

Introduction

So, you're shortlisted, now what? Firstly, well done, you have overcome the first hurdle and have been shortlisted for an interview. The interview is an opportunity for you to further demonstrate to both the university and the service, that you are the best candidate for the job. This chapter will look at the interview process in detail from both a University and Service perspective. Interview panels for Trainee CBT positions will usually consist of senior clinicians/managers from the service and a tutor from the course. Both will be looking at your overall performance at interview, but from slightly different perspectives.

Cheryl (service perspective)

This might sound obvious but the most important thing you can do is prepare for the interview. The questions will differ from service to service, year to year, but will have similar themes. There are likely to be questions on

- risk;
- managing the demands of the training;
- your experience of supervision;
- your clinical experience;
- your awareness and engagement in the CBT literature.

Make sure you are familiar with some key CBT texts; however, you won't be expected to be able to provide a full reference or to talk about them in any great depth but consider a specific chapter that you found interesting or useful. This knowledge demonstrates that you already have a basic knowledge of what CBT is and that you have done some reading in this area which shows a genuine interest in CBT. The Roth and Pilling CBT competencies (2008) is a good starting point. This outlines the core competencies required to deliver effective CBT, and whilst some of these are related to theoretical knowledge and clinical skills that you will develop during the training year, many of these are skills you will already have

DOI: 10.4324/9781003428527-6

from your current work experiences that can be demonstrated or referred to during the interview process. The panel is aware this is an interview for a trainee position, so there won't be any in-depth theoretical questions, but there is an expectation that you are able to demonstrate a good understanding of the role and what being a CBT therapist entails.

> **Top tips:** Prior to the interview, spend some time thinking about the experience and skills you already have and ensure you convey this in the answers to the interview questions.
>
> Take every opportunity during the interview to demonstrate you have these transferrable skills.

Making your answers count

After each interview, the panel will review the responses given and award a score for each question and task. The higher the score, the more likely you are to be appointed. This is why it is very important that you give as much detail as possible in your answers. The trainee CBT positions are highly sought after, and services often receive a high volume of applicants and interview multiple applicants for each position. In some cases, there are only a few points between the person that is appointed and those that are not successful at interview (see examples of high- and low-scoring answers).

> **Example Question:** How will you manage the demands of both the clinical and academic elements of the role?
>
> ### Poor answer
>
> *I have completed my psychological wellbeing practitioner (PWP) training, so I have studied and had a placement before. I am well organised; I won't miss any lectures and I have a lot of clinical experience so I can build on those skills. I think I will manage this well.*

This answer is poor because it's vague and lacks detail. There are so many transferrable skills from the PWP training, and this response does not use this as an opportunity to highlight these. It also does not mention any personal strategies you have to manage stress outside the workplace, and this is crucial to let the interviewers know you are aware of the importance of self-care and managing your own wellbeing.

Good answer

I have previously completed my PWP training which involved studying whilst on placement. I know from this experience that I need to keep on top of the academic assignments and reading. I make sure I know when the upcoming deadlines are and make sure I use my time effectively to ensure I don't fall behind with anything. I understand how important it is to take on board what is taught at university and to implement this into my clinical work on the placement so I can develop my clinical skills in line with the academic learning. I know how important it is to engage in regular supervision and how important supervision is in my development. I have a lot of skills that will help me manage these demands including good organisational skills, and good IT skills. I have studied at post graduate level previously, so I am confident about my academic writing ability. My PWP experience has given me a good foundation to build and develop my clinical skills from and has made me feel confident I will be able to undertake further academic training whilst on placement. I also have some good personal strategies in place that help me prioritise my wellbeing and manage stress. I have a good social network and I enjoy walking my dog and doing Yoga.

Conversely, the second example demonstrates a good answer. This answer goes into much more detail about transferrable skills and how the candidate has learnt from past experiences. It includes information on managing both the academic and clinical elements of the role, it refers to how supervision was utilised to assist learning and development, it considers some more general skills such as information technology (IT) and organisation, and it includes personal strategies. There are lots of different factors that have been considered and this answer will score more points at interview.

Engage with the panel

Whilst it's important to be prepared for the interview, it's not advisable to take any notes into the interview with you. Some services will allow this if you ask. Firstly, you don't know what the questions are going to be, so notes won't really help during the interview. Secondly, you will spend time looking through them and won't be fully engaged in the interview process. Finally, all this is demonstrating to the panel is that you can read things off a piece of paper! The panel are looking for you to demonstrate your ability to answer the questions based on your past experiences and knowledge which you should be able to do without notes to prompt you. Remember, you won't be able to look through notes when you have you are in a room with your first CBT client! You need to be able to demonstrate your ability to answer questions that you have not prepared for, drawing from the knowledge you have. It may also be useful to consider the function of the notes – is this a safety behaviour (Thwaites & Freeston, 2005) to help you feel more able to manage the process? Having some prompts to read before you go into the interview may be helpful, so you have things you want to ensure you mention in mind, but don't bring them into the interview with you.

> **Top tip:** If a panel member asks if there is anything you want to add or expand on, you should always say yes as this is the panel members way of saying you need to give us more detail. If you are not sure of what else to add, ask to hear the question again and think about what you could elaborate on.

The interview task

Most Trainee CBT interviews are likely to involve a short role-play. Like the interview questions, this will differ across services. You may be given details of the role-play in advance to give you time to prepare, or you may be given the specific details of the role-play when you arrive and some time to prepare before the interview commences.

> **Top tip:** Ensure you carefully consider what the role-play is asking for. Is it an assessment? Sharing a formulation or undertaking/introducing a change method? Ensure you demonstrate what is being asked. Some interview panels will request that you explain the formulation to a client, yet the interviewee has spent the time assessing the client and not sharing the formulation, therefore not completing the correct task during the role-play.

If you are asked to share or draw out a formulation, ensure you use a model that you are familiar with. It's better to demonstrate good use of a five aspects model (Padesky & Mooney, 1990) than deliver a bad demonstration of a depression or panic model. During the role-play, the panel is not just looking at your clinical/theoretical knowledge; they are looking for other core competencies such as interpersonal skills, body language, collaboration, checking understanding, summarising, and pacing. Remember, the panel members are willing for you to do well, and we have all been in your position previously!

The importance of self-reflection

In most cases, you will be asked to reflect on the role-play. This is a great opportunity for you to demonstrate your reflective skills. The ability to do so is essential for any CBT therapist as it's a means for you to continually develop and improve your clinical skills over the training course and throughout your CBT career (Haarhoff & Thwaites, 2015). Try and be balanced in your role-play reflection, highlighting both strengths and weaknesses. Don't be worried about drawing the panel's attention to the parts you did not do well (they also probably picked up on this). Having an awareness of this, and saying what you could do to improve will be seen as a positive (see examples of good and not so good reflective answers)

Poor reflection

I think it went well. I explained the model clearly and they seemed to understand it. I demonstrated empathy well. I would like to have asked more questions but didn't have time to. I use the five areas model all the time, so I felt confident in using it. The client seemed to be on board with what we were doing.

Good reflection

I used a five areas model as I am very familiar with using this, it's also easy for the client to understand and introduces the main area's CBT focuses on. I think I demonstrated good interpersonal skills and nonverbal communication and put the client at ease. I made sure I checked the clients understanding of how the different areas were related. I could have done this better and spent more time explaining this. I normalised some of the symptoms they mentioned and tried to give some brief psychoeducation. I could have asked more questions to get more detail of some of the things they mentioned. For example, they mentioned worrying a lot and I could have asked more about this, for example the content of the worry, how long they worry for and any specific times of day this is better or worse. I think I rushed some parts of it, but I was trying to ensure I got everything into the time given. When they were talking about the physical anxiety and how distressing they find some of the symptoms, I could have used a rating scale and asked how bad it is on a scale of 1 to 10 to give me a clearer understanding of the patients experience. They referred to some thoughts that they felt hopeless, in practice I would have explored these in much more detail and completed a full risk assessment, but I did not do that in the role-play as I wanted to stay focused on the task and not use the time completing a full risk assessment.

Final thoughts

When I am a member of an interview panel, I am not only looking for the interviewee to answer the questions well and demonstrate a good basic knowledge of CBT (although this is essential), I am also thinking:

- Did they demonstrate the key skills required to develop a good therapeutic relationship?
- Will they fit into my team of staff well?
- If I were a client and I attended an assessment or first treatment appointment with this person, would I be happy that they were my therapist and would I want to go back for my second appointment?

Top tip: The value of the therapeutic relationship is so important to engagement and therapy outcomes that demonstrating these skills effectively in an interview will be advantageous. Be yourself, be genuine, be empathic. The interview is your opportunity to make the panel members see that you are someone they would want on their team of clinicians.

Sarah (tutor's perspective)

It may be that you have not had an interview for a whilst, or perhaps you have had several interviews but have not had any offers. Nevertheless, it's important to spend time on your interview technique. This section looks at specific ways to improve your answers.

Improving your interview answers

It is common for prospective trainees to apply to various services to gain a place on the training using a scattergun approach. Although this can increase your chances of being offered a post, it can also carry risks as interviewers may question your commitment to their service. To help mitigate against this and to simply demonstrate your passion, make sure you do your research on where your placement will be and be ready for questions such as 'why do you want to work for us?' Although some of the placements may be in the NHS, others are NHS commissioned, and therefore, you will be working for a separate organisation with potentially different values and working conditions. Make sure you do your research and consider speaking to others who work within the service to see if it is the right fit for you.

Another consideration is that you may attend separate interviews for different services but have the same university panel members. This isn't necessarily a problem; however, it's important to show them that you have taken the feedback on board from previous interviews if you were not offered a post. Within CBT training, you will be provided with ongoing, constructive feedback through various assignments. For example, you will have to record clinical sessions with your clients and watch these back whilst your service and university supervisors provide a critique of your clinical competencies. It is important that you can put the feedback you receive into practice! See this interview as an opportunity to demonstrate this skill.

Interview skills

You might want to consider using the STAR technique (see Figure 4.1) to help you structure your interview answers. This is a helpful technique that is commonly used by candidates, particularly when addressing competency-based questions. The components of STAR will help you demonstrate your skills clearly and succinctly.

Virtual interviews

During the pandemic, we shifted lots of working practices online, including interviews. For many services, this shift has become permanent. This works particularly well when services recruit alongside universities as the panel do not have to be together in the same location. It is also possible to conduct more interviews within a set timeframe when they are virtual compared to face to face. However, virtual interviews can lead to issues for the interviewee.

Additional challenges to consider online

1. Poor audio or video quality can be time-consuming within an interview, and it certainly does not give a great impression to the interview panel. This might also cause concerns if the service offers virtual appointments to their clients; they may question whether you will be able to do the job. It is therefore important to test your technology beforehand and ensure that you have the correct software installed.
2. For a trainee position, it is important for you to demonstrate effective interpersonal skills within the interview. This can be difficult when interviewing

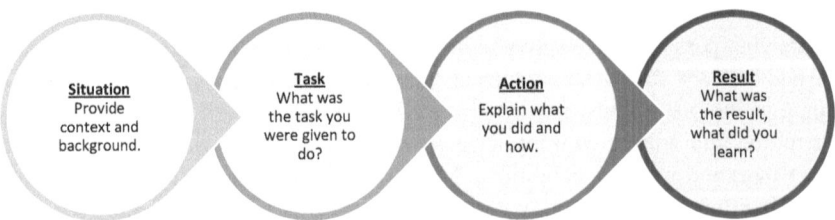

Figure 4.1 STAR technique

virtually, for example, depending on the set up of your camera there could be a lack of eye contact limiting your connection with the panel. It is therefore important to be mindful of how you might compensate for this.

3. There may also be several other interviews on the same day, so it is important that you stand out from the crowd. Ensure that you talk about your individual qualities and experience/s and demonstrate clearly how they make you suitable for *this* role.

Example of using the STAR technique

Interview question: *Tell me about a time when you have managed risk.*

Situation: *When I worked as a PWP, I screened new clients coming into the service to determine whether they were eligible for the service, and to determine the urgency of allocation.*

Task: *As part of each screening, I completed a risk assessment to evaluate the potential risk/s the client posed to themselves and/or others. A few weeks ago, one particular client stated that they were having frequent thoughts of harming themselves.*

Action: *I followed the Trust protocol and completed a full risk assessment as I had been trained to do. I asked about the specifics of these thoughts, that is, what were these thoughts, how often did they have them, and were they going to act on them. The client told me that although they were having these thoughts frequently, they knew they would not act on them. I asked them what was stopping them from acting on them and asked questions around historic self-harm and suicidal ideation. We then completed a safety plan within the appointment, which identified who the client would contact if their thoughts became more frequent or intense. I also informed the client's GP (the referrer) via letter so that they were also fully informed of the situation.*

Result: *Following the screening, I took the client to clinical supervision to talk through the case and ensure that I had followed procedure correctly. Unfortunately, I had to wait for supervision as my supervisor was on annual leave. I recognised that this was not ideal and identified that it could have been particularly problematic if anything had been missed during the screening. I therefore set up weekly post screening clinics that were facilitated by a Senior PWP, so that all screenings could be discussed within 5 working days.*

Making use of technology to enhance interview skills: case study – David (pseudonym)

I knew that I wanted to do my CBT training. I'd been working in mental health for years as a Registered Mental Health Nurse (RMN) and I was tired of firefighting and wanted to help clients manage their mental health conditions and get 'better'. I had applied for several CBT training posts, and I always got offered an interview. Unfortunately, this never came to anything, so I knew I needed to do something different.

I had completed mock interviews before, but this time my supervisor suggested that we record our interview so that we could watch it back. This was relatively easy to set up as most of our work had moved online due to the pandemic. It wasn't a comfortable exercise, but it was certainly eye-opening. My supervisor and I watched it back together, one question at a time. We were able to critique my answers, and my general demeanour. Overall, it was clear that I needed to give more examples to demonstrate my skills and experience, and to slow down! The proof is in the pudding as they say, as following this I was offered a training post. It was also helpful in preparing me for watching clinical sessions and critiquing my skills in CBT as part of the course.

Final thoughts

Do you have any questions?

You will usually be given the opportunity to ask the panel questions at the end of your interview. You might wonder, if you do not ask a question, could this come across as arrogant? If you do ask questions, what sort of questions should they be?

Examples of helpful questions:

* How is the timetable structured?
* What days would I be studying at university and which days would I be in service?

Ask for support

If you are aware that you may need specific support, for example with academic writing, it can be helpful to ask a question to identify what is available should you be offered a place. This demonstrates your self-awareness and may also provide you with some assurances that support is available.

Remember, this is probably the last part of the interview and therefore the lasting image that the panel will have of you. It is important to leave a good impression!

Top tips

- Research the organisation and university where you will be studying.
- Do some reading of key CBT texts.
- Have an awareness of the core CBT competencies you can demonstrate in the interview.

  - Talk to others who have been through the training.
  - Have a mock interview to gain informal feedback

- Listen to the questions and think before you answer.

  - It's ok to pause whilst you think.
  - You might want to ask the panel to repeat the question or write down the question to help you process it better.
  - Give lots of detail in your answers but don't waffle!
  - Consider using the STAR technique.
  - Show the panel how you are suitable for the role.

- Lastly, be authentic, the panel want to see the real you!

Conclusion

This chapter has looked at the interview process in detail, outlining useful ways to prepare. It has given an insight into what panel members are looking for, considered how to deal with the interview task, highlighted techniques to ensure you answer interview questions well, and has given some guidance on how to manage remote interviews. It is now up to you to put this into practice and deliver a good interview on the day, but you can be sure that the whole panel is rooting for you to do well. Finally, if you are not successful at interview, ensure you ask for feedback. This is an opportunity for you to get the panels perspective on what you did well and areas for improvement. If you have applied for several positions, this will help you hone your interview skills in preparation for future interviews. Make sure you take time to reflect on this feedback in preparation for your next interview.

Further reading

Higgins, M. (2014). Using the star technique to shine at job interviews: A how-to guide. *The Guardian*.

References

Haarhoff, B., & Thwaites, R. (2015). *Reflection in CBT*. Sage.
Padesky, C. A., & Mooney, K. A. (1990). Clinical tip: Presenting the cognitive model to clients. *International Cognitive Therapy Newsletter*, 6(1), 13–14.

Roth, A. D., & Pilling, S. (2008). Using an evidence-based methodology to identify the competences required to deliver effective cognitive and behavioural therapy for depression and anxiety disorders. *Behavioural and Cognitive Psychotherapy*, *36*(2), 129–147.

Thwaites, R., & Freeston, M. H. (2005). Safety-seeking behaviours: Fact or function? How can we clinically differentiate between safety behaviours and adaptive coping strategies across anxiety disorders?. *Behavioural and Cognitive Psychotherapy*, *33*(2), 177–188.

Chapter 5

Leaving behind your 'previous professional self' – the challenges of role transition

Mathew Wilcockson

Introduction

Becoming a cognitive behavioural therapist involves personal change. It is easy for us to overlook obvious questions professionally, such as 'Where am I now?', 'How did I get to this point?', 'How am I changing?', and 'How am I coping with the change?' Consideration of such questions in the context of self-practice and self-reflection (SP-SR) is critical for development and ongoing growth of the cognitive behavioural therapist (Bennett-Levy et al., 2014). I have likened these changes to having a baby – whilst I can describe the changes in words, the words make no sense until the change occurs in the context of your own experience. The aim of this chapter is to assist the facilitation of transition from practising a core profession to practising cognitive behavioural therapy (CBT), addressing the key factors in the transition process both generically, and specific to each core profession. We will address the process of changing attitudes and behaviours, using CBT and sometimes existing skills from core professions.

Understanding change

Change is not a simple matter of acquiring knowledge but also acquiring beliefs and behaviours. Even just acquiring new knowledge will change our attitude to ourselves, to those around us, and how others may relate to us, including investment in and allegiance to this knowledge, ideals, and behaviours (e.g. Van Zomeren et al., 2010). Theory and research in a range of situations where transition occurs from fields as diverse as changing jobs (Ashforth, 2000) to changing cultures (Kim, 2001) show that the process is not simply a matter of substituting one behaviour and attitude for another, there are many possible outcomes when new and old paradigms conflict.

Managing conflict within our previous selves

We react to change in different ways, depending on the nature of the change, the nature of the loss, and personal factors, including some demographic characteristics and personality factors. We have invested time and resources in our core

DOI: 10.4324/9781003428527-7

professional backgrounds, which we are now choosing to leave behind. Ashforth describes that roles being transitioned from and to both have reinforcers, which are typically delivered through:

> Symbolic management, including mission statements, strategies, stories, rituals, advertising, physical settings, and role models.
>
> (Ashforth, 2000; p. 154)

Becoming a CBT professional (as with the practice of CBT itself) does not simply involve acquisition of knowledge, beliefs, and behaviours; it also involves dealing with conflicts in these beliefs and behaviours and sometimes a leaving behind of former practices which you may have invested in. This is corroborated by several research studies on transition (e.g. Currie et al., 2012). Leahy (2012) addresses some of the reasons for resistance to change in a therapeutic context, including for example, 'Sunk costs'. If you have learned anything about CBT, it may be that existing beliefs and behaviours can be quite resistant to change.

Reflective exercise

What is exciting you about CBT? What are your hopes for the training?
What do you really not want to think about/engage with?
What is comfortable about your core professional background that you really don't want to change?
What is motivating you to be a CBT therapist rather than stay in your core profession?

What are core professions?

Professions historically have been typified by rituals (e.g. Ward rounds), recognisable features (e.g. attire), a body of knowledge, and protecting freedom of entry through education and standards (Friedson, 1994; Salhani & Coulter, 2009). For any profession to be successful, identification from its members needs to be strong, and the process of knowledge and skills development and testing in core professions inducts the clinician into the profession. It also causes them to invest in it through factors such as repetition, peer pressure/support, and cognitive dissonance.[1] Each profession brings with it assets which will assist the practice of, and transition to CBT, but also factors that will conflict with it and impede the transition (Robinson et al., 2012; Wilcockson, 2022).

Key Point: Changing from your current position to CBT can involve unexpected as well as anticipated change. Being 'human' as well as 'professional' is part of the role, as is a need to be aware of the personal factors affecting the therapeutic intervention itself. In many other health related roles, it is broadly possible to 'act' a professional role and keep personal lives separate (e.g. Bray, 1999). There is not a lot of room to hide in CBT. This is described in the context of 'competing selves' in Roscoe et al. (2022) and described at a more personal level in the case study of Binnie (2008).

Universal features in transitioning from previous roles

There appear to be several universal processes in transition across all core professions. These are as follows:

- **Stressors are present and greater than originally anticipated.** Even though the student is told or reads about the difficulties in the training year, there is not a full grasp of it at a personal level. The dissonance between the expectation and the reality and the responses does vary between the professions but is universally present.
- **Avoidance of more uncomfortable parts of CBT, such as observed practice, rarely resolves through self-reflection, and often cognitive dissonance is required.** It is natural that we would want to avoid that which is uncomfortable, and delaying, excusing, or avoiding altogether are common management strategies. Course requirements of being rated and judged generates a tension that resolves in favour of investing in this behaviour, re-setting beliefs in the context of valuing the learning and committing to self-reflection.
- **Self-practice is important in transition, and a protective factor.** There is a dearth of literature on how self-practice is used by CBT therapists, particularly in relation to role transition. Wilcockson (2017) found that therapists used self-practice/self-reflection (SP/SR) to replace previous stress management strategies and managing crises of various descriptions during training.
- **Supervision is important.** It is easy to avoid opening-up discussion of your practice to avoid judgement; however, supervision provides both support and wisdom to make self-practice sustainable in addition to client- and therapy-based learning.
- **Positive experiences with clients are important.** Feeling a sense of skill and achievement is sometimes cited as a turning point for CBT therapists in training.
- **Integration of personality with CBT.** Trying to keep CBT as a role that is acted in professional life, and separate from the personal life, is not feasible, as too many intrapersonal conflicts are experienced.

Core professional reactions to skill-based assessment through observation

As students, you may develop a difficult relationship with the Cognitive Therapy Scale (Revised) (CTS-R) during your course (Blackburn et al., 2001). The CTS-R, originally developed as a reflective tool for trainees and clinicians, has become the primary measure of CBT competency in the United Kingdom (UK). A supervisor rates the competence of the clinician across 12 domains, using a 0–6 scale (Half marks are allowed) for the assessment. Research by Wilcockson (2017) suggests that 35–40% (Depending on the test used) of the overall variance in scores across four core professions (Nursing, Counselling and Psychotherapy, Occupational therapy, and Knowledge, Skills, and Attitudes or KSA route as it's commonly referred to) could be accounted for by the core profession itself, with >99.9% confidence ($n = 76$). At the level of the individual items, 10–40% of the variance could be accounted for by core profession, with 11 of the 12 items demonstrating significant difference by core profession at the 99.5% confidence level.

The same research also looked at therapist self-ratings and concluded that the self-rating of some core professional groups is considerably higher than the actual levels of skill. This difference became more marked the more professionalised the core profession was, especially for mental health nurses, counsellors, and psychotherapists. This is more marked at lower levels of competence. Nursing and Counselling/Psychotherapy, for example, contain empathy as a professional value, leading the student to identify with that value as a member of that profession. If that student was not competent in that area, they often failed to recognise it due to their professional affiliation 'I must be empathic because I am a Nurse'. It was a surprising finding that membership of these healthcare groupings can reduce self-awareness under certain circumstances.

Reflective exercise

What assumptions do you hold about yourself based on your core profession? What are the ideal characteristics of your core profession? Do you ascribe to these values?

. . . .

How receptive to feedback are you if this was to contradict your prior beliefs?

. . . .

An overview of some key issues by core profession

Mental health nursing

Mental health nursing has two dominant ideologies, the medical model and the humanistic, or caring model, which often conflict with each other. The medical model is dominated by a positivist approach where a single reality is assumed ('This patient has Schizophrenia'), often through formal assessment processes such as diagnosis, and prescribed treatment focuses on evidence-based treatment, based on outcomes from trials of clients exhibiting similar symptoms, usually for medications or psychotherapies according to diagnoses (e.g. Townsend & Morgan, 2017). A symptom-focus shares features with CBT for categorisation purposes, but, from a CBT perspective, reducing symptoms may not address the problem – like pushing a ball underwater, it only masks the problem and is likely to come back if maintaining factors are not addressed.

The humanistic model draws on the work of Rogers (1957) and others. It primarily postulates that building a strong relationship with the client, through the core conditions of empathy, genuineness, and unconditional positive regard, is the most important condition to affect client change. Several studies have confirmed that these conditions are at least necessary for change (see Watson et al., 2014). Unlike the medical model, the humanistic model is much more interested in the individual experience of the client, resisting the categorisation process. This model, often nominally taught in training, is much more consistent with the ideals of the profession (e.g. caring).

Where medical and humanistic models conflict, the medical model tends to take priority (Bray, 1999). Even when humanistic work is carried out, it tends to be through a task discrete lens 'I'm just going to spend 15 minutes on my named nurse session'. Because the nursing profession makes up by far the largest number of clinicians in the NHS, there is a need for roles to be task discrete to manage the overall structure of the organisation. Therefore, even activities related to the humanistic model, such as spending time with patients and supervision, are filtered through a task discrete lens, diluting the humanistic experience aspired to by nurses.

Top tip: Be flexible and prepared for personal change. Although CBT is usually aspirational to mental health nurses, resistance to aspects of CBT can delay development, which has much more support during the training year.

- Be prepared to bring your personal self into the training.

This creates several problems in transition to CBT. CBT at a high-intensity level is not a task, done by an expert to a client. It also involves a process, connecting with the client and facing self- and client-based emotion. A second problem is that coping strategies to manage stress used in nursing are less permitted in CBT (e.g. professional distancing/and structured categorisation; Wilcockson, 2020). Consequently, nurses risk higher levels of dysregulation of stress for a whilst when previous coping strategies are removed.

> **Reflective question for mental health nurses**
>
> What attracted you to Mental Health Nursing? Why is it no longer sufficient for you at a personal level?
>
> . . . .

Protective strategies in nursing

Nursing models of practice differ in several important ways to CBT, and coping strategies often fall within these frameworks.

Fragmented collectivism

As a rule, prevailing training and roles ensure that nursing views the client as in some way broken or insufficient, fitting within constructs of the nurse as a 'professional' that 'does to' the client according to their expertise. Given that nurses tend to be witness to the most extreme levels of mental distress on a frequent basis, appropriate strategies are necessary since nursing approaches do not allow time for more reflective options. Labelling the patient as having a problem and the nurse as professional allows for a separation between nurse and client that is likely to be protective for the nurse. The fact that the nurse 'plays' a professional role allows for separation between personal and professional selves, which is also protective. The labelling of the problem means that the nurse can respond to the perceived problem with 'evidence-based solutions' for that problem, means that the problem edits the client's distress and provides a solution that manages the symptoms rapidly for client and therapist, but does not necessarily resolve the problem. Fragmenting the problem into separate roles (medication, housing, etc.) also provides distance from distress.

Counselling and psychotherapy

Counselling and psychotherapy is broadly identified as a core profession, typically through accreditation and registration with several professional bodies. Training may be in one modality or be integrative to include CBT but filtered through a lens which may not fully fit with the application of CBT in practice.

There are features of this approach that both fit with and jar with CBT, even if included within the training. Most other psychotherapies emphasise the right of the therapist to go where the client believes they need most support, rather than where the evidence directs. This allows the therapist freedom to act according to their therapeutic skill, and if appropriate, be rich and diverse in their interventions. It also means that the therapist can avoid performance judgement as there is not necessarily a 'correct' intervention.

Top tips

As you experience CBT 'from the inside', make notes about the client experience. How do the clients experience CBT? What adaptations do you need to make to authentically respond to the client's needs in your own way? Are there any understandings of the client experience that is relevant to your own life? How can CBT be applied to this?

A key factor in resolution for psychotherapists is to experience CBT through the eyes of a client, develop an empathy, for the process, and adjust in your own practice.

Being confronted with judgement can be difficult for some counsellors and psychotherapists. The centrality of the core conditions being challenged (even with therapists practising CBT) can be experienced as a significant loss to many. Furthermore, CBT is unusual as a psychotherapy as emotions are often not the primary focus of treatment. Much more than nursing, psychotherapists do not always find that CBT simply adds to or eventually replaces existing skills, often they can be held in ideological conflict.

Reflective questions for counsellors and psychotherapists

Counsellors and psychotherapists: What brings you here to CBT?

. . . .

How would letting go of unconditional positive regard feel for you?

. . . .

What could interfere with you engaging in the process of CBT learning?

. . . .

Counselling and psychotherapy self-care

Whilst not coherently one model, counselling and psychotherapy employ several coping strategies. One strategy that has already been alluded to is independence and the freedom to practise according to the needs of the client. This has side effect of making the therapist feel valued by the client and may have a protective function from criticism and therefore stress. Also, freedom to practise according to the therapist's perceived needs of the client exempts them from judgement by others ('Doing it wrong'), which is also a protective factor. Both features of counselling are reduced significantly in CBT, increasing the burden of stress initially.

Most psychotherapies recognise the need for self-practice and self-reflection. Counselling and psychotherapy models do vary but typically the community of therapists support each other, through informal supervision and personal therapy. A certain richness from being contained within a community is likely to be protective.

CBT – or at least NHS Talking Therapies CBT – appears to place a difference in emphasis on the responsibility for self-reflection. Supervision supports the process of reflection but may also promote adherence to frameworks of working. A significant emphasis is placed on individual responsibility for self-reflection in CBT; the therapist may see the process of self-reflection as 'work' rather than 'Recuperation'.

Social work

Social work as a profession has not experienced much ethnographic research lately; however, exposure to extremely distressing information and a desire to advocate for the client both have significant impacts on stress, with sickness rates very high as a profession (Frieiro Padin et al., 2021). Supervision and support structures do exist but are considered by some practitioners to be reactionary. As with mental health nurses, there are few structures in training to facilitate self-management of stress in a reflective way.

Reflective questions for social workers

What draws you away from social work?

. . . .

. . . .

What draws you towards CBT?

. . . .

. . . .

Occupational Therapy (OT)

Although the model of human occupation has been around since 1980 (Kielhofner & Burke, 1980; O'Brien et al., 2017), the ability to implement a theoretical model in practice has been difficult, due to being small in number within services, sometimes leading to filling gaps in service provision in order to find space for the role. Generic concepts of British healthcare practice, such as relationship focus and multidisciplinary working is strongly identified with and a solid foundation for CBT training.

This author compared CTS-R scores at initial stages of training and found that, although a small sample ($n = 76$ overall), OTs consistently scored higher on the CTS-R across most domains when compared with Nursing and Psychotherapy and had more accurate perceptions of their own therapeutic ability. Although professional identification is strong, the lack of ownership of ideals and the familiarity of adapting roles to wider teams seems to have kept transferrable skills high in this profession and this may facilitate the transition process. There remain universal issues of transition to this new role, however. Working with and adherence to specific models may be a challenge for some.

Reflective questions for occupational therapists

What originally motivated you to be an occupational therapist? In what ways is this no longer sufficient for you now?

. . . .
. . . .
. . . .
. . . .
. . . .

KSA (Knowledge, Skills, and Attitudes)

This group is defined by them having no core profession, and they must demonstrate equivalence through cumulative professional skills (BABCP, 2020). A surprising finding of Wilcockson (2017) was that individuals completing the KSA route showed high competence and reflective ability at initial stages. One study (Liness et al., 2019) suggests that this group requires more support resources in transition; however, the competence noted above and the qualitative exploration of this by Wilcockson (2020) would suggest that the demand for this extra support is more indicative of confidence rather than competence.

Since these studies, this group has become dominated by psychological wellbeing practitioners (PWPs) who utilise 'low-intensity' CBT interventions and formulations.

Top tips

Try and avoid assuming that you already know CBT. There is a different perspective that it is hard to grasp without exposure to high-intensity training.
Attempts to preserve PWP practice are likely to undermine development.

The role of lessening structure present in PWP roles and greater emphasis on process in high-intensity therapy, and the process of 'being with' rather than 'Doing to', is unfamiliar to many of this group (see Roscoe et al., 2022).

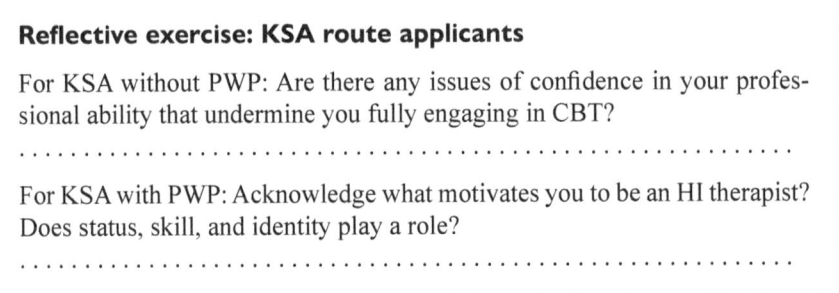

Reflective exercise: KSA route applicants

For KSA without PWP: Are there any issues of confidence in your professional ability that undermine you fully engaging in CBT?

....

For KSA with PWP: Acknowledge what motivates you to be an HI therapist? Does status, skill, and identity play a role?

....

There is limited ethnographic evidence about coping strategies in several of the main core professions. PWPs identify work pressures as a major source of stress, but partly cope by focusing on their values, and sharing the experience of adversity (Vivolo, 2022). One difficulty with this role is that a strategy provided by employers to help manage stress (management supervision) is also a source of stress, reinforcing aspects of the role that generate stress (Painter, 2018).

Social workers use coping strategies broadly similar to nurses (Ben-Zur & Michael, 2007), some of which include disengagement, demand reduction, and compensation (Astvik et al., 2014). Occupational therapists use more conscious or pre-emptive strategies such as management of work–life strategies and self-reflection (Gupta et al., 2012).

For social workers, occupational therapists, and PWPs/KSA applicants

How do you cope with stress? Is it similar to the research or do you not fit into your profession's typical patterns? What issues come up if you were to drop these strategies? What challenges are involved with adopting self-practice of CBT and self-reflection as the main coping strategy?

Top tip:

Start self-practice and self-reflection early. You will be grateful it is in place when existing coping strategies are removed.

For all backgrounds

Take stock of where you are now. How have you changed from the start of the course?
What did you just not understand at the start?

What are you working on now that you had no idea about at the start?
What have you left behind?
What remains uncomfortable?
What are you looking forward to at the end of the course?
Are there other ways of representing the changes (stories, metaphors, and images)?

Taking stock in the middle of the avalanche

Being in the process of change involves uncertainty and discomfort for everyone at some stage. It can sometimes to be helpful to see the bigger picture, acknowledging what you are in the middle of. Here is a list of questions to help you acknowledge where you are currently at in terms of how things are changing for you, in the middle of your training:

Towards the end of training

Self-practice and self-reflection are not something you 'achieve'; ideally, it is an ongoing balanced state, continuing your development and awareness in the face of ongoing insights into your own five areas through therapy and personal commitments.

Shifting the goalposts exercise

It's easy to take where you are for granted and acknowledge the most significant changes for you over this training year from core profession to CBT therapist.

How does acknowledging these changes impact your understanding of them. What implications does this have for your clinical work in the context of understanding the client's needs?

How do you build on the changes that you have made in your training year? What are the next steps in your journey?

Top tips

- Embrace the crisis and the uncertainty
- Self-practice flexibly
- Embrace being your own client
- Notice successes
- Absorb support
- Offer support

Conclusion

The development of the CBT therapist from the core professional is a complex process not guaranteed to succeed. There are some universal challenges, and some specific to each core profession. Embracing challenges to core professional theory and practice early assists the transition process, as does the adoption of SP/SR. SP/SR requires long-term commitment in the context of CBT as it provides profession-congruent protection from and management of the risk of stress and burnout into the long term.

Note

1   In essence, Cognitive Dissonance predicts that, if you undertake a behaviour which is contrary to your beliefs, a process of dissonance occurs which under most predictable circumstances resolves in favour of the behaviour (Festinger, 1957; Cooper, 2007).

Further reading

Binnie, J. (2008). From CPN to CBT: A reflective account of the transition from community psychiatric nurse to cognitive behavioural therapist. *Issues in Mental Health Nursing*, *29*(12), 1273–1276.

Robinson, S., Kellett, S., King, I., & Keating, V. (2012). Role transition from mental health nurse to IAPT high intensity psychological therapist. *Behavioural and Cognitive Psychotherapy*, *40*(3), 351–366.

Wilcockson, M. D. (2020). Transition to cognitive behavioural therapy from different core professional backgrounds: Three grounded theory studies. *The Cognitive Behaviour Therapist*, *13*, e35.

References

Ashforth, B. (2000). *Role transitions in organizational life: An identity-based perspective.* Routledge.

Astvik, W., Melin, M., & Allvin, M. (2014). Survival strategies in social work: A study of how coping strategies affect service quality, professionalism, and employee health. *Nordic Social Work Research*, *4*(1), 52–66.

Bennett-Levy, J., Thwaites, R., Haarhoff, B., & Perry, H. (2014). *Experiencing CBT from the inside out: A self-practice/self-reflection workbook for therapists.* Guilford Publications.

Ben-Zur, H., & Michael, K. (2007). Burnout, social support, and coping at work among social workers, psychologists, and nurses. *Social Work in Health Care*, *45*(4), 63–82. https://doi.org/10.1300/J010v45n04_04

Binnie, J. (2008). From CPN to CBT: A reflective account of the transition from community psychiatric nurse to cognitive behavioural therapist. *Issues in Mental Health Nursing*, *29*(12), 1273–1276.

Blackburn, I., James, I., Milne, D., & Baker, C. (2001). The revised cognitive therapy scale (CTS-R) psychometric properties. *Behavioural and Cognitive Psychotherapy*, *29*(4), 431–446.

Bray. (1999). An ethnographic study of psychiatric nursing. *Journal of Psychiatric and Mental Health Nursing*, *6*(4), 297–305.

British Association for Behavioural and Cognitive Psychotherapies. (2020). *Guidelines for assembling and assessing KSA portfolios or evidence for course assessment.* https://babcp.com/Knowledge-Skills-Attitudes

Currie, G., Lockett, A., Finn, R., Martin, G., & Waring, J. (2012). Institutional work to maintain professional power: Recreating the model of medical professionalism. *Organization Studies*, *33*(7), 937–962.

Friedson, E. (1994). *Professionalism reborn: Theory, prophecy and policy*. University of Chicago Press.

Frieiro Padin, P., Verde-Diego, C., Arias, T. F., & González-Rodríguez, R. (2021). Burnout in health social work: An international systematic review (2000–2020). *European Journal of Social Work*, *24*(6), 1051–1065.

Gupta, S., Paterson, M. L., Lysaght, R. M., von Zweck, C. M. (2012). Experiences of burnout and coping strategies utilized by occupational therapists. *Canadian Journal of Occupational Therapy*, *79*(2), 86–95. https://doi.org/10.2182/cjot.2012.79.2.4

Kielhofner, G., & Burke, J. P. (1980). A model of human occupation, part 1. Conceptual framework and content. *The American Journal of Occupational Therapy*, *34*(9), 572–581.

Kim, Y. Y. (2001). *Becoming intercultural: An integrative theory of communication and cross-cultural adaptation*. Sage.

Leahy, R. L. (2012). *Overcoming resistance in cognitive therapy*. Guilford Press.

Liness, S., Beale, S., Lea, S., Byrne, S., Hirsch, C. R., & Clark, D. M. (2019). Multi-professional IAPT CBT training: Clinical competence and patient outcomes. *Behavioural and Cognitive Psychotherapy*, *47*(6), 672–685.

O'Brien, J. C., Hinojosa, J., Kramer, P., & Royeen, C. B. (2017). Model of human occupation. In Hinojosa, J., Kramer, P., & Royeen, C. B. (Eds.), *Perspectives on human occupation: Theories underlying practice* (pp. 93–136). F.A. Davis Company.

Painter, A. (2018). *Processing people! The purpose and pitfalls of case management supervision provided for psychological wellbeing practitioners, working within improving access to psychological therapies (IAPT) services: A thematic analysis* [Doctoral dissertation, University of the West of England].

Robinson, S., Kellett, S., King, I., & Keating, V. (2012). Role transition from mental health nurse to IAPT high intensity psychological therapist. *Behavioural and Cognitive Psychotherapy*, *40*(3), 351–366.

Rogers, C. R. (1957). The necessary and sufficient conditions of therapeutic personality change. *Journal of Consulting Psychology*, *21*(2), 95.

Roscoe, J., Bates, E. A., & Blackley, R. (2022). 'It was like the unicorn of the therapeutic world': CBT trainee experiences of acquiring skills in guided discovery. *The Cognitive Behaviour Therapist*, *15*, e32.

Salhani, D., & Coulter, I. (2009). The politics of interprofessional working and the struggle for professional autonomy in nursing. *Social Science & Medicine*, *68*(7), 1221–1228.

Townsend, M. C., & Morgan, K. I. (2017). *Psychiatric mental health nursing: Concepts of care in evidence-based practice*. FA Davis.

Van Zomeren, M., Leach, C. W., & Spears, R. (2010). Does group efficacy increase group identification? Resolving their paradoxical relationship. *Journal of Experimental Social Psychology*, *46*(6), 1055–1060.

Vivolo, M. (2022). *The process of building resilience in the IAPT psychological wellbeing practitioner role: A qualitative grounded theory study* [Doctoral dissertation, University of East Anglia].

Watson, J. C., Steckley, P. L., & McMullen, E. J. (2014). The role of empathy in promoting change. *Psychotherapy Research*, *24*(3), 286–298.

Wilcockson, M. D. (2017). *The contribution of the core professions to the IAPT high intensity role* [Unpublished PhD University of Coventry].

Wilcockson, M. D. (2020). Transition to cognitive behavioural therapy from different core professional backgrounds: Three grounded theory studies. *The Cognitive Behaviour Therapist*, *13*, e35.

Wilcockson, M. D. (2022). Conflicts of identity – how counsellors practice CBT 5 years post qualification. *Sciences*, *11*(2), 42–50.

Chapter 6

Am I well suited to the role?

Understanding some of the factors that influence our 'alignment' with CBT

Jason Roscoe and Elaine Davies

Introduction

What causes mental illness? Do separate mental disorders exist or are they socially constructed? How should we treat them, with medication or through talking treatments alone? These are questions that are rarely asked during CBT training selection yet have the potential to influence how we engage with cognitive behavioural theories and interventions.

The intention of this chapter is to help you consider how well suited you are to working as a CBT therapist, or in the case of clinical psychologists, adopting this as your main modality. Building on the profession-specific challenges that were introduced in Chapter 5, this chapter will help you to consider the degree to which you are currently aligned with the core principles and practices of CBT and, what you can do to improve your alignment.

Rather than viewing your suitability as a simple 'yes' or 'no', we can think of it as a sliding scale of alignment with the theories and practices associated with CBT (Roscoe & Wilbraham, 2024).

> **Key Point:** Passing an interview for a CBT training course is no guarantee of how good a 'fit' this modality will be for you as a career. This chapter will help you reflect on factors that might influence your natural alignment with CBT theories and ways of working.

Research indicates that there might be an interaction between who we are prior to training (our personal self) and the job role we were in (our previous professional self) that might predispose us to certain difficulties during CBT training (see Deacon et al., 2013; Meyer et al., 2014; Roscoe et al., 2022; Wilcockson, 2020). These predisposing factors can impede skill acquisition (e.g. resisting CBT as a way of conceptualising client difficulties) or influence what we are willing to do in our treatment sessions (e.g. helping clients face difficult memories, emotions or situations). Furthermore, personal and/or previous professional selves might continue

DOI: 10.4324/9781003428527-8

to influence how we practice therapy or use supervision once qualified if we fail to continually reflect on their influences (Roscoe & Taylor, 2023).

Reflective exercise

Imagine a scale from 0 to 10 where 10 is the most 'aligned' you could be to CBT theories, interventions, and ways of working with clients and 0 represents complete rejection of all of these. Be honest with yourself, what number would you give yourself right now and why?

NOTE: This number is likely to change during training as you gain more knowledge and skill, and common misconceptions may also be corrected.

'Personal self' (PS) factors and their impact on our CBT alignment

This section looks at a range of personal characteristics that may affect our alignment with CBT. Before examining personal characteristics, it is useful to briefly introduce a model that helps us understand how CBT therapists acquire knowledge and skills.

How therapists develop their knowledge and skills?

The declarative procedural reflective (DPR) model (Bennett-Levy, 2006) proposes that therapist skill development arises through the accrual of technical knowledge of CBT (declarative knowledge) and knowing how to deliver an intervention in a range of contexts (Procedural knowledge and skills). Whilst different training methods are used to support the development of the 'Therapist self' (see Bennett-Levy et al., 2009), our reflective system helps us to compare learning from clinical experiences with our declarative and procedural knowledge of CBT and vice versa. Of significance here is the concept of two 'selves' that interact during CBT skill acquisition – the 'personal self' which contains all the trainees' life experiences and beliefs prior to training and the emerging 'therapist self'. Below is a non-exhaustive list of 'personal self' facets that we bring with us into our training:

- core beliefs about ourselves and others (I am . . ./Others are . . .);
- rules (Shoulds/Musts) & Assumptions (If . . . then);
- level of meta-cognitive awareness;
- pre-existing mental health problems;
- tolerance for uncertainty;
- affect regulation;

- propensity towards experiential avoidance;
- self-esteem;
- self-consciousness;
- interpersonal relational skills (e.g. compassion, warmth empathy, charisma);
- capacity for self-care.

The influence of your 'previous professional self' (PPS)

Whilst Chapter 5 has explored the profession-specific challenges of role transition, Roscoe et al. (2022) hypothesised the existence of a third 'self' that competes with the emerging 'CBT therapist self' during training. The development of a CBT pathway within clinical psychology doctorates complicates this process further (see Lack et al., 2024; Rodwell et al., 2023). For example, the trainee clinical psychologist has, in theory, two emerging 'therapist selves' – 'clinical psychologist' and 'CBT therapist' in addition to their previous professional self.

Multiple selves with multiple motivations?

When we factor in our 'personal self' characteristics such as one's tolerance for uncertainty that pre-date CBT training, there are a multitude of complex factors that have the potential to affect the trainees engagement with core CBT interventions (e.g. exposure). As Figure 6.1 shows, our 'personal self' influences our choice of previous professional role, and this then reinforces or changes existing schemas. These can act as barriers to the input from lectures, role-play, and clinical experiences in the formation of our 'CBT therapist self'.

Forewarned is forearmed

Experience on interview panels suggests that many of these 'facets of self' do not feature in most CBT interview questions except for self-care strategies. The

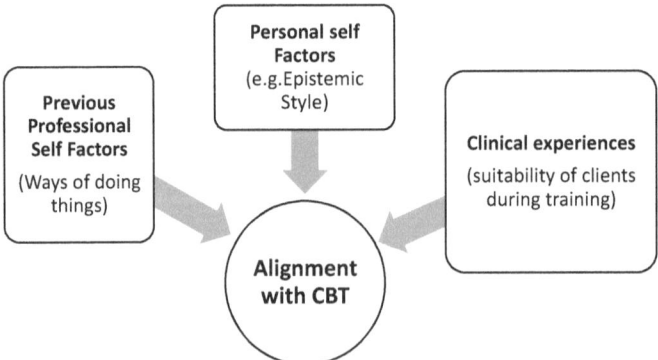

Figure 6.1 Factors hypothesised to influence our alignment with CBT

consequence of this is that ordinarily they do not come to your attention until well into the training programme. For example, a minority of trainees find self-practice or modelling of certain interventions (especially in the treatment of anxiety disorders) highly aversive (Haarhoff et al., 2015). Some examples of what you are expected to do during CBT training might include

- engaging in 'bandwidth broadening' experiments when treating Social Phobia (e.g. asking a stranger where the library is whilst stood in front of the entrance to it; see Wells, 1997);
- writing down or saying out loud unpleasant words or scenarios about your own loved ones (e.g. *I want Chloe to die in a car crash*) to help demonstrate Thought-Action-Fusion experiments to clients (see Bream et al., 2017).

Reflective exercise

Are there any CBT interventions that you would feel hesitant or unwilling to deliver?

How do you anticipate overcoming these personal hurdles?

In summary, our personal, previous professional, or co-existing therapist 'selves' may collectively influence

- our beliefs about what constitutes CBT;
- our therapeutic style (Didactic vs. Socratic; level of emphasis on therapeutic relationship);
- how we use supervision;
- our beliefs about the origins and maintenance of mental health problems;
- how we define and measure progress;
- how 'triggered' we become by certain clients or clinical presentations.

The impact of specific 'therapist schemas'

Leahy (2001) proposed that a number of 'Therapist Schemas' exist and that they interfere with CBT skill acquisition and practice yet they remain poorly understood (Haarhoff, 2006; Roscoe et al., 2022; Roscoe & Taylor, 2023). Whilst schemas are usually thought of as intrapsychic processes, it is important to consider how contextual factors shape and maintain certain beliefs and behaviours (Rameswari et al., 2021). One example might be how a profession such as nursing creates a 'contextual schema' about how we think about the origins and treatment of mental health problems and how we interact with clients and how we use supervision (Robinson et al., 2012).

Understanding your 'epistemic style'

It is beyond the scope of this chapter to explore this concept in depth; however, it is useful to be aware of how your epistemic style might influence yours (and your clients) level of engagement with CBT (Moorey, 2023). Some research suggests that people may be drawn to therapies that closely match their way of understanding the world (Lee et al., 2013; Neimeyer et al., 1997). Most therapists can be thought of as falling under one of three epistemic styles known as positivism, constructivism, and pragmatism (Moorey, 2023). In short, CBT is typically considered to be aligned with positivism, a philosophical position that argues for there being an objective reality that can be discovered and measured (Hughes, 2018; Roscoe & Wilbraham, 2024). Other modalities such as person-centred counselling are thought to be more closely aligned with a constructivist worldview which proposes that there is no single reality and that individuals construct their own reality based on their life experiences and the meaning they ascribe to them. Lastly, pragmatists concern themselves with 'what is useful to my clients?' rather than the pursuit of objective truths.

Reflective exercise

Whether we recognise it or not, we all have an epistemological position, and this acts as a lens through which we view the world.

Q. Would you identify more with positivism, constructionism, or pragmatism? On what basis?

Q. How do you think this might affect your use of certain CBT methods?

Alignment difficulties

Intrapersonal conflicts during training

The trainee faces cognitive dissonance due to the input from lectures and clinical experiences where the emerging 'CBT therapist self' is often torn between assimilating, accommodating or rejecting this new information due to a schematic mismatch with existing beliefs (Moloney & Kelly, 2004; Piaget, 1948; Wilcockson, 2020).

The vignettes describing the experiences of Sarah and Miguel highlight common 'intrapersonal conflicts' arising due to tensions between one's epistemic style and the concepts that are presented during CBT training (e.g. where cognitive dissonance occurs).

Training vignettes

1. *Whilst being introduced to the CBT interventions for depression, Sarah felt strongly that cognitive restructuring appeared to blame the client for their thinking instead of recognising the socio-economic difficulties that were contributing to their low mood.*
2. *Miguel thought that behavioural activation would only work when clients had the money to do pleasurable activities. He struggled to see how those on state benefits could access enough positive reinforcement to lift their depression.*

Potential consequences of unresolved intrapersonal conflicts

These examples are representative of common objections to CBT where its core ideas and methods are seen as reductionistic (Dalal, 2018). It is worth noting that whilst these trainees are fictional, the content of their objections to aspects of CBT are common. Given all the input from our PPS and PS, some degree of trainee resistance to CBT is highly likely. However, without adequate attention, this might lead to avoidance of certain techniques or formulations resulting in what we call 'therapist drift' (Waller, 2009). Alternatively, one might experience a shift towards (e.g. training in another modality) or back to a different way of working (Ball & Corrie, 2024; Roscoe et al., 2022).

> **Key Point:** If there is a considerable mismatch between your own epistemic style and that most closely associated with CBT, it is likely that during training or later in your career, you will encounter tensions between what you are learning and what you have believed about the world until this point.

In the next section, Elaine describes how she manages to work across two modalities that may appear to be conflicted at first glance, without too much intrapersonal conflict.

Elaine's story

Before I begin, I want to tell you a bit about myself. I am a British White, 63-year-old cis-gendered heterosexual Welsh woman who has lived and worked in the same town for 40 years and then moving two miles from that town for the last 20 years. I have been employed by a local GP surgery, then the NHS for more than 35 years. I have worked in training and education for more than 25 years in England and Wales for Universities and Further Education, teaching Counselling and CBT. At the time of writing this chapter, I work for a university in England teaching on the NHS England Talking Therapies postgraduate diploma in CBT. I have a face to face and online private practice for the other days based in a small mining village in South Wales. I am also active with British Association for Behavioural and Cognitive Psychotherapies (BABCP), the UK-based charity organisation that regulates CBT members. I come from working-class roots and through education and hard work, mobilised myself into middle class working and living. Why do I need to tell you all of this; well, if I am going to be part of a chapter that asks about the suitability to train in CBT, it is probably important for you to gain sense of who is doing the writing. From this, you might derive some assumptions of the values and beliefs I might hold which may inform you of the validity in what I say.

I describe myself lately as a cognitive behavioural psychotherapist and counsellor. These terms are used interchangeably, although I hope to show in this chapter how I have found a way of differentiating both when I am teaching, in supervision for others and training. I am accredited with BABCP, BACP (British Association for Counselling and Psychotherapy), and am also a member of ACTO (Association for Counselling and Therapy Online). In an unregulated psychotherapy field, these accrediting bodies support me to work in an ethical and professional manner. The arguments and debates go on as to who is the best, but I try to stay impartial to the nuances but will speak up for both counselling and CBT if myths are told. With such diversity, there is inevitable *schoolism*, a term coined by Clarkson (2000) in which different schools defend their 'truths', and even within the same schools, there will be attacks. I have witnessed this in many forums, the attacks on CBT from counselling and vice versa. I have also witnessed in the school of cognitive and behavioural interventions conflicts surrounding technique and intervention and of late, protocol driven models. For new trainees of any psychotherapy including CBT, this must be confusing and overwhelming. Not forgetting the client, if this goes on, how can we best help the client to decide what works and for what?

Straddling philosophical and theoretical positions

For years, I have been straddling philosophical and theoretical positions of CBT and Counselling, and I believe in what works for whom at different points in their life. The philosophical position of CBT dates to the role of Stoicism. Socrates was a Greek philosopher (469–399 BC) who had a student Plato, who wrote of Socrates questioning style for others to discover their own answers on life's meanings. Being a stoic means to view the world logically and objectively, seeing what comes, and responding to outcomes calmly and without excess emotion. Easier said than done! Helpful though to think about the roots of CBT before embarking on training. Both Aaron Beck (the founder of CBT) and Albert Ellis before him were influenced by stoicism and Epictetus, another Greek philosopher that it is not events but our opinions about events that cause us suffering. This is another way to think about whether one is suitable to train in CBT. Of course, I am aware during my writing that I am taking a reductionist view of the history of philosophy and the links with CBT.

The philosophical and theoretical epistemology of counselling is untidy due to the nature of drawing on a range of lived experience, philosophers, and new developments in the field. The UK lags the rest of the world in their philosophers or philosophical counsellors where there is no such recognised profession (Baggini, 2018). Philosophy is not taught on counselling or CBT courses, but you might find it part of an existential counselling course. For me, some of our life decisions are deep-rooted in philosophical underpinnings and perhaps we ought to give more time to reflect on this prior and during training.

Comparing and contrasting CBT and counselling

What does all this mean? Is counselling the same as CBT? Can you be a counsellor and use CBT? Can you move away from counselling and become a CBT therapist? I would ask a similar question if you had a core profession for example a social worker, a nurse, and a health visitor. Do you want to transition to a psychotherapist or do you want to keep your primary role and become CBT informed to enhance your primary role. These are all good first questions when starting to train as a CBT therapist which I hope by the end of this chapter your own answers will emerge.

Shared origins

All talking therapies were started by a role of some alignment to the definition of doctor or a person to help, maintain, and restore health in the context of disease. Undoubtedly even if some therapies have moved away from the 'medical model', all forms of help start somewhere. It is impossible to talk about CBT without some reference to the term 'medical model'. The physician is seen as the expert, dominant, and trained in diagnosis and treatment. CBT does align itself with the medical model, and when I was working primarily in the NHS with brief therapy models of intervention of problem-solving and being solution focused, CBT was an early attraction. It is helpful, therefore, to think about the context of employment alongside the curious questions of CBT suitability.

Before committing to any training as a psychotherapist, counsellor, or indeed CBT therapist, it is best to understand the factors that have influenced the self and the chosen training (see comments earlier in this chapter). Personality, values, early experiences, culture, previous professional experience, sudden life changes or events, finances, social class mobility, and even experiencing therapy are commonly cited as reasons people chose to train in talking therapies. In some parts of the UK where counselling was taken off the table to help others and only CBT was offered, this has disadvantaged some clients who are not suited to CBT. So, whilst we are asking the question from a new trainee perspective 'am I suitable to CBT?' it is also helpful to ask this from a client viewpoint.

The role of therapist

In both CBT and counselling, we bring *the self* to the work. The professional self being the frameworks and the skills in our role. The personal self involves drawing on our values and experiences, which helps us connect with others. The private self we might keep hidden. In Counselling, more so with person-centred therapy, it is likely that all three are as one, often using personal therapy and supervision regularly to address any hidden bias, judgement, or lack of authenticity towards another. Where personal therapy is not mandated during CBT training, the personal self is typically accessed through self-practice/self-reflection (SP/SR) (Bennett-Levy et al., 2014).

Client preferences

Helping clients decide on whether counselling or CBT will be the right intervention for them is not easy, nor should it be. Finding out about the client, what their own world views are, their values, culture, and life philosophy will help (Moorey, 2023). Helping the client decide if they know what their problem is or what they need help about can all set the scene for helping interventions, whether it be Counselling or CBT. Assessment and formulation of the problem, how the client views their problem, what goals they might set themselves, and what context the therapist and client meet under are important factors. Clients may choose counselling if they don't like labels or are not seeking a diagnosis, or if they want to discover aspects of themselves with no timeframe or if they are not ready for immediate change.

Counselling can include CBT as part of an overarching model described earlier (which is how I have adopted my counselling). I use three modalities; person-centred, cognitive behavioural, and cognitive analytical to inform my work with clients. I also use CBT as a standalone treatment of choice. CBT still stands out in many presenting issues as the 'go to' therapy. I think this is right that we continue to ask the client what might work for them but also inform them of long-standing evidence-based treatments. This is an area where we are doing better on letting the client have the say (Subramaniam, 2021).

Self-rating your 'alignment' with CBT principles and practices

Hopefully the information in the previous sections will have helped you to get some idea of where your default alignment to CBT 'sits' at present. The CBT alignment scale (see Appendix 1) has been developed by Roscoe (2023) to help potential CBT therapists gauge their personal suitability to engage in this role. Items have been derived from research, a review of the relevant literature and experience from training multiple cohorts of therapists and from discussions with colleagues at other training institutions. The scale has five sections which broadly relate to the style, structure, and epistemological and ontological positioning of CBT. It uses a Likert scale to gauge the strength of alignment to each category, and the intention is to use this to self-identify your current level of alignment. You can then reflect on how each item changes throughout your training and post-qualification. Low scores might indicate a need to address any negative beliefs about CBT, misconceptions about theory or interventions or other personal characteristics that have the potential to inhibit skill acquisition (e.g. experiential avoidance).

Improving your alignment

Having reviewed your scores for each section, it is important to reflect on areas where scores were lower and the reasons for this.

- Perhaps there are some 'personal self' rules and assumptions about interrupting clients, and this can be overcome during supervision.
- Perhaps you notice that there are some fundamental aspects of CBT practice that don't fit with how you want to deliver therapy.

Roscoe and Wilbraham (2024) propose a checklist for use in CBT supervision to help trainers and trainees keep an eye on alignment and how this might change during training. There are some suggestions about potential barriers to CBT alignment and what aspects of skills training might help. This checklist could be used at the start, halfway through, and towards the end of one's course.

Conclusion

Learning theories (e.g. Piaget, 1948) suggest that we do not simply absorb new information like sponges; instead, new knowledge is compared with existing templates of 'how things are done'. As described in Chapter 5, there are different intrapersonal conflicts for trainees depending on their previous role. This chapter has considered how, in tandem with our previous professional selves, our personal characteristics shape our alignment with CBT. It is beyond the scope of this chapter to examine every therapist characteristic that might affect our alignment with CBT; however, our capacity to tolerate our own and others' distress and our willingness to impose structure at the expense of free association (amongst other things) will impact how we engage with CBT models and methods. The good news is that research suggests that some maladaptive therapist beliefs are amenable to targeted training practices. For example, Leahy (2001) identified a range of therapist schemas that can be identified and worked on throughout training and supervision (Haarhoff, 2006). SP/SR is also a helpful vehicle for understanding ourselves better whilst deepening our knowledge of CBT simultaneously, and whilst currently underutilised, deliberate practice offers a promising medium for managing blocks to learning (McLeod, 2022).

Acknowledgements

Thanks to Rhiannon Blackley for helpful comments on earlier versions of this chapter.

Further reading

Moorey, S. (2023). Three ways to change your mind: An epistemic framework for cognitive interventions. *Behavioural and Cognitive Psychotherapy, 51*, 187–199.
Neimeyer, G. J., Robert, J., & Morton, R. J. (1997). Personal epistemologies and preferences for rationalist versus constructivist psychotherapies. *Journal of Constructivist Psychology, 10*(2), 109–123. https://doi.org/10.1080/10720539708404616
Roscoe, J., & Wilbraham, S. (2024). 'When it goes well, it works fantastically': Motivations to train and their impact on the practice of CBT. *The Cognitive Behaviour Therapist, 17*, e6.

References

Baggini, J. (2018, March). The philosophy gap: There's no treatment for life. *BACP University and College Counselling, 6*(1).
Ball, C., & Corrie, S. (2024). "Bridging the gap": A reflexive thematic analysis of the experiences of therapy trainees transitioning from psychodynamic counselling to cognitive behavioural therapy. *Counselling and Psychotherapy Research, 24*(2), 631–641.
Bennett-Levy, J. (2006). Therapist skills: A cognitive model of their acquisition and refinement. *Behavioural and Cognitive Psychotherapy, 34*, 57–78.
Bennett-Levy, J., McManus, F., Westling, B. E., & Fennell, M. (2009). Acquiring and refining CBT skills and competencies: Which training methods are perceived to be most effective?. *Behavioural and Cognitive Psychotherapy, 37*(5), 571–583.
Bennett-Levy, J., Thwaites, R., Haarhoff, B., & Perry, H. (2014). *Experiencing CBT from the inside out: A self-practice/self-reflection workbook for therapists*. Guilford Publications.
Bream, V., Challacombe, F., Palmer, A., & Salkovskis, P. (2017). *Cognitive behaviour therapy for obsessive-compulsive disorder*. Oxford University Press.
Clarkson, P. (2000). Eclectic, integrative and integrating psychotherapy and beyond schoolism. In S. Palmer & R. Woolfe (Eds.), *Integrative and eclectic counselling and psychotherapy*. Sage.
Dalal, F. (2018). *CBT: The cognitive behavioural tsunami: Managerialism, politics and the corruptions of science*. Routledge.
Deacon, B. J., Farrell, N. R., Kemp, J. J., Dixon, L. J., Sy, J. T., Zhang, A. R., & McGrath, P. B. (2013). Assessing therapist reservations about exposure therapy for anxiety disorders: The therapist beliefs about exposure scale. *Journal of Anxiety Disorders, 27*(8), 772–780. https://doi.org/10.1016/j.janxdis.2013.04.006
Haarhoff, B. A. (2006). The importance of identifying and understanding therapist schema in cognitive therapy training and supervision. *New Zealand Journal of Psychology, 35*, 126–131.
Haarhoff, B., Thwaites, R., & Bennett-levy, J. (2015). Engagement with self-practice/self-reflection as a professional development activity: The role of therapist beliefs. *Australian Psychologist, 50*(5), 322–328. https://doi.org/10.1111/ap.12152
Hughes, S. (2018). A brief introduction to the philosophy of science as it applies to clinical psychology. In S. C. Hayes & S. G. Hofmann (Eds.), *Process-based CBT: The science and core clinical competencies of cognitive behavioral therapy*. New Harbinger Publications.
Lack, S., Handley, R., Barr, L., Rivers, M., Patel, A., Coe, M., & Hale, L. (2024). CBT accreditation for clinical psychologists: A limitation or an opportunity to apply and

maintain our organisational and systemic influence and leadership? *Clinical Psychology Forum, 375*. https://doi.org/10.53841/bpscpf.2023.1.371.4

Leahy, R. (2001). *Overcoming resistance in cognitive therapy*. Guilford Press.

Lee, J. A., Neimeyer, G. J., & Rice, K. G. (2013). The relationship between therapist epistemology, therapy style, working alliance, and interventions use. *American Journal of Psychotherapy, 67*(4), 323–345.

McLeod, J. (2022). How students use deliberate practice during the first stage of counsellor training. *Counselling and Psychotherapy Research, 22*(1), 207–218.

Meyer, J. M., Farrell, N. R., Kemp, J. J., Blakey, S. M., & Deacon, B. J. (2014). Why do clinicians exclude anxious clients from exposure therapy? *Behaviour Research and Therapy, 54*, 49–53. https://doi.org/10. 1016/j.brat.2014.01.004

Moloney, P., & Kelly, P. (2004). Beck never lived in Birmingham: Why CBT may be a less useful treatment for psychological distress than is often supposed. *Clinical Psychology-Leicester*, 4–10.

Moorey, S. (2023). Three ways to change your mind: An epistemic framework for cognitive interventions. *Behavioural and Cognitive Psychotherapy, 51*, 187–199.

Neimeyer, G. J., Robert, J., & Morton, R. J. (1997). Personal epistemologies and preferences for rationalist versus constructivist psychotherapies. *Journal of Constructivist Psychology, 10*(2), 109–123.

Piaget, J. (1948). *The moral judgment of the child* (M. Gabain, trans.). Free Press.

Rameswari, T., Hayes, B., & Perera-Delcourt, R. (2021). Measuring therapist cognitions contributing to therapist drift: A qualitative study. *The Cognitive Behaviour Therapist, 14*, e7. https://doi.org/10.1017/S1754470X21000039

Robinson, S., Kellett, S., King, I., & Keating, V. (2012). Role transition from mental health nurse to IAPT high intensity psychological therapist. *Behavioural and Cognitive Psychotherapy, 40*, 351–366. https://doi.org/10.1017/S1352465811000683

Rodwell, D., Kent, T., & Hale, L. (2023). Trainee clinical psychologists' views on the facilitators and barriers to cognitive behavioural practice: A thematic exploration. *Clinical Psychology Forum, 362*, 64–70. https://doi.org/10.53841/bpscpf.2023.1.362.64

Roscoe, J. (2023, July). *Therapist schemas: What they are, why they matter and what we can do about them*. BABCP Annual Conference, Cardiff, Skills Class.

Roscoe, J., Bates, E. A., & Blackley, R. (2022). 'It was like the unicorn of the therapeutic world': CBT trainee experiences of acquiring skills in guided discovery. *The Cognitive Behaviour Therapist, 15*, E32. https://doi.org/10.1017/S1754470X22000277

Roscoe, J., & Taylor, J. (2023). Maladaptive therapist schemas in CBT practice, training and supervision: A scoping review. *Clinical Psychology & Psychotherapy*, 1–18. https://doi.org/10.1002/cpp.2802

Roscoe, J., & Wilbraham, S. (2024). 'When it goes well, it works fantastically': Motivations to train and their impact on the practice of CBT. *The Cognitive Behaviour Therapist, 17*, e6.

Subramaniam, A. (2021, September 29). Why lived experience matters. The limits of empathy. [Blog]. *Psychology Today*. www.psychologytoday.com/us/blog/parenting-neuroscience-perspective/202109/whylived-experience-matters

Waller, G. (2009). Evidence-based treatment and therapist drift. *Behaviour Research and Therapy, 47*, 119–127. https://doi.org/10.1016/j.brat. 2008.10.018

Wells, A. (1997). *Cognitive therapy of anxiety disorders: A practice manual and conceptual guide*. Wiley.

Wilcockson, M. D. (2020). Transition to cognitive behavioural therapy from different core professional backgrounds: Three grounded theory studies. *The Cognitive Behaviour Therapist, 13*, E35. https://doi.org/10.1017/S1754470X20000331

Chapter 7

Managing as a trainee with lived experience of mental health difficulties

Julia Limper-Menapace

Introduction

'You need to look after yourself first before you can help others'. As therapists, we have probably all said this sentence at least once. There is truth in this statement – research shows that therapists who are burnt out and stressed struggle to support their clients to the best of their ability (Everall & Paulson, 2004). Nevertheless, managing our own mental health seems to be a challenge for many of us. Surveys conducted amongst UK therapists suggest that 29% experience symptoms of stress, depression, or burnout, a state characterised by emotional and physical exhaustion (Pines & Aronson, 1983; Tay et al., 2018).

Managing your own mental health during training will be one of the most important things that you can do, especially for trainees who have a pre-existing mental health difficulty. From research, we know that stress leads to us being less effective therapists (Bearse et al., 2013; Neff & Germer, 2022). It can also cause difficulties in building and maintaining therapeutic alliances, attention deficits, and memory impairments (Arnsten, 1998; Flückiger et al., 2018; Hersoug et al., 2018; Liston et al., 2006). This not only affects patients but the training experience and how much we learn. Most importantly, we should not need a rationale for prioritising our mental health.

Reflecting on personal challenges

You may have come into this career with a long history of working in mental health and have already learned some ways of maintaining your wellbeing. This chapter will focus on those who have lived experiences of mental health difficulties, though the principles apply to all. It could be that you face a challenge in your personal life during the course, that previous symptoms are triggered, that you struggle with the role transition, real or perceived criticism, the education system, or with some of the patients and presentations you work with. Whatever your background is, it is likely that training will bring about new challenges.

DOI: 10.4324/9781003428527-9

This chapter will also investigate the impact of lived experience from a strength perspective, discussing strategies to manage your mental health and potential options for support. To avoid a list of generic experiences and strategies, it is important to look at this from your personal point of view, which is where this chapter will start.

Reflective exercise: reflecting on challenges

Which challenges do you anticipate facing during CBT training? Think back to what may have previously triggered lapses or relapses for you – what might you experience during the course? These challenges could be academic, personal, and clinical. These may not be adverse life events but could be times of high pressure (e.g. house moves and weddings) that may combine with academic and clinical challenges. Make a list of these challenges.

Look over the list you have written. Perhaps some of these challenges are ahead of you, and some planning may help reduce some stress associated with them. However, we can't anticipate all our challenges.

An overview of challenges during the training year

Therapist burnout and compassion fatigue

Burnout, as defined by Freudenberger (1975), is thought to have three key components: exhaustion, depersonalisation (loss of empathy and caring – also referred to as compassion fatigue), and a decreased sense of accomplishment. The impact on a therapist's personal life and professional practice can be far-reaching. There are other concepts that have been used to describe therapists' experiences, though some constructs, such as vicarious trauma, lack validation, and there is a lot of overlap between these different constructs (Kadambi & Ennis, 2004). Vicarious trauma in therapists is defined as an acute response to distressing material, with symptoms closely mirroring the experience of PTSD (Sodeke-Gregson et al., 2013). A key message, however, is that whilst concepts may have some differences, experiences of vicarious trauma, compassion fatigue, or burnout are not unique to trauma therapists (Kadambi & Ennis, 2004) and can lead to disconnection from our support network and our patients and isolation (Deighton et al., 2007; Poulsen et al., 2014). The potential negative impact of these symptoms may appear obvious; however, in high-stress situations, we may still miss the early warning signs.

Case study (Julia)

When I started the CBT training, I had worked as a psychological wellbeing practitioner (PWP) and PWP lead for a few years. During my PWP training, I had received treatment for PTSD but I felt in a good place to start this high-intensity training.

Within a month of starting this training, my relationship ended and my living situation significantly changed. I then failed two different video recording submissions. In the panic that followed, I felt I had to prove to everyone that I could cope but struggled to admit how challenging I was finding the course, especially working with PTSD.

When I failed for the second time late in the course, I was exhausted and every word of criticism seemed to tell me that 'you are not a good enough therapist' despite evidence suggesting otherwise. I blamed the CTS-R (Cognitive Therapy Scale-Revised; Blackburn et al., 2001), university staff, teaching sessions, my personal life, the course pressures and mostly, myself.

My own experience powerfully demonstrated to me that even if you have carefully thought about the timing of the course and organised your life around it, you cannot prepare for all challenges that you face. There was not a single thing that supported me in getting through this challenge – it was about reaching out to my peers and my line manager for support, consciously spending time not thinking about university, getting further therapy, and discussing with my supervisor how I was managing PTSD patients. Though challenging, I still think back to my time on the course as one of the most impactful times in my life, not just in terms of what I learned about myself as a therapist but also how I developed in my personal life.

Amongst challenges common in the helping professions, such as burnout and compassion fatigue (Ondrejková & Halamová, 2022), the course also involves academic challenges. This can come alongside external challenges, such as stressors in our day-to-day life, or major life events, such as bereavement, significant illness, house moves, or weddings. These factors, especially combined, can very easily become overwhelming and lead to burnout.

Top tip: detecting signs of burnout

To be mindful of your own distress and levels of compassion fatigue, measures, such as Maslach's Burnout Inventory (MBI; Maslach & Jackson, 1981), can help us gain some insight. Equally, it is a good idea to agree on goals with your supervisor to manage and be mindful of these symptoms together (e.g. at the beginning or mid-point of your training year).

Lived experiences – handicap or superpower?

Lived experience within therapists is a topic that lacks discussion and research, with therapists often avoiding disclosure due to the fear of being stigmatised (Harris et al., 2016; Huet & Holttum, 2016). As a result of both self-stigmatisation and stigma amongst others, we often struggle to look at our lived experience from a place of strength (King et al., 2020). It is important to understand that lived experience, if managed well, can be a unique asset. When we think about these difficult experiences, we tend to question our capacity as therapists, seeing ourselves as 'impaired professionals' (King et al., 2020). Of course, how we look after ourselves and manage these emotions is important to consider. However, evidence points towards the potential of lived experience being a positive contributor to a therapist's practice (Boyd et al., 2016; Cleary & Armour, 2022; Harris et al., 2016).

Reflective exercise – lived experience as a strength

Take a moment to reflect on some of the significant experiences you have had in your life. How have they helped you make sense of difficult circumstances in the past? What did you learn from them? How could they be helpful when you are working with patients or studying?

Maintaining wellbeing during the course

When mental health difficulties resurface, it can be exceedingly difficult to think about where you might turn for support. Therefore, it is important to be prepared, and consider the potential options to explore if you feel things are getting difficult or you are experiencing a setback, lapse or relapse.

Setbacks, lapses, and relapses are part of recovery, and recovery does not tend to be linear (Slade & Longden, 2015). Therefore, you have likely already experienced ups and downs in your mental health and may have significant knowledge about managing these. However, it can be difficult to keep your mental wellbeing at the forefront during the course whilst you are managing your clinical workload, course requirements, and your personal life.

Key Point: If you notice your lived experience impacting your personal and/or therapeutic practice, it is important to reach out for further support, with a list of options shared later in the chapter. Equally, your lived experience has the potential to support your journey as a therapist and help you manage other challenges, which the reflective exercise will encourage you to reflect on.

To monitor your mental health and understand which symptoms to watch out for, it can be useful to understand our mental health difficulties as a continuum (Keyes, 2002). Looking at our mental health as a continuum allows us to respond to changes accordingly. Table 7.1 provides an example of what this might look like:

As you can see from Table 7.1, both symptoms and potential actions are clearly outlined. You may already have a good idea of what works for you when you are struggling, or you can draw on different chapters of this book to get an idea of potential actions. It is important to be prepared and write these down clearly, so that when you are struggling, you do not need to invest the few resources you have in thinking about what helpful steps you can take.

A note on extensions, suspensions, and withdrawals

Thinking about asking for more time, suspending, or even withdrawing from the course can be challenging, especially if we struggle with perfectionism. However, there are several issues that we need to hold in mind when we approach these topics:

1. **There is no shame in needing more time**
   You can apply for extensions when you have a genuine and evidenced reason that you are not able to submit an assignment on time. These processes exist at university, as it is understood that difficult circumstances can happen. Asking for an extension is not a personal shortcoming – it shows your insight and that you understand that your mental health (or other reasons) may mean that at present you cannot deliver your usual standard of work. A recent alumna worded this well when asked what advice she would give anyone starting the course:

   > To not be afraid to take extensions when you have extenuating circumstances, like struggling with your mental health. There is no shame in needing extra time, and as therapists, we need to be looking after ourselves and make sure what we are trying to do is realistic and in our own best interest and our patient's best interest.

2. **Suspending just means pausing the course**
   The term suspension often triggers anxiety for students. When I recently explained this option to a student, they found a better term for this 'hitting the pause button'. Ultimately, suspension means that you need to pause all learning and assessment activities on the course as continuing to study is not in your best interest.

3. **Withdrawal does not mean the end of your journey as a therapist**
   You may consider withdrawal as an option if you do not feel that returning to study will be a realistic target to achieve within the maximum suspension period. Withdrawal may also be discussed if you have failed an assignment multiple times and are unable to apply for further attempts. This is of course

Table 7.1 Continuum of Mental Health Difficulties

Unwell (0–10%)	Struggling (10–25%)	Surviving (25–60%)	Doing well (60–80%)	Thriving (80–100%)
Symptoms: Thoughts: thoughts of being a failure (80% of the time) Emotions: feeling sad and hopeless most of the day Physical: sleeplessness and nightmares most nights, no appetite Behaviours: Avoiding friends and family, not exercising, falling behind on university and patient work.	**Symptoms:** Thoughts: thoughts of being a failure (50% of the time) Emotions: feeling sad and numb Physical: sleeplessness, tension Behaviours: Only seeing friends and family once a month, rarely exercising, falling behind on university work.	**Symptoms:** Thoughts: thoughts of not doing well enough (30–50% of the time) Emotions: anxiety, overwhelmed Physical: 1–2 nights with disrupted sleep a week, increased appetite Behaviours: Only seeing friends and family once a month, rarely exercising, procrastinating university work most of the time.	**Symptoms:** Thoughts: occasional negative thoughts that are easily challenged. Emotions: mix of happy, anxious, excited. Physical: some tension and disrupted sleep a few times a month. Behaviours: Seeing friends and family regularly, occasionally avoiding exercise, occasionally procrastinating work	**Symptoms:** Mostly just excited for the course, enjoying things, feeling refreshed and happy Behaviours: on top of all my work, exercising regularly, seeing friends and family frequently
Actions to take: Consider significant extensions, suspension or withdrawal – speak to academic tutor and manager immediately Attend therapy regularly	**Actions to take:** Reach out to academic tutor and discuss. Extensions may be helpful. Speak to manager about workload if applicable. Start therapy again – speak to GP, consider the university counselling service or Employee Assistance Programme	**Actions to take:** schedule regular self-practice/ self-reflection (SP/SR) time, prioritise wellbeing activities like exercise. Check in with tutor and manager and consider if reasonable adjustments are sufficient. Let friends and peers know about challenges and share next steps with them	**Actions to take:** continue to practise SP/ SR, keep a good routine, be kind to myself Make sure I am registered with Disability Advisory Services and know to go for support if needed.	**Actions to take:** Ensure I don't overdo it and allow for breaks Make sure I am aware of all the support options and registered with relevant support services at university, Make tutor aware of previous difficulties.

a significant decision. However, even if this is the route you take, this does not automatically mark the end of the journey as a therapist (or even as a CBT therapist). If you have completed significant parts of the course, you may later decide to attempt to apply for British Association for Behavioural and Cognitive Psychotherapies (BABCP) accreditation by completing outstanding components via a self-funding route or similar (see BABCP, 2023). You may also reapply for the training again (but should be mindful that funding restrictions can apply). Finally, you may also decide that you prefer to pursue a different therapy modality.

> **Key Point:** Ultimately, it is important to remember that whilst these are significant and challenging decisions to make, to put it plainly, it is just a course and your mental health should take priority. It can be difficult to hold this in mind whilst you are in the middle of it – the next section will discuss tips and tricks to manage this.

Putting things into perspective: you are more than a CBT therapist

It's very easy for CBT training to seep into all areas of your life. After all, if you are attending the course full time, you are spending three days working and two days studying at minimum, plus you may be spending weekends or evenings on assignments.

If you come from a place of lived experience, being a good therapist is likely an especially important part of your identity. Therefore, experiences of falling short of your standards or failing can be difficult to process and may feel overwhelming. Ruminating on those experiences can take over other areas of your life and repeated experiences of failure can start to feel personal. As a therapist, we probably also know how unhelpful this is and how we need a balance in our lives.

> ### Reflective exercise – creating a continuum and action plan
>
> Using the example in Table 7.1 as a template, create your own continuum and think about potential actions you might take if you are struggling. You may use different percentages or titles for each column, depending on what you find helpful.
>
> You can continue adding to this plan during the course. Some find it helpful to share this document with others, so others may make them aware of early warning signs we could miss ourselves.

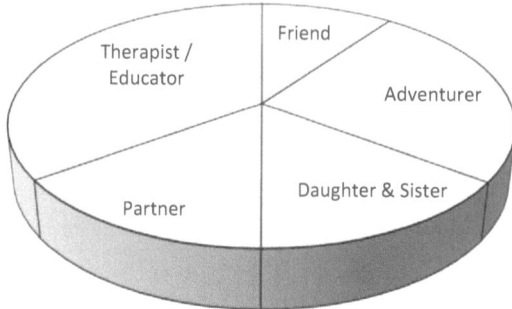

Figure 7.1 The different roles we undertake in our lives

Roles and sources of strength

We can strengthen our perspective taking capacity by writing down the roles that are important to us on a day-to-day basis. These do not all have to be big roles – some may refer to your hobbies and doing things you enjoy. In Figure 7.1, I have provided my own example with percentages allocated to each of my different roles – *therapist/educator, partner, friend, sister and daughter, and adventurer (travelling, DIY, exercising, and spending time with the dogs).*

> ### Reflective exercise
>
> Have a go at listing your own roles then draw out your own pie chart. Following this, fill in the percentages and draw this up in the circle. Try to place your professional identity last. Keep in mind some of your identities may overlap.

From the example, we can see that my career as an educator and therapist is a significant part of my identity but there are many other roles that are important to me. At times in the course, however, it felt like 90–100% of my identity was being a therapist and student. This very much explains why failing course components felt so difficult. Because I was investing almost all my time into the course, I had the additional pressure of feeling like I was falling short in most other areas of my life too. Understandably, this led to a lot of anxiety.

Overidentifying with our work as a therapist can have some negative consequences. Whilst it is inevitable that at times the course takes over, there are also times when we need to (and might have to) take a step back and re-examine. A starting point might be looking at other areas in our lives and spending some time looking after other important parts of our identity. For me, after failing my final CTS-R submission, this meant asking for an extension and taking off on a surfing holiday for a few weeks before returning to studying and therefore spending some time on the 'adventurous' side of my identity that had been neglected.

There may however also be points in time when you are not sure if the course is the right thing for you right now or altogether. It is important to ask ourselves these questions and consider that being a good therapist does not necessarily equal passing the course or even being a CBT therapist. Whilst these considerations can be difficult at the time, they are nonetheless important learning experiences (and parts of the journey of being a therapist).

Key Point: It can be difficult to remember other parts of our identity when we feel overwhelmed by the course. The following reflective exercise looks at reminding ourselves that we are more than 'just' CBT therapists and encourages you to reflect on other roles and sources of strength within your life.

Top tips to manage your mental health during the training year

- Reflect on challenges early and anticipate and prepare for what you can.
- Reflect on your experiences to date and consider how you can draw on your strengths during the training year.
- Do not be afraid to ask for support from friends, peers, the university or your employer.
- Plan ahead: set goals in supervision to monitor and manage your wellbeing.
- Consider extensions when needed. Plan study days and annual leave carefully.
- Being a responsible therapist means acting in the best interest of our clients, which in serious cases can mean suspension or withdrawal.
- Remember that this is a challenging course and many people struggle.
- Remember that you are more than a CBT therapist.

Conclusion

CBT training presents a unique set of challenges that can quickly become overwhelming. A key consideration for trainees is understanding the impact that these challenges can have on our personal and professional lives, anticipating them where possible and reaching out for support quickly. When we notice difficulties, it is important to also spend time focusing on other areas of our lives that are key to maintaining our wellbeing.

Previous experiences of challenges and lived experience, if well managed, can result in a unique set of strengths that can help trainees connect with their clients and manage difficult situations whilst on the course (King et al., 2020). Being a responsible therapist can also mean taking a step back, taking a shorter or longer-term break from the course and/or our therapeutic practice to preserve the interest of our patients. In these moments, it is key to remember that we are more than 'just' CBT therapists and call to mind the other identities that we hold.

Further reading

Andersson, G., Björklind, A., Bennett-Levy, J., & Bohman, B. (2020). Use, and perceived usefulness, of cognitive behavioural therapy techniques for self-care among therapists. *The Cognitive Behaviour Therapist, 13*, e42.

Limper-Menapace, J. (2023). Supporting CBT trainees with lived experience of mental health difficulties. *CBT Today, 51*(2).

Norcross, J. C., & Vandenbos, G. R. (2018). *Leaving it at the office: A guide to psychotherapist self-care*. Guilford Publications.

References

Arnsten, A. F. (1998). The biology of being frazzled. *Science, 280*(5370), 1711–1712.

Bearse, J. L., McMinn, M. R., Seegobin, W., & Free, K. (2013). Barriers to psychologists seeking mental health care. *Professional Psychology: Research and Practice, 44*(3), 150.

Blackburn, I. M., James, I. A., Milne, D. L., Reichelt, F. K., Garland, A., Baker, C., & Claydon, A. (2001). *Cognitive therapy scale-revised (CTS-R)*. Newcastle Cognitive and Behavioural Therapies Centre.

Boyd, J. E., Zeiss, A., Reddy, S., & Skinner, S. (2016). Accomplishments of 77 VA mental health professionals with a lived experience of mental illness. *American Journal of Orthopsychiatry, 86*(6), 610.

British Association for Behavioural and Cognitive Psychotherapies. (2023). *BABCP minimum training standards for the practice of cognitive behavioural therapy*. https://babcp.com/Minimum-Training-Standards

Cleary, R., & Armour, C. (2022). Exploring the role of practitioner lived experience of mental health issues in counselling and psychotherapy. *Counselling and Psychotherapy Research, 22*(4), 1100–1111.

Deighton, R. M., Gurris, N., & Traue, H. (2007). Factors affecting burnout and compassion fatigue in psychotherapists treating torture survivors: Is the therapist's attitude to working through trauma relevant?. *Journal of Traumatic Stress, 20*(1), 63–75.

Everall, R. D., & Paulson, B. L. (2004). Burnout and secondary traumatic stress: Impact on ethical behaviour. *Canadian Journal of Counselling, 38*(1), 25–35.

Flückiger, C., Del Re, A. C., Wampold, B. E., & Horvath, A. O. (2018). The alliance in adult psychotherapy: A meta-analytic synthesis. *Psychotherapy, 55*(4), 316.

Freudenberger, H. J. (1975). The staff burn-out syndrome in alternative institutions. *Psychotherapy: Theory, Research & Practice, 12*(1), 73.

Harris, J. I., Leskela, J., & Hoffman-Konn, L. (2016). Provider lived experience and stigma. *American Journal of Orthopsychiatry, 86*(6), 604.

Hersoug, A. G., Wærsted, M., & Lau, B. (2018). Nondirective meditation used in stress management. *Nordic Psychology, 70*(4), 290–303.

Huet, V., & Holttum, S. (2016). Art therapists with experience of mental distress: Implications for art therapy training and practice. *International Journal of Art Therapy, 21*(3), 95–103.

Kadambi, M. A., & Ennis, L. (2004). Reconsidering vicarious trauma: A review of the literature and its' limitations. *Journal of Trauma Practice, 3*(2), 1–21.

Keyes, C. L. (2002). The mental health continuum: From languishing to flourishing in life. *Journal of Health and Social Behavior*, 207–222.

King, A. J., Brophy, L. M., Fortune, T. L., & Byrne, L. (2020). Factors affecting mental health professionals' sharing of their lived experience in the workplace: A scoping review. *Psychiatric Services, 71*(10), 1047–1064.

Liston, C., Miller, M. M., Goldwater, D. S., Radley, J. J., Rocher, A. B., Hof, P. R., Morrison, J. H., & McEwen, B. S. (2006). Stress-induced alterations in prefrontal cortical dendritic morphology predict selective impairments in perceptual attentional set-shifting. *Journal of Neuroscience, 26*(30), 7870–7874.

Maslach, C., & Jackson, S. E. (1981). *Maslach burnout inventory – ES form (MBI)* [Database record]. APA PsycTests.

Neff, K., & Germer, C. (2022). The role of self-compassion in psychotherapy. *World Psychiatry, 21*(1), 58.

Ondrejková, N., & Halamová, J. (2022). Prevalence of compassion fatigue among helping professions and relationship to compassion for others, self-compassion and self-criticism. *Health & Social Care in the Community, 30*(5), 1680–1694.

Pines, A., & Aronson, E. (1983). Combatting burnout. *Children and Youth Services Review, 5*(3), 263–275.

Poulsen, A. A., Meredith, P., Khan, A., Henderson, J., Castrisos, V., & Khan, S. R. (2014). Burnout and work engagement in occupational therapists. *British Journal of Occupational Therapy, 77*(3), 156–164.

Slade, M., & Longden, E. (2015). Empirical evidence about recovery and mental health. *BMC Psychiatry, 15*, 1–14.

Sodeke-Gregson, E. A., Holttum, S., & Billings, J. (2013). Compassion satisfaction, burnout, and secondary traumatic stress in UK therapists who work with adult trauma clients. *European Journal of Psychotraumatology, 4*(1), 21869.

Tay, S., Alcock, K., & Scior, K. (2018). Mental health problems among clinical psychologists: Stigma and its impact on disclosure and help-seeking. *Journal of Clinical Psychology, 74*(9), 1545–1555.

Part II

Acquiring and consolidating your CBT knowledge and skills

Chapter 8

How to thrive during training?

A tutor's perspective

Gavin Lawton

Introduction

The start of a cognitive behavioural therapy (CBT) training programme is an exciting time for trainee therapists. Typically, this will be the culmination of many years of hard work during which time the trainee will have developed the necessary academic and clinical experience before embarking on the next stage of their professional career. It is a time filled with hope and optimism. It can also be a time where self-doubt and anxiety are understandably common experiences. In particular, the demands of the course are a significant challenge. This chapter will focus on the experiences of one trainee cognitive behavioural therapist (Jessica*) to set out some of the course-related challenges before reflecting some of the best ways to combat course-related stress. The details within the vignette are an accurate reflection of one person's experience. The name of the individual and some of the details have been changed at their request*.

Anticipating the challenges

The trainee therapist might encounter several potential stressors during the training period. Bennett-Levy and Beedie (2007) and Jenkins et al. (2018) highlight how the transition from a position of relative competence in the current healthcare role to a trainee role can be a challenging experience. Personal life events and existing mental health problems are another potential source of stress. The challenges of gaining CBT competencies and course-related demands such as workload and assessment deadlines are also identified as potential sources of stress. This chapter will utilise the stress vulnerability model and the Stress Bucket analogy (Brabban & Turkington, 2002) as a framework for making sense of this before looking at the impact that stress can have on trainees. It will focus specifically on some examples of course-related stressors with more specific examples set out in the vignette.

The trainee stress bucket

The stress vulnerability model was originally developed by Zubin and Spring (1977), with the stress bucket analogy being developed by (Brabban & Turkington,

DOI: 10.4324/9781003428527-11

2002). The model highlights that vulnerability to stress or an individual's capacity for tolerating stress can differ greatly from person to person. Once the threshold for stress is breached, there will be a wide range of potential stress reactions. For example, some people may start to be more self-critical whereas others might start to worry more. Others might notice more physical sensations commonly associated with anxiety. The model also proposes that we can reduce our stress levels by engaging in activities or coping mechanisms that create some breathing space so that we feel that we are able to face the different challenges without becoming overwhelmed. Increased stress and anxiety along with a reduced ability to cope have been linked to less effective learning (Delany et al., 2015). For this reason, it is vital that we can recognise and manage the signs of stress (see Figure 8.1).

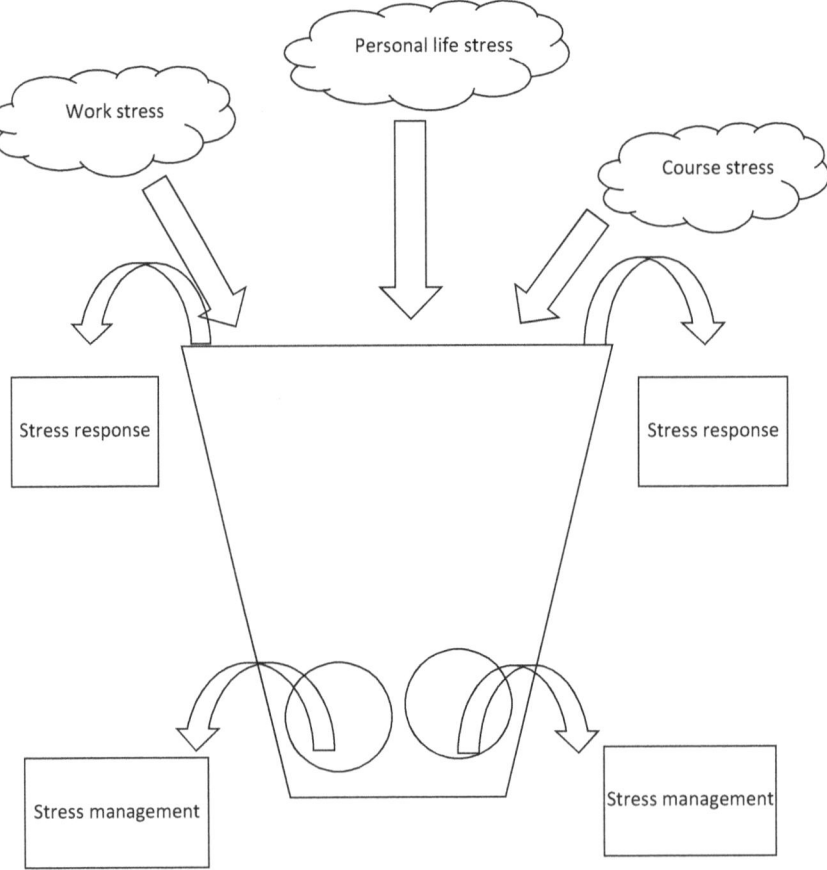

Figure 8.1 The trainee stress bucket

Course-related sources of stress

Bennett-Levy and Beedie (2007) developed a model to help us understand the trainee experience of self-perception around CBT competency which identified three main sources of stress. These are categorised as **workplace stress, home or personal life stress** and **course-related stress**. Whilst it is inevitable that these three components will overlap, we will be focusing here on issues related to competency development and meeting the requirements of the course which might be best considered from a workplace and a course perspective.

Workplace stress

Bennett-Levy and Lee (2014) identified that a sense of safety is crucial for a trainee's confidence to engage with the process of competency development. The experience of Jessica highlights some of the factors that might impact on this sense of safety. For Jessica, there were some practical stressors around learning some of the organisational and client requirements for recording sessions. Jessica also refers to the actual recording of sessions being an uncomfortable situation. All of this is set against waning confidence levels as she adapted to a new role and a sense of feeling de-skilled and less competent. Robinson et al. (2012) highlight this common experience of feeling de-skilled when transitioning from a core profession to a trainee therapist role. They identify that role identity and identity shift as well as the learning of new clinical skills being some of the biggest challenges. We can see that this is also reflected in the experience of Jessica who struggled with the transition from mental health nurse and team manager to a much less experienced trainee therapist.

Jessica's experience

What happened?

I was a student on a two-year Post Graduate Diploma in CBT course. I had found the first year more stressful than I had anticipated. I had come from a nursing background and left behind a successful career where I was a team manager. As a trainee therapist I felt de-skilled, and this had a big impact on my confidence. This meant that role-play, OSCE (objective structured clinical examination) and other skill-based tasks were quite anxiety provoking. On top of this there were written assignments and it had been a whilst since I had last studied, so academic deadlines became a source of stress. Despite all of this I struggled on feeling like I was just about hanging in there. The biggest setback came at the end of the first year when we were required to submit our first live therapy session for assessment. The recording of therapy sessions had become another source of stress.

Finding clients who would consent to being recorded and then some clients withdrawing consent was a challenge. In addition there were a number of organisational barriers around access recording software. With hindsight I can see that I avoided addressing these issues early on which delayed the recording of sessions. This meant that I hadn't had much feedback through live supervision. I failed the assessment by some way. As this was the final assessment of the year the resubmission point was at the start of the next academic year which meant that I could not progress onto the second year with the rest of my cohort.

Course-related stress

Competency-based training programmes can be challenging, particularly when you align the course expectations around competency development with the in-service expectations around caseload management and clinical outcomes (Bennett-Levy & Lee, 2014). There is a lot of information to process as well as technical skills to acquire. Courses will often provide handbooks, tutorials, and workshops to help trainees to come to terms with what is required but this can still feel overwhelming. Jessica refers to the stressful demands of the academic requirements, particularly having not studied for some time. Skill-based exercises (e.g. role-plays) and assessments are also identified as a source of stress (Bennett-Levy & Beedie, 2007). Jessica describes these experiences set against a background of lacking in confidence.

Whilst meeting academic deadlines is stressful, Jessica highlights a particular critical incident centred around formal competency assessment as being a main contributor to her experience of stress. Another potential source of course-related stress is the practice portfolio. The practice portfolio, often required for NHS Talking Therapies courses can look unachievable at the start of the course, and when we add this into the stress bucket it is a significant aspect of the course-related stress. Muse et al. (2022) refer to the multi-faceted Practice Portfolio document as a key tool for pulling together evidence of competency across the whole programme. This means that in some way, all aspects of theoretical knowledge acquisition and clinical skill competency development are evidenced through the portfolio.

The impact of course-related stress

How did this affect you?

I was devastated. The failed assessment fed into the belief that I was not cut out to be a therapist. My mood fluctuated from feeling sad to angry about the course team to anxious and worried about my future. I also felt embarrassed. I didn't feel like meeting up with friends and would avoid social situations. Instead, I spent time dwelling on the situation. I was quite hard on myself, I felt a sense of injustice towards the course team and I would often drift into worrying about my future playing out scenarios around returning to nursing and the embarrassment of returning a failure. The embarrassment and sense of injustice also stopped me from reaching out for help and I would avoid the office as I had felt like I had let my colleagues down.

It is important to be able to recognise the signs of when we are nearing the threshold for our capacity for tolerating stress. Below are some examples of the signs of stress but generally we might consider these to be the emotional impact, physical sensations, dysfunctional thinking processes, and unhelpful ways of responding to the problem or the stress.

Emotional impact

Jessica describes feeling devastated, embarrassed, sad, angry, and anxious.

Physical

We often experience emotional discomfort through physical sensations. These could be: restlessness, gastrointestinal symptoms, palpitations, tension, and headaches (to name just a few).

Dysfunctional thinking

Common cognitive responses to stress are worry, catastrophising, intolerance of uncertainty, sense of injustice, mindreading, jumping to conclusions, and self-criticism. Jessica was able to recognise negative thinking about herself, the situation and her future. There was also negative thinking about the course which created a sense of injustice.

Unhelpful responses

When feeling overwhelmed by stress, people will make attempts to cope and to make themselves feel better. Procrastination and avoidance (sometimes around reaching out for help) are examples of short-term coping rather than a longer-term solution to the problem. Again, Jessica was able to reflect on how embarrassment, a sense of injustice and feeling down all impacted on her not accessing support networks. This allowed the emotional impact of the course and the setback to build pushing Jessica further away from more helpful longer-term solutions to her problems.

Helpful ways of responding to course-related stress

You managed to make it through the course so what did you do?

I was lucky to have friends and family who encouraged me to keeping going with the course but also to find some balance between the course require-ments and my personal life. I had a great supervisor in service who was able to normalise some of my thoughts and feelings. It turned out that she too had failed a competency assessment. Also the initial emotional impact les-soned over time and I started to think differently. Once I had gained some balance and perspective, I was able to engage better with the University support structures. I reached out to my academic supervisor who was a great source of support, again normalising a lot of what I had been going through. I spent time with the lecturer who had marked my assessment and they helped me to make sense of the feedback. This enabled me to reflect on some of the progress that I had made and realise that with a few small improvements I could achieve a pass. This enabled me to develop an action plan. I still felt some resentment that I had not been able to progress onto the second year with my peers but I was able to look at the situation from a positive angle. The failed assessment was a depression case, so over the next year I worked with a number of depression cases. This improved my competency significantly and enabled me to pass the resubmission.

Unhelpful ways of responding to challenges as set out above can leave a person stuck in the problem. Here we will consider more helpful ways of responding to course-related stress. We can consider the experience of Jessica and helpful ways of responding to stress in three parts. These are **achieving balance in her personal life, accessing clinical supervision,** and **accessing academic supervision.**

Utilising supervision

The importance of clinical supervision in CBT training is well evidenced (Milne et al., 2010; Rakovshik et al., 2016). 'Live' supervision is highlighted as a crucial part of trainee competency development as it allows for direct competency-focused feedback (Alfonsson et al., 2018). The feedback provided through supervision sup-ports the learning process set out by Bennett-Levy (2006) where clinical knowl-edge and skill acquisition is implemented. Feedback provided through supervision provides the trainee with a focus for reflection and further skill development.

This feedback process is reflected in the experience of Jessica. Specific feedback enabled Jessica to target certain clinical skills to promote competency improvement. Both academic and clinical supervision also seem to have had other positive influences on Jessica's management of course-related stress. Jessica refers to the normalising of setbacks during competency development, and also there seems to have been a therapeutic benefit to engaging with supervision and starting to look for solutions to problems rather than avoiding support networks. Self-practice of CBT methods and also reflective practice are discussed in Chapter 18 so won't be discussed in detail here. It is however worth highlighting the wealth of evidence behind the application of both of these wellbeing processes (Bennett-Levy & Lee, 2014) and both are therefore worth consideration when thinking about the management of course-related stress.

Reflection points and advice for managing course-related stress

What are your reflections on the experience and what advice do you have for trainee therapists?

The most important lesson that I have learned having now also supervised trainee therapists is that when it comes to competency assessment, failure is common. Whilst it might feel like a setback, I believe that receiving constructive feedback helps to build competency. Another piece of advice that I pass onto trainees is to make sure that you are accessing support and also to not compare yourself to other trainees. The course and the assessment requirements can be an emotional rollercoaster. Accessing the support of peers, service supervisors and the course team can help to manage these emotions and ensure that we are facing challenges in a helpful manner. If the course stressors are managed in a constructive manner, then they will intrude less in your personal life. The final piece of advice would be to look into the recording of sessions as early as possible. This will enable the trainee to overcome and organisational or practical issues enabling the trainee to start recording sessions much earlier. Recording sessions is great for confidence building but also getting direct feedback through live supervision is the best way to build competency.

Conclusion

This chapter has focused on workplace and course-related stressors. The stress vulnerability model provides a framework for understanding how stress can affect us, and through the experience of Jessica, we can see how stress and emotions can impact on the way that we think about a problem. Unhelpful thinking styles can lead to unhelpful behaviour responses. In the case of Jessica, we can see how rumination, worry, self-criticism, and avoidance resulted in Jessica not accessing support and remaining stuck in the problem. This chapter has also highlighted how a loss of role identity and feeling de-skilled can be a potential stressor. Caseload management, recording of therapy sessions, CBT competency development, academic requirements and the practice portfolio are other potential challenges. We have seen through the experience of Jessica how important supervision is. Clinical supervision plays a crucial role in supporting the training through competency development and can also be a valuable source of support for other workplace stressors. The role of the academic supervisor has also been highlighted. Whatever stress the trainee might be going through, there is usually a solution to this and the academic supervisor is crucial in this regard. The training period can be personally, clinically, and academically challenging, but if the trainee makes full use of the support networks, then the training can be a positive and rewarding experience.

Further reading

Bennett-Levy, J., & Beedie, A. (2007). The ups and downs of cognitive therapy training: What happens to trainees' perception of their competence during a cognitive therapy training course? *Behavioural and Cognitive Psychotherapy, 35*, 61–75.

Jenkins, H., Waddington, L., Thomas, N., & Hare, D. J. (2018). Trainees' experience of cognitive behavioural therapy training: A mixed methods systematic review. *The Cognitive Behaviour Therapist, 11*, e2.

Robinson, S., Kellett, S., King, I., & Keating, V. (2012). Role transition from mental health nurse to IAPT high intensity psychological therapist. *Behavioural and Cognitive Psychotherapy, 40*(3), 351–366. https://doi.org/10.1017/S1352465811000683

References

Alfonsson, S., Parling, T., Spännargård, Å., Andersson, G., & Lundgren, T. (2018). The effects of clinical supervision on supervisees and patients in cognitive behavioral therapy: A systematic review. *Cognitive Behaviour Therapy, 47*(3), 206–228. https://doi.org/10.1080/16506073.2017.1369559

Bennett-Levy, J. (2006). Therapist skills: A cognitive model of their acquisition and refinement. *Behavioural and Cognitive Psychotherapy, 34*(1), 57–78.

Bennett-Levy, J., & Beedie, A. (2007). The ups and downs of cognitive therapy training: What happens to trainees' perception of their competence during a cognitive therapy training course? *Behavioural and Cognitive Psychotherapy, 35*, 61–75.

Bennett-Levy, J., & Lee, N. K. (2014). Self-Practice and self-reflection in cognitive behaviour therapy training: What factors influence trainees' engagement and experience of benefit? *Behavioural and Cognitive Psychotherapy, 42*(1), 48–64. https://doi.org/10.1017/S135246581200078

Brabban, A., & Turkington, D. (2002). The search for meaning: Detecting congruence between life events, underlying schema and psychotic symptoms. In A. P. Morrison (Ed.), *A casebook of cognitive therapy for psychosis* (Vol. 59, p. 76). Routledge.

Delany, C., Miller, K. J., El-Ansary, D., Remedios, L., Hosseini, A., & McLeod, S. (2015). Replacing stressful challenges with positive coping strategies: A resilience program for clinical placement learning. *Advances in Health Sciences Education, 20*, 1303–1324.

Jenkins, H., Waddington, L., Thomas, N., & Hare, D. J. (2018). Trainees' experience of cognitive behavioural therapy training: A mixed methods systematic review. *The Cognitive Behaviour Therapist*, *11*, e2.

Milne, D., Reiser, R., Aylott, H., Dunkerley, C., Fitzpatrick, H., & Wharton, S. (2010). The systematic review as an empirical approach to improving CBT supervision. *International Journal of Cognitive Therapy*, *3*(3), 278–294.

Muse, K., Kennerley, H., & McManus, F. (2022). The why, what, when, who and how of assessing CBT competence to support lifelong learning. *The Cognitive Behaviour Therapist*, *15*, e57.

Rakovshik, S. G., McManus, F., Vazquez-Montes, M., Muse, K., & Ougrin, D. (2016). Is supervision necessary? Examining the effects of internet-based CBT training with and without supervision. *Journal of Consulting and Clinical Psychology*, *84*(3), 191–199. https://doi.org/10.1037/ccp0000079

Robinson, S., Kellett, S., King, I., & Keating, V. (2012). Role transition from mental health nurse to IAPT high intensity psychological therapist. *Behavioural and Cognitive Psychotherapy*, *40*(3), 351–366. https://doi.org/10.1017/S1352465811000683

Zubin, J., & Spring, B. (1977). Vulnerability: A new view of schizophrenia. *Journal of Abnormal Psychology*, *86*(2), 103.

Chapter 9

Making the most of supervision

Joanne Myers and Sam Thompson

Introduction

Supervision will be a crucial aspect of your training experience, both in helping you learn to provide good-quality therapy to your clients and to support you through your course. This chapter has been written by Sam Thompson, a Clinical Supervisor, with extensive supervision experience of CBT and Joanne Myers, a Supervisee, who has experienced supervision in a range of different formats from various individual supervisors. Speaking from a supervisor's perspective, Sam sets the scene by discussing the purpose of supervision and outlining the complexities of the supervisory relationship. He talks about supervision goals, supervision questions (accompanied with a case study) and the importance of live observations and giving feedback. Joanne, from her supervisee's experience, talks you through how to prepare for supervision, make the most of each session (with a poignant case study), and overcome any obstacles around giving feedback to your supervisor. The top tips and conclusion highlight some of the common themes from both perspectives which will stand you in good stead for your training and beyond, as you thrive as a CBT therapist.

The supervisor's perspective

Clinical supervision is not just imperative to the training of CBT therapists but there is also the emphasis on ensuring that there is an adherence to delivering evidence-based practice (Roscoe et al., 2022; Roth & Pilling, 2008). The role of your clinical supervisor is to ensure that they are meeting your learning needs, as well as developing your necessary and appropriate clinical skills (Roscoe, 2021). Your supervisor will need to see and observe sufficient quality in your practice and to ensure that you are fulfilling your competencies (Roth & Pilling, 2008). If you are studying on a British Association for Behavioural and Cognitive Psychotherapies (BABCP)-accredited course, then your supervisor will have been through the CBT training process and so will have a clear understanding on how you can achieve these competencies and work towards appropriate goals. You may feel a

DOI: 10.4324/9781003428527-12

considerable amount of pressure and expectation to meet the requirements of your training course, as well as being expected to have suitable clinical training cases, the time to write assignments and to ensure that your portfolio is complete. The list can go on, but it is important that your supervisor is able to support you through this process.

The supervisee/supervisor relationship

There are various elements which can influence the supervisee and supervisor relationship, such as supervisory style, transference/countertransference, supervisee anxiety, and issues related to difference and diversity (Beinart, 2012; Rodenhauser, 1997, Toldson & Utsey, 2008; Watkins, 2011). As a supervisor, developing and maintaining a healthy supervisory relationship are imperative to effective supervision and ensuring that the supervisee can make the most of the time. One of the most common ways we might explain the functions and process of supervision is the 'tandem model' as outlined below (Milne & James, 2005; Milne, 2009).

In this model, supervision is liked to a tandem bike where the front wheel of the bike is the supervisor who steers and the supervisee who follows close behind. We all know how a tandem bike works and you can't go in different directions which is why this analogy works well to highlight the importance of working together on a journey of learning and development. The supervisor (lead cyclist) is responsible for the assessment of the supervisees needs, agreeing learning objectives, the use of methods to facilitate learning and evaluation. Whereas you (the second cyclist) focus on the Kolb (1984) model of experiential learning: experience, reflection, conceptualisation, and planning. Supervision therefore is a continuous journey of learning and development.

The importance of supervision questions

One of the most important aspects of supervision for a trainee is to bring a supervision question yet, as a supervisor, I often find that supervisees don't bring a clear question. Whilst this may mean there are no current concerns or issues (perhaps this is unlikely on a training course), we may miss the opportunity to discuss future difficulties. A supervision question helps to facilitate the supervision session and journey of learning. Sometimes you may find it difficult to bring a supervision question or you are not sure how to ask what you want to ask.

Key Point: Don't be surprised if your supervisor asks you some curious questions if you haven't brought a question to your supervision session.

We may also see a lot of information being presented about a particular case which can impact on the quality of the question. As a supervisor, I often want to unpick the following questions:

- What is the meaning of the supervisee's question?
- Are they asking for guidance with a clinical intervention? Or experiencing difficulties with engagement?
- Are they unsure about a service-related issue?

It is important to consolidate the client information into a suitable and reasonable question. If your supervisor asked you to repeat the question again, would you be able to? Or would there be too much information? Below is an anonymised example of one of my supervisees who is having difficulty formulating a supervision question.

Case study

Supervisor: Hi Violet, I just wanted to check in really and see how you are finding things?

Violet: Yeah, not too bad thank you

Supervisor: Good. How are you finding the course?

Violet: Yeah all good. Very full on but enjoying it.

Supervisor: That's understandable. What questions have you brought for supervision today?

Violet: Erm . . . well. . . . I wasn't entirely sure. There is this case, they have panic symptoms and I am not sure what to do. I have followed this protocol

Supervisor: Ok, so what's your supervision question?

Violet: Well, I don't know. Is it panic or generalised anxiety or both. Sorry, I forgot to bring a supervision question

Supervisor: It's alright Violet, no problem at all. I just wanted to check that everything is ok. I know you mentioned earlier that you were finding the course 'full on' and hadn't brought a supervision question. The course can be demanding and often supervisees feel the pressure of bringing supervision questions, whilst managing a caseload and wanting to pass the course.

Violet: Yeah, you're right. I am finding it hard now, especially with certain cases. This case is stressful as I don't know what their presenting need is.

Supervisor: Ok, so am I right in thinking that you have a particular case where you are not sure how to formulate their difficulties and this is causing further confusion?

Violet: *Yeah that's right*
Supervisor: *I wonder if we could possibly explore a bit further as to why you*
              think the client may have panic, generalised anxiety or both and
              then we can formulate a supervision question after that.
Violet: *Thank you. That would be helpful.*

The importance of live supervision

Bring recordings/clips to every supervision

You will know at the beginning of your course that there will be a requirement to show recordings from your clinical sessions during supervision, as well as gaining consent from your patients to do so. From my experience, the more clips you record and show in supervision, the easier it will be. Like with any great CBT intervention; exposure! Exposure!

Exposure! It can feel daunting to see clips of yourself, especially when training as a therapist but it is the perfect opportunity to learn and reflect.

> **Top tip:** When you're watching your clip in supervision, make a note of one aspect you enjoyed and one you would like to improve. Showing clips can really enhance your learning as a trainee! I still share recordings in my supervision now and it continues to enhance my practice.

Whilst being a trainee, there is often a significant amount of pressure to get the most out of supervision. You will have a combination of university and workplace supervision to enhance your development into being a competent therapist. Often during the supervision process, we may not feel entirely comfortable sharing our true beliefs about how we are finding supervision. Below is an example of how a trainee may come across during supervision but there are significant beliefs about this which may impact on their experience.

We may use the iceberg analogy in our clinical work with our clients, especially when exploring the emotions that may lie underneath the surface. In the example above, the iceberg shows a situation in which a trainee states '*I am fine*' when they are not; their real thoughts can be seen in the diagram below the ocean surface. We know there is a lot of pressure with undertaking a CBT course.

> ### Reflective exercise
>
> If you thought your supervisor was having difficulty missing or not understanding how you are thinking and feeling, would you be able to express your views to them?

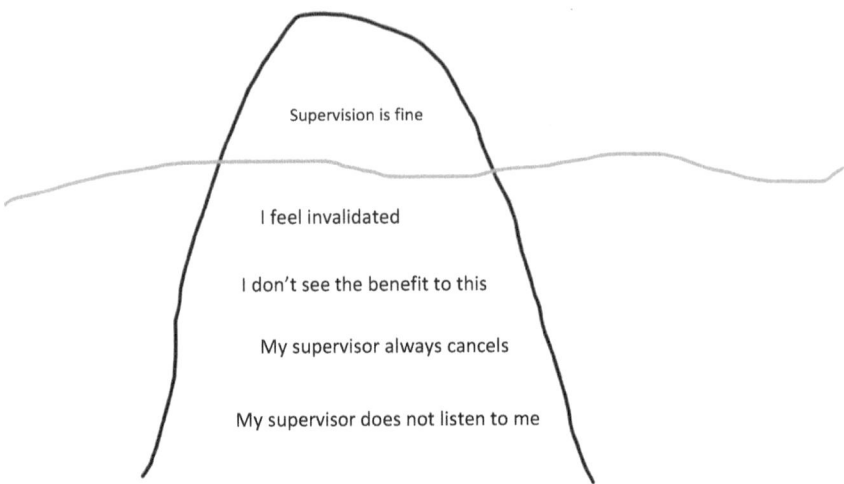

Figure 9.1 The iceberg analogy: what the supervisee may think and not say during supervision

As a supervisor, I always collect feedback from my supervisees as it is a continuous path of learning and development. Your supervisor should be curious to elicit your thoughts and feelings on certain topics; however, supervisors can 'drift'. What we mean by 'drift', especially in the context of supervision, is that we may unintentionally miss certain aspects (see Roscoe, 2021). After all, we are only humans, so, if possible, explain how you are really feeling about your course and about your clients.

Reviewing your supervision goals

Although supervision adheres to a certain structure, it is important to emphasise the importance of supervisees making the most of their time. Regularly discussing and reviewing supervision goals whilst referring to the supervision contract can be beneficial to you. As a supervisor I often see trainees not being organised and prepared for supervision, for example not completing the paperwork or having a specific supervision question (as mentioned before) which can mean that they waste the allocated time in supervision. This can then lead to a 'knock on' effect where you may need to ask your supervisor further questions later on which could have been addressed earlier in supervision. Due to the structure of supervision, especially in a group setting, a significant part of their time can be used up just defining the question so be organised and prepared as much as you possibly can. It will help you and your clients, and I am sure you will see the benefits in your therapeutic work. As a supervisor, I will always give time and space to trainees to support them with any of these difficulties and I am sure your respected supervisor will do the same for you.

Completing feedback forms

We know in our practice there is a copious amount of paperwork to complete but completing feedback forms can be incredibly beneficial to our learning and development. You may find that your supervisor asks you to complete certain forms such as a 'supervisory relationship questionnaire' (e.g. Wainwright, 2010). Please be as open and honest as possible. A good supervisor will appreciate your feedback, and this will enhance their learning and development too! It can be tempting just to give 'positive' feedback to avoid uncomfortable conversations but as a supervisor, I would like to know what areas I can improve as well.

Top tips from a supervisor

- Receiving a lot of supervision can feel overwhelming at times but try to make the most of that time. Your supervisor will want you to develop and do well, especially on a demanding course.
- Try and bring a supervision question if you can. If you are finding things difficult, then please reach out to your supervisor. They are there to help you!
- The CBT training course often comes with a lot of paperwork, having a folder and page dividers at the beginning will help keep all your paperwork organised.
- Review supervision goals when you feel it is appropriate to do so.
- Bring recordings/clips to every supervision session if you can (sometimes gaining consent may be tricky)
- Utilise feedback forms and be honest with your feedback!

The supervisee's perspective

Now we've heard from Sam, with the supervisor's perspective, let's hear from Joanne with the supervisee's experience.

Preparing for supervision

Before beginning supervision both on your course and in your placements, it can be helpful to think about any previous experiences of supervision you've had and how this has shaped your expectations. If you are asked to complete a supervision induction questionnaire, be as honest as you can as this will help your supervisor understand what works well for you. If there is a mismatch between what you are expecting from supervision (from what you have been told on your course) and your actual course or workplace supervision, then discuss this with your supervisor as early as possible or seek advice from your manager or tutor.

Whilst taking a different client to supervision, each session is quite common; this can mean that supervision sessions feel quite discrete from each other. Giving careful consideration to your supervision goals (in the supervision contract), and reviewing them regularly (Kennerley & Clohessy, 2010) and taking responsibility for them will help you develop your skills and confidence over time by providing an overarching theme for supervision.

Let's move on to preparing for each session. As mentioned earlier, do get into the habit of preparing a supervision question (a suggestion made by Padesky, 2014). From my experience, I and fellow trainees tended to ask questions along the lines of 'I'm stuck; what shall I do next with client X?' Table 9.1 provides some examples of how to firm up your supervision question. Whilst the essence of this will often be an appropriate question, please be aware that you can also ask process-based questions in supervision. They allow an opportunity to discuss how you might feel or think about a client and whether this is getting in the way of treatment. You can also celebrate successes in supervision by taking a case that is going well!

Table 9.1 Making Supervision Questions More Specific

Supervision focus	Specific question
You are dreading seeing a particular client next week	How can I manage my emotional reactions towards this client?
You have a client that you feel quite uncomfortable working with	Please can we explore how I feel about this client to identify the source of my uncomfortable feeling and then plan to address this?
You have had a difficult time with clients recently and are losing your confidence and recognise you need to focus on your successes too	Please can we review what has been going well with client X and what skills and characteristics I have been drawing on to help with their treatment?
I always seem to bring new/different clients to supervision. It would be nice to revisit a previous case.	Can we return to discuss client Y. I was really struggling with them a few weeks ago and things have improved significantly recently. I would like us to review what has changed and what we think may have helped with their progress so I can reflect on this and apply this learning for my other clients.

Reflective exercise: *Preparation for asking a broader range of supervision questions.*

Please can I invite you to consider what issues or difficulties you ideally would like to discuss in supervision. Using the examples above, see if you can generate a specific question from the focus for supervision you have identified.

Making the most of each session

Just as therapists can drift (Waller & Turner, 2016), as we heard earlier, supervisors can drift (e.g. drifting from using the active methods recommended for supervision to using mainly discussion; Pugh & Margetts, 2020). As a supervisee, you have some responsibility for identifying and responding to this if necessary (responsibility also sits with the supervisor themselves, your supervisor's supervisor and line manager, Roscoe, 2021).

Our supervisor's attitudes, amongst many other factors, can lead to supervisory drift (Pugh & Margetts, 2020). Imagine, for example, a supervisor, who believes 'everyone must hate listening to their session clips', and they think 'we've done the minimum number of clips for their training course, I won't ask them to do anymore'. This thought may influence supervision if they discourage their supervisee from bringing as many clips as they want. The impact of this may be that a trainee who is struggling to deliver consistently good-quality CBT goes unnoticed and this could have negative consequences for themselves (Ladany et al., 2013) and their clients (Milne, 2020).

Of course, our own beliefs can affect supervision as well (Roscoe, 2021). Thinking about the above example, if you believe 'I cannot question anyone in authority', then you may not have the courage to ask that you listen to live clips regularly in supervision.

> **Top tip:** You could use self-practice/self-reflection (SP/SR) which was developed by James Bennett-Levy (see Sanders & Bennett-Levy, 2010) to notice your own beliefs, thoughts, feelings, and behaviour and act accordingly. In this example, you may test out a new guideline; *'I can make a valid suggestion to my supervisor about something important'* by raising the issue assertively and problem-solving any obstacles.

Making sense of your own avoidance

Let's flip this scenario around now; you may have a supervisor who is keen on using active methods of supervision (e.g. regular live observation, role-play, chair work). This is excellent and is what is recommended for CBT supervision (Pugh & Margetts, 2020). However, you may find role-play excruciating and end up resisting these methods. This would be another opportunity to use SP/SR; for example, what is it that you fear, and can you take part to test out this fear? Using SP/SR during training is a timely opportunity because it helps you with an issue and gives insight into what doing CBT is like for your clients (see Barnes, 2022).

If you are willing to embrace active methods of supervision, there are many advantages:

- Supervision is more interesting.
- Supervision becomes an immersive experiential learning experience which is more powerful than discussion (e.g. trainee therapists allocated to active-based

supervision improved in their overall competency compared to those who attended discussed-based supervision; Bearman et al., 2017).

- Increased empathy towards your clients and being able to take their perspective which not only helps your clients but can shift any of your uncomfortable feelings (Pugh, 2020). An example of the latter can be seen below.

Case study – The advantages of active supervision methods

Carol, a very experienced supervisor, has been supervising Georgina, a trainee therapist, for several months. Quite early on into Georgina's training, one of her clients severely harmed themselves (with no indication of this possibility after a thorough assessment) and Georgina experienced an intense reaction to this. As well as blaming herself for the situation, Georgina was convinced that the client's Mum (who she had seen once with the client in a local shop) would blame her if they bumped into each other again. Georgina had started avoiding the shop and was becoming anxious when working with her other clients. Georgina, aware that she needed to address her thoughts and feelings, had been using responsibility pie charts and self-compassion techniques (which she knew from her previous profession); however, she had not been able to shift her guilt or the fear of the Mum. During supervision, after some guided discovery (which elicited the many factors that had contributed to the client's self-harm and that the right course of action had been taken by Georgina based on the information she knew), Carol suggested that they role played Georgina bumping into the Mum and her blaming Georgina. Both the supervisor and supervisee knew this was an imagined scenario because Georgina would not have been able to break her client's confidentiality by talking to her mother anyway. Georgina was willing to take part in the role play and she practised saying, 'I am sorry to hear about what happened to your daughter'. Carol, playing the Mum and having permission to do so, then raised her voice at Georgina and blamed her for what happened. In that moment, Georgina asserted herself, saying that she was not to blame. During reflection, Georgina stated that whilst she would not have responded exactly that way in real life to the mother (if she had permission to speak to her), the act of asserting herself and stating that she had no reason to feel guilty shifted her emotion constructively in a way that previous discussions and exercises had not. Consequently, she felt more confident carrying on with her training course and treating her clients.

Using active methods in supervision takes longer than discussion. If you believe 'I need to explain everything so that my supervisor fully understands' and you take a long time describing your client, then time for active methods will be limited. If this applies to you then try following Padesky's (2014) tip of summarising the client in two minutes by using an egg timer. If you are concerned that this will reduce the benefits of supervision then try experimenting with a long, full description versus a brief description and compare the outcomes of supervision.

Finally, tune into how you feel and what you believe about receiving and giving feedback. Your supervisor should provide regular feedback and ask you for feedback on each supervision session. If you have any hesitancies about giving negative feedback or you struggle hearing negative feedback then try to address this early on in supervision. A useful idea might be to give feedback to your supervisor around how you like to receive constructive feedback.

Top tips from a supervisee

- Prepare well for your first supervision session and each session thereafter.
- Be aware of your own beliefs, thoughts, feelings, and behaviour and if they are negatively impacting on supervision.
- Use SP/SR to challenge your beliefs/rules and test out new ones and to practise new behaviours.
- Be assertive with your supervisor if you are aware that any of their beliefs or behaviours are negatively impacting your supervision.
- Embrace active methods of supervision!

Conclusion

It's unlikely to be a coincidence if you have noticed some common themes between the supervisor and supervisee's perspectives and top tips. As we've heard from both perspectives, the supervisory relationship is complicated and can be affected by both the supervisor's and supervisee's thoughts, beliefs, emotions, and behaviour. Being aware of these factors and addressing any issues by being honest and providing feedback to your supervisor have been a common theme. We've also heard from both perspectives about the importance of setting and reviewing goals, preparing well for supervision and making the most of every session (by taking clips and engaging with active methods of supervision). A final theme has been around using CBT ourselves, whether that is using exposure or behavioural experiments, to make the most of supervision.

If you prepare well for supervision and engage in its key components, then you stand to gain interesting, powerful, and effective supervision. If you are willing to consider the supervisory relationship and your role within it then you are likely to benefit from even more meaningful supervision. We hope this guidance helps you with your course and your current clients. Following it can set you up with good habits for supervision that will extend well beyond your training, as you move on to thrive as a CBT therapist.

Acknowledgements

Thank you to Kate Tilbury for providing excellent supervision and proofreading our chapter. We would also like to thank our many supervisees and supervisors over the years who have helped inspire the backbone of this chapter.

Suggested further reading

Gordon, P. (2012). Ten steps to cognitive behavioural supervision. *The Cognitive Behaviour Therapist*, *5*(4), 71–82. https://doi.org/10.1017/S1754470X12000050

Padesky, C. (2014, June 27). *Better supervision.* www.padesky.com/making-supervision-better/

Scaife, J. (2013). *Supervision in clinical practice: A practitioner's guide.* Routledge.

References

Barnes, N. (2022). Incorporating SP-SR into a high intensity cognitive behavioural training course within IAPT. *CBT Today.*

Bearman, S. K., Schneiderman, R. L., & Zoloth, E. (2017). Building an evidence base for effective supervision practices: An analogue experiment of supervision to increase EBT fidelity. *Administration and Policy in Mental Health*, *44*(2), 293–307. https://doi.org/10.1007/s10488-016-0723-8

Beinart, H. (2012). Models of supervision and the supervisory relationship. *Supervision and Clinical Psychology: Theory, Practice and Perspectives*, *2*, 36–50.

Kennerley, H., & Clohessy, S. (2010). Becoming a supervisor. In M. Mueller, H. Kennerley, F. McManus, & D. Westbrook (Eds.), *Oxford guide to surviving as a CBT therapist* (pp. 323–371). Oxford University Press.

Kolb, D. A. (1984). *Experiential learning: Experience as the source of learning and development.* Prentice-Hall.

Ladany, N., Mori, Y., & Mehr, K. E. (2013). Effective and ineffective supervision. *The Counseling Psychologist*, *41*, 28–47.

Milne, D. L. (2009). *Evidence-based clinical supervision: Principles and practice.* John Wiley & Sons.

Milne, D. (2020). Preventing harm related to CBT supervision: A theoretical review and preliminary framework. *The Cognitive Behaviour Therapist*, *13*, E54. https://doi.org/10.1017/S1754470X20000550

Milne, D., & James, I. (2005). Clinical supervision: Ten tests of the tandem model. In *Clinical psychology forum* (Vol. 151, pp. 6–10).

Padesky, C. (2014, June 27). *Better supervision.* Retrieved January 23, 2024, from www.padesky.com/making-supervision-better/

Pugh, M. (2020). *Cognitive behavioural chairwork distinctive features.* Routledge.

Pugh, M., & Margetts, A. (2020). Are you sitting un(comfortably)? Action based supervision and supervision drift. *The Cognitive Behaviour Therapist*, *13*, E17. https://doi.org/10.1017/S1754470X20000185

Rodenhauser, P. (1997). Psychotherapy supervision: Prerequisites and problems in the process. In C. E. Watkins, Jr. (Ed.), *Handbook of psychotherapy supervision* (pp. 527–548). Wiley.

Roscoe, J. (2021). Conceptualising and managing supervision drift. *The Cognitive Behavioural Therapist*, *14*, E37. https://doi.org/10.1017/S1754470X21000350

Roscoe, J., Taylor, J., Harrington, R., & Wilbraham, S. (2022). CBT supervision behind closed doors: Supervisor and supervisee reflections on their expectations and use of clinical supervision. *Counselling and Psychotherapy Research, 22*(4), 1056–1067. https://doi.org/10.1002/capr.12572

Roth, A. D., & Pilling, S. (2008). Using an evidence-based methodology to identify the competences required to deliver effective cognitive and behavioural therapy for depression and anxiety disorders. *Behavioural and Cognitive Psychotherapy, 36*(2), 129–147.

Sanders, D., & Bennett-Levy, J. (2010). When therapists have problems: What can CBT do for us? In M. Mueller, H. Kennerley, F. McManus, & D. Westbrook (Eds.), *Oxford guide to surviving as a CBT therapist* (pp. 457–480). Oxford University Press.

Toldson, I. A., & Utsey, S. (2008). Racial and cultural aspects of psychotherapy and supervision. In A. K. Hess, K. D. Hess, & T. H. Hess (Eds.), *Psychotherapy supervision: Theory, research, and practice* (pp. 537–559). Wiley.

Wainwright, N. A. (2010). *The development of the Leeds Alliance in supervision scale (LASS): A brief sessional measure of the supervisory alliance.* https://etheses.whiterose.ac.uk/1118/

Waller, G., & Turner, H. (2016). Therapist drift redux: Why well-meaning clinicians fail to deliver evidence-based therapy, and how to get back on track. *Behaviour Research and Therapy, 77*, 129–137.

Watkins, C. E., Jr. (2011). Toward a tripartite vision of supervision for psychoanalysis and psychoanalytic psychotherapies: Alliance, transference-countertransference configuration, and real relationship. *The Psychoanalytic Review, 98*, 557–590.

Chapter 10

Maximising the training year through shadowing and 'in vivo' work

Alex Preston

Introduction

One of the key features that sets CBT aside from other modalities is the emphasis that it places on the 'active' or behavioural component of treatment. In this instance, what we mean by this is the 'doing' phase of therapy, changing behaviours, and implementing different strategies based on the discussion we've had and the new appraisals that we have potentially been able to reach.

Traditionally, therapy sessions may have been considered to be limited to the clinic room, with the main mechanism of change being the exploration and interactive dialogue that the therapist has with the patient. This is still a method that it would be hard to imagine ever becoming redundant; however, cognitive therapy seeks to expand the realm of learning available by extending exploration beyond these confines (Bennett-Levy et al., 2004). It achieves this with the identification and practical testing of hypotheses and with scientific exploration and experimentation. Following this, it seeks to introduce new information and promote a subsequent change of behaviours which research suggests is one of the most powerful tools within the therapeutic arsenal and allows the modification and challenge of the potentially dysfunctional or distressing thoughts and beliefs through experiential learning (Wells, 1997).

Working together with your patient

Beck et al. (1979) place a fundamental need for the therapist and patient to develop a sense of 'collaborative empiricism' towards the therapeutic process, in essence a teamwork strategy for learning and curiosity to discover new information. What better way to do this than to actively test out theories together and discover evidence that may yield the very change that the patient has sought treatment for? This chapter seeks to explore some of the benefits to the inclusion of experiments and learning experiences within the therapy session but maybe those which are enhanced by being outside of the clinic room. It briefly considers the differing design and types of such, the approaches, and factors we may need to have considered before stepping into the outside world and how the observation of others allows therapists to compare and contrast their own approaches.

DOI: 10.4324/9781003428527-13

What does it look like in practice?

Firstly, let us be clear what we are referring to with a brief definition of a behavioural experiment (BE). Functionally, BEs are the identification of a hypothesis or belief to be tested. Then we explore the specifics and pertinent factors, especially those which may inhibit the process, such as 'safety behaviours' which may inhibit learning or the availability of new information (Salkovskis, 1991). Next are the collaborative agreement and implementation of action and the subsequent review of any new information available with the reflection as to whether this supports the initial hypothesis or whether we may need to reappraise.

In the excellent *Guide to Behavioural Experiments in Cognitive Therapy* (Bennett-Levy et al., 2004), we are given a multitude of rich and detailed examples of BEs, and very helpfully, a few times whereupon they did not go to plan. It also gives us insight into the differing design types of BEs, namely the 'hypothesis testing' experiments and the more general 'discovery' experiments. In the former, we have a belief or theory that may be held by the patient that we may need to learn some more information about.

Hypothesis testing

This may take the form of a single hypothesis (e.g. Theory A), for example within obsessive-compulsive disorder (OCD), 'If I have a thought that something bad is going to happen then it will'. Alternatively, we may wish to compare and contrast the initial theory against another alternative (Theory B), for example, 'these thoughts about bad things occurring are linked to my anxiety level and don't necessary mean harm in reality'. In session, we may encourage the individual to invoke a thought that fits with this notion such as their therapist becoming unwell and then we may ask them to avoid the 'neutralisation' of such consequential anxiety (not engaging in the compulsive response). Therefore, learning what occurs when indeed we do not respond. By designing experiments in this manner, we are able to be scientific in our exploration of evidence and later using the theory A/B worksheets to log all of our newly available data, helping both therapist and patient to reach a more evidence-based appraisal.

Discovery

'Discovery' experiments on the other hand may not be quite as clearly defined in terms of what the individual is seeking to learn about. They may well actually be utilised when a negative prediction is not quite as available, for instance in cases where behavioural patterns have been engaged in for a longer period of time, possibly even when the patient no longer recalls what the perceived threat originally was.

A discovery experiment might be something quite simple that tests any alternative to what the individual has always done and when they honesty can't conceive of what would happen if they behaved differently. An example I may have done could be work around social phobia where I ask the patient to listen to me reading a chapter of a book with all the previous safety behaviours in place and the focus to be internal as usual, then read another chapter where they focus externally on my voice and the detail. The discovery element would be that they notice that they take in more of the information and that through not focusing on interoceptive cues, they actually feel less anxious.

Another alternative might be 'ABABA' approach for checking behaviours in health anxiety, having a day on with all the checks or scans that they feel compelled to complete then noting how anxious they feel; then a day whereupon they don't engage in the checking/scanning with anxiety rated after that day. It's set up to test an outcome, but a clear prediction isn't made – just an experiment to see the impact of checking.

These types of experiments may also assist the therapist and patient in the process of case formulation, especially when the individual has difficulty predicting how they may feel or indeed has limited insight, having never previously engaged with these new approaches or behaviours before (Bennett-Levy et al., 2004).

Moving beyond the comfort zone

For therapists more accustomed to primarily designing BEs for the patients to complete out of session, the temptation may be to stay with what feels comfortable. Therefore, experimenting in the room or indeed, stepping out of the clinic room, for some represents a significant dynamic shift in role and at times of new skill development or uncertainty, the temptation may well be to go with what feels familiar (Roscoe et al., 2022). However, the evidence overwhelmingly supports the use of these practical and experiential techniques, so much so that it is within clinic guidance from NICE (Liness et al., 2017). This creative inclusion can be responsible for 'rapid belief change', something that cognitive work alone may struggle to achieve (O'Keeffe et al., 2016).

> ### Reflective exercise
>
> Consider your own barriers to attempting out-of-session work; what do you potentially have to gain from getting out of the clinic room with your patient?
>
> Consider designing an experiment that you might conduct; could we write out a cost/benefit analysis for giving it a go verses staying in clinic room?

Interventions that can be supported by the therapist and conducted in real-world settings are far more effective at promoting belief change than those that rely more primarily on written exercises, worksheets, or discussion (Bennett-Levy, 2003; McManus et al., 2012). However, despite this, the evidence suggests that as a profession, we may not be using what we understand to be more effective and the greatest promoter of change.

When questioning qualified CBT therapists regarding the interventions that they use on a regular basis, Liness et al. (2017) found that less than 10% of individuals utilised any outside of therapy room interventions with any degree of regularity. The rationale for this paucity of use was linked to time constraints from services (specifically clinician's balancing contact hour demands with the extra time required to get out of the clinic room), service policy, and therapists' lack of confidence. Meyer et al. (2020) also disturbingly found that some services declined to permit the use of intervention outside of the clinic room; however, thankfully this was only reported by one respondent. I have also heard it mentioned that pressures to maintain 'recovery rates' mean that clinicians become more rigid in approaches and lack motivation or drive to be creative with experiments, or alternatively that they believe BEs will result in increased dropout from treatment. Paradoxically therefore they avoid the BEs, which undermines the efficacy of treatment and actually increases the likelihood of individuals leaving the treatment episode without a significant reduction of symptoms. Meyer et al. (2020) also note that there is no correlation between increased use of well-constructed BEs and dropout, quite the opposite in fact, and therapists may need to challenge this belief and others about intervention efficacy.

Walking into the unknown

We should also be aware that taking those first steps can be a daunting experience and at times both parties may also be unclear as to the specifics of the feared situations. For instance, if the individual has been engaging in highly avoidant behaviour for a long time, they may find themselves in unquestioned and habitual behavioural patterns, no longer entirely certain of the specifics of the feared consequence. The therapist is often asking the patient to move towards a feared stimulus and to reverse the behaviours that have been negatively reinforced for a significant period of time. At this point, having a collaborator on side to support and guide may be the difference between engagement and continued distress/avoidance (Harris et al., 2021). Introducing a more cognitive or learning approach to experimentation or exposure work allows the therapist and patient to identify the specifics together, with one providing the detail and the other facilitating objective questioning.

Presley et al. (2023) also note that we may discover by-proxy information from these experiments, in that both the therapist and patient can learn about their own tolerance for distress and the ability to cope with such. If we avoid distress, then we effectively learn very little about such states and as such, this 'experiential avoidance' can create a self-fulfilling prophecy. Once tackled, however, often within a therapist-supported session, we can take the information and learn about coping with distress and emotional tolerance and potentially consider generalising into other areas, creating further opportunities for new information and increased self-efficacy (Macatee et al., 2016).

Below is an example of such with an individual suffering from obsessive-compulsive disorder (OCD).

Case vignette

Michael was a 46-year-old White British male, who self-referred to his local 'Talking Therapies' service for the treatment of OCD. Michael was seen face to face at his request due to feeling uncomfortable discussing his issues in his own home for concern that his family would hear. This was in spite of the symptoms being life limiting and overt within the household. By his own admission the severe OCD symptoms had permeated into pretty much all facets of his life and at first it was difficult for us to assess which were more distressing. As such, the hierarchy developed for treatment had high anxiety ratings across the board and Michael reported limited belief in the ability to be able to address these. Michael also had experience with significant physical health issues (Crohn's), and in the observation of direct family members becoming unwell. He had observed the impact when his brother developed health issues and how his family had responded with heightened distress and fear. This had led to a sense of responsibility for harm/illness and the excessive management of his Crohn's disorder (which had been previously diagnosed as an eating disorder but which we subsequently eventually hypothesised was a misinterpreted symptom of the OCD – compulsive management of food intake to reduce risk of illness).

Following a clear formulation stage, inclusive of longitudinal aspects of the OCD development, time was spent exploring the rationale for CBT, developing insight into the disorder and discussion around how treatment may progress. After this, a hierarchy utilising subjective units of distress (SUDS) was developed between therapist and patient (see excerpt in Table 10.1), connecting behaviours to illness symptoms, but as mentioned, it was encumbered by difficulties in identifying differences in distress. An agreement around what might be completed outside of session was however reached in session 4, with the expectation to review the new information in the following session.

When this session came around Michael reported that he was unable to complete this work independently due to the anticipated level of distress and ability to cope. This left the session with no new information to review; therefore, a discussion was had about how we might proceed. It was suggested to Michael that the time be used to practically test out the beliefs. Following some initial reluctance, collaborative agreement was reached that we would leave the clinic room, drive to Michael's house, and then drive back the same way, an experience that was highly linked to becoming unwell with a belief rating of 90%.

> *With therapist support it was possible to not only conduct this experiment and reach a significantly reduced reappraisal (10%), but it was also what Michael referred to as the 'turning point' of his curiosity in addressing some of his OCD-based beliefs. A less planned benefit of this experiment was that in doing so, and possibly due to the anxiety experienced, Michael also neglected to turn on the Satnav or notice what volume the radio was on, meaning we were able to tackle three items in one go.*
>
> *The outcome of this was not only the new information available to reach an alternate hypothesis, but also the learning about self-efficacy for Michael to engage in future experiments.*

Table 10.1 Hierarchy Excerpt

Situation/behaviour that avoids anxiety or fears	Distress
Driving the same way to and from a place	60%
Putting the Satnav on when going anywhere in the car	55%
Having the radio on even numbers	55%

McMillan and Lee (2010) suggest in-session experiments are used less in depression than anxiety disorders, potentially due to a greater wealth of literature and evidence to support the intervention or examples of such for anxiety issues. However, for a good example, see Skilbeck et al. (2020), which demonstrates the use of a spontaneous BE with a depressed individual and how they may overcome perceived barriers within the session. Another significant point of note from this example is that the experiment does not necessarily need to be complicated or elaborate but can also be more a simple focus on self-efficacy to return to previously enjoyed experiences such as the reading of a book chapter and maintaining focus.

Therapists can be implementing these smaller in-session experiments at an early stage to promote 'quick wins', and indeed, the earlier we can introduce them, the greater the likelihood that our patients start to increase their confidence and potentially their hope for the therapeutic process (Skilbeck et al., 2020). Whether it is a smaller gain or significant hierarchy work, both of these case-study examples come from a situation whereupon the individual felt unable to complete the experiment independently, and as such they became in-session experiments in a spontaneous manner. However, for this to be possible, clear case conceptualisation was necessary and an awareness of what the individual needed to potentially learn in order to challenge the beliefs that were a barrier to completion.

Shadowing

As noted earlier, in the process of training as a cognitive behavioural therapist, we have established means in which to assimilate the necessary theory, but maybe none quite so impactful as the opportunity to 'shadow' colleagues and qualified therapists (Bennett-Levy et al., 2009). It is a truly unique learning experience that encourages 'direct observation' and can also offer valuable insight into practical and adaptive skills development, bridging the gap between classroom and clinic room in what may well be considered the trainees own 'interactive' BE. As such, the rationale for shadowing is that it can improve confidence in technique implementation of trainee therapists (Wray et al., 2022) as they observe and learn in an active manner.

It allows first-hand exposure to subtle nuances and intricacies of 'live' sessions and may indeed be a far richer experience than 'direct observation' in alternate forms, such as watching or listening to session recordings. However, even this latter option has been reported in the literature to be utilised glaringly infrequently, with Townend et al. (2002) reporting only 6% of individuals utilising this method, improving only to 37% more recently (Reiser & Milne, 2016).

If we compare and contrast these approaches, although session recordings may be easier to facilitate and have access to, they may not give an entirely accurate representation of the therapeutic process. Loades and Myles (2016) suggest that at times recordings can suffer from a selection bias, where the therapist being observed may only be willing to disclose sessions whereupon everything 'went well' or when the intervention 'ran smoothly'. It may take considerable comfort in your abilities or aptitude to feel at ease with the sharing of evidence of fallibility, especially when individuals may be more accustomed to sharing recordings that are sufficient for CTS-R pass (Blackburn et al., 2001). For the trainee therapist, however, it might actually be of more benefit to observe sessions when the therapist needed to think on their feet or had to respond to some barriers or challenges.

Applying learning theory to the process

If we use Kolb's (1984) learning cycle as a framework to look at the notion of shadowing, we can see the 'concrete experience' may be the opportunity to be in the room and observe the interactions between therapist and patient. The 'reflective observation' may occur following the session whereupon the trainee is able to explore with the therapist what was happening at certain points, why they explored specific avenues in favour of others, and why they may have utilised a specific intervention. 'Abstract conceptualisation' follows where the trainee explores how this may apply to their own caseload or more general approach within the therapy room, and then we enter the phase of applying this learning practically via means of 'Active experimentation'. The trainee therapist tests out their new learning to build association and therefore grounding or consolidating the new theory.

> **Top tips**
>
> - Use your time well – repeat if possible because it takes time and planning to get out of the clinic room.
> - Know what you need to achieve so that you can be adaptive to opportunity – Conceptualise clearly – '*What does your patient need to learn to be able to alter existing beliefs?*'
> - Always use your formulation as the basis for your experiments.
> - BEs are most effective at the start of therapy as this is when the biggest change is occurring.
> - Start asking colleagues about 'Shadowing' straight away (be persistent with requests as despite their reluctance, qualified therapists need to have recordings for their own British Association for Behavioural and Cognitive Psychotherapies [BABCP] accreditation).
> - For Talking Therapies for Anxiety and Depression courses in England shadowing and 'co-delivery' with experienced therapists is now mandatory.
> - Volunteer for 'stooge' work – always useful for a 'quid pro quo'.

Key points

- Behavioural experiments can elicit the most effective change.
- Being outside of the clinic room grounds theory within real-life experiences.
- Observing colleagues provides the nuance that textbooks may struggle to explain.
- 'The Seeing', in both the therapy session and the trainee's learning process, is a far more effective motivator of change and development – for all parties involved.

Conclusion

In conclusion, we might marry the two topics of this chapter in one ideal framework – namely the aspiration to be able to shadow a colleague conducting an in-session BE with a consenting patient. In both of these topics (BEs and shadowing), there is a need for individuals to practically learn something new through experience that they may have only theorised or discussed previously. In each instance, there may well have been an exploration that has prompted an element of curiosity as to what might be the case if we adopt a differing behavioural approach, which for the trainee, this may mean the transition of role to a more active facilitator of learning. The end result is that we are able to marry the head/heart divide to promote belief change and build confidence for further exploration and learning (Eustis et al., 2020).

Further reading

Bennett-Levy, J., Butler, G., Fennell, M., Hackman, A., Mueller, M., & Westbrook, D. (2004). *Oxford guide to behavioural experiments in cognitive therapy*. Oxford University Press.

McManus, F., Van Doorn, K., & Yiend, J. (2012). Examining the effects of thought records and behavioral experiments in instigating belief change. *Journal of Behavior Therapy and Experimental Psychiatry*, *43*(1), 540–547.

Skilbeck, L., Spanton, C., & Roylance, I. (2020). Helping clients 'restart their engine'– use of in-session cognitive behavioural therapy behavioural experiments for engagement and treatment in persistent depression: A case study. *The Cognitive Behaviour Therapist*, *13*, e5.

References

Beck, A. T., Shaw, B. F., Rush, A. J., & Emery, G. (1979). *Cognitive therapy for depression*. Guildford Press.

Bennett-Levy, J. (2003). Mechanisms of change in cognitive therapy: The case of automatic thought records and behavioural experiments. *Behavioural and Cognitive Psychotherapy*, *31*(3), 261–277.

Bennett-Levy, J., Butler, G., Fennell, M., Hackman, A., Mueller, M., & Westbrook, D. (2004). *Oxford guide to behavioural experiments in cognitive therapy*. Oxford University Press.

Bennett-Levy, J., McManus, F., Westling, B. E., & Fennell, M. (2009). Acquiring and refining CBT skills and competencies: Which training methods are perceived to be most effective?. *Behavioural and Cognitive Psychotherapy*, *37*(5), 571–583.

Blackburn, I. M., James, I. A., Milne, D. L., Baker, C., Standart, S., Garland, A., & Reichelt, F. K. (2001). The revised cognitive therapy scale (CTS-R): Psychometric properties. *Behavioural and Cognitive Psychotherapy*, *29*(4), 431–446.

Eustis, E. H., Cardona, N., Nauphal, M., Sauer-Zavala, S., Rosellini, A. J., Farchione, T. J., & Barlow, D. H. (2020). Experiential avoidance as a mechanism of change across cognitive-behavioral therapy in a sample of participants with heterogeneous anxiety disorders. *Cognitive Therapy and Research*, *44*, 275–286.

Harris, O., Kustner, C., Paskell, R., & Hannay, C. (2021). Using targeted cognitive behavioural therapy in clinical work: A case study. *The Cognitive Behaviour Therapist*, *14*, e2.

Kolb, D. A. (1984). *Experiential learning: Experience as the source of learning and development*. Prentice Hall.

Liness, S., Lea, S., Nestler, S., Parker, H., & Clark, D. M. (2017). What IAPT CBT high-intensity trainees do after training. *Behavioural and Cognitive Psychotherapy*, *45*(1), 16–30.

Loades, M. E., & Myles, P. J. (2016). Does a therapist's reflective ability predict the accuracy of their self-evaluation of competence in cognitive behavioural therapy?. *The Cognitive Behaviour Therapist*, *9*, e6.

Macatee, R. J., Allan, N. P., Gajewska, A., Norr, A. M., Raines, A. M., Albanese, B. J., Boffa, J. W., Schmidt, N. B., & Cougle, J. R. (2016). Shared and distinct cognitive/affective mechanisms in intrusive cognition: An examination of worry and obsessions. *Cognitive Therapy and Research*, *40*, 80–91.

McManus, F., Van Doorn, K., & Yiend, J. (2012). Examining the effects of thought records and behavioral experiments in instigating belief change. *Journal of Behavior Therapy and Experimental Psychiatry, 43*(1), 540–547.

McMillan, D., & Lee, R. (2010). A systematic review of behavioral experiments vs. exposure alone in the treatment of anxiety disorders: A case of exposure while wearing the emperor's new clothes?. *Clinical Psychology Review, 30*(5), 467–478.

Meyer, J. M., Kelly, P. J., & Deacon, B. J. (2020). Therapist beliefs about exposure therapy implementation. *The Cognitive Behaviour Therapist, 13*, e10.

O'Keeffe, F., Watson, S., & Linke, S. (2016). Training novice clinical psychologist trainees to implement effective CBT for anxiety disorders: Training model and clinic outcomes. *The Cognitive Behaviour Therapist, 9*, e38.

Presley, V. L., Jones, G., & Marczak, M. (2023). The relationship between therapist experiential avoidance and observed CBT competence during training: A preliminary investigation. *The Cognitive Behaviour Therapist, 16*, e15.

Reiser, R. P., & Milne, D. L. (2016). A survey of CBT supervision in the UK: Methods, satisfaction and training, as viewed by a selected sample of CBT supervision leaders. *The Cognitive Behaviour Therapist, 9*, e20.

Roscoe, J., Bates, E. A., & Blackley, R. (2022). 'It was like the unicorn of the therapeutic world': CBT trainee experiences of acquiring skills in guided discovery. *The Cognitive Behaviour Therapist, 15*, e32.

Salkovskis, P. M. (1991). The importance of behaviour in the maintenance of anxiety and panic: A cognitive account. *Behavioural and Cognitive Psychotherapy, 19*(1), 6–19.

Skilbeck, L., Spanton, C., & Roylance, I. (2020). Helping clients 'restart their engine'– use of in-session cognitive behavioural therapy behavioural experiments for engagement and treatment in persistent depression: A case study. *The Cognitive Behaviour Therapist, 13*, e5.

Townend, M., Iannetta, L., & Freeston, M. H. (2002). Clinical supervision in practice: A survey of UK cognitive behavioural psychotherapists accredited by the BABCP. *Behavioural and Cognitive Psychotherapy, 30*(4), 485–500.

Wells, A. (1997). *Cognitive therapy of anxiety disorders: A practice manual and conceptual guide.* Wiley & Sons.

Wray, A., Kellett, S., Bee, C., Smithies, J., Aadahl, V., Simmonds-Buckley, M., & McElhatton, C. (2022). The acceptability of cognitive analytic guided self-help in an improving access to psychological therapies service. *Behavioural and Cognitive Psychotherapy, 50*(5), 493–507.

Chapter 11

Developing essential competencies in culturally inclusive practice

Shah Alam

Introduction

To begin, I'd like to emphasise the need to see this topic as an ethos and way of working to embody. Culturally inclusive practice is essential and not optional; therefore, this should not be seen as a standalone chapter, to avoid 'othering', in the sense that we need a separate chapter or set of skills to work with minoritised communities. These skills should be weaved throughout everything we do, which is the standard of good practice.

I mention language and use the term 'racially minoritised' rather than 'BAME' (Black, Asian, and Minority Ethnic) which has been used in the United Kingdom (UK). I am part of this demographic, and this term can be oppressive by grouping people into one category. There is vast diversity that is not captured by this term. Instead, 'racially minoritised' is used to acknowledge how people are actively minoritised by others as a social process (Predelli et al., 2012). For too long, racially minoritised people have been underserved (Alam et al., 2024), and rather than seeing communities as 'hard to reach' (Begum, 2006), practitioners must ask, are we reaching out hard enough?

Throughout this chapter, I draw on my own lived experience as a British-Bangladeshi Muslim man from East London, my clinical and research experience as a CBT therapist and clinical psychologist, my role as a co-chair of the British Association for Behavioural and Cognitive Psychotherapies (BABCP) Anti-Racism Special Interest Group (SIG; formerly Equality and Culture), and lastly, my involvement within academic courses which train CBT therapists and clinical psychologists. I reference key papers and use a fictional case example of 'Hussain'.

Mental health needs of racially minoritised communities

Long-standing health inequalities exist within the UK, with racially minoritised communities having a higher likelihood of greater mortality, poorer health outcomes, and barriers in accessing healthcare (Raleigh & Holmes, 2021). There is a higher prevalence of anxiety and depression in South Asian women at 63.5%

DOI: 10.4324/9781003428527-14

compared to 28.5% of White women (Weich et al., 2004). Additionally, the risk of psychosis in Black Caribbean people is estimated to be nearly seven times higher than in the White population (Fearon et al., 2006). To avoid locating a problem within an individual or community, it is important to shine a spotlight on the role of social and economic inequalities, racism, and discrimination on wellbeing (Gibbons et al., 2012). For example, Bisby et al. (2003) identify the impact of low income, unemployment, family stress, housing, gender differences, racism, language difficulties, and low integration into society, within the British-Bangladeshi population. Bhui et al. (2018) state that there is growing evidence that the experience of racism leads to a greater chance of an individual developing mental health difficulties, such as depression. Racially minoritised people also had an increased risk of dying from the COVID-19 pandemic, which unfortunately further highlighted disparities (Williamson et al., 2020).

There are clear mental health needs of racially minoritised communities, considering the adversity in society that people face. Unfortunately, there are also disparities in access to mental health care as NHS Digital (2020) highlights on the use of Talking Therapies (previously known as Improving Access to Psychological Therapies [IAPT]) services in England, where fewer racially minoritised people are referred to Talking Therapies services compared to the White British population. Furthermore, racially minoritised people have lower recovery rates as 50% of people identifying as White moved to recovery, compared with 46% of those identifying as Black or Black British and 44% Asian or Asian British (Baker, 2018). It is continued to be reported that racially minoritised people are still under-represented in Talking Therapies services, as Asian British people are 14% less likely than the White British population to be in contact with services (Baker, 2020).

More recently, NHS Race and Health Observatory (2023) reported positive progress with improved outcomes for some racially minoritised groups such as 'Black African' and 'Black Caribbean' communities. However, accessing therapy continues to be difficult for Black and Asian communities, and there are continued inequalities between groups, with much more work needed to focus on specific communities and intersectionality (e.g. age, gender, and socio-economic status). Recommendations are made such as continued implementation of the BAME Positive Practice Guide (Beck et al., 2019) and training, recruiting, and retaining a diverse and skilled workforce. Services should also meet the aims of the Patient and Carer Race Equality Framework (NHS England, 2023), which is a participatory approach to anti-racism that mental health trusts and staff should take to improve the access, experience, and outcomes of racially minoritised communities.

Barriers to mental health support and the need to remove these

There are many barriers at different levels that make it harder for racially minoritised communities to access formal mental health support. Rathod et al. (2015) identify key barriers such as mistrust of services/practitioners, worries about a breach of confidentiality, poor information on psychological therapies/accessibility, language and terminology leading to being misunderstood, fear of being stigmatised, previous experience, stereotyping by therapists, doubt regarding CBT being empowering enough, lack of understanding of cultural norms and values by the therapist, perception of cultural incompetence, clinician's belief in the power of drugs, faith/spirituality and religion, individualism versus collectivism, gender issues, racism/colonial history, interpretation problems, financial burden, and practical matters (e.g. environment for therapy and transport issues). Therefore, it is even more vital that practitioners and services do more to reach out and support communities.

Within my own research, I completed a systematic review looking at the barriers to mental health support for racially minoritised communities within the UK. Several barriers make it harder for people to access mental health support, such as stigma, having a 'non-Western' understanding of mental distress, the competence of services in meeting people's needs, and accessibility. Action must be taken at all levels by commissioners, services, professionals, and others to eliminate barriers in mental health care, improve experiences, and actively work more collaboratively with communities (Alam et al., 2024).

Reflective exercise – improving access

In order to improve access to mental health care for racially minoritised populations, an initial step would be for services and practitioners to map the communities in the local area and see if this represents the populations accessing the service. It's important to listen to communities, identify shortfalls, and make changes (Beck et al., 2019).

What percentage (%) of people in the area your team serves are from racially minoritised groups?

What are the patterns of migration in your area? Who are the most recent immigrant groups?

What are the main faith groups in your area?

Does your staff group reflect the area you serve?

Who can you go to for a consult about the cultures and communities in your area?

Are staff being given protected time for community engagement work?

The need to develop culturally inclusive practice

Mental health Talking Therapies services have aimed to increase the availability of NICE-recommended psychological therapies in the NHS (Beck et al., 2019). However, as previously stated, racially minoritised communities have been under-represented in services, with poorer outcomes (Baker, 2018). Memon et al. (2016) suggest ways to overcome these barriers, such as improved service access pathways, training for healthcare providers in culturally sensitive care, and improved engagement with racially minoritised people within service development. Services must be visible, accessible, and responsive to the needs of the community.

Faheem (2023) interviewed racially minoritised services users who had accessed Talking Therapies services and found that therapy was experienced as helpful, but people felt that their experience could be improved. There was a need for therapists to recognise cultural dissonance (conflict people experience with their culture and environment) within therapy and to develop cultural competence. The BAME Positive Practice Guide (BAME PPG, Beck et al., 2019) was developed with service users and clinicians to provide a framework for Talking Therapies commissioners, service managers, supervisors, and clinicians to improve access and outcomes for racially minoritised communities. There is an audit tool which should be used to consider how the needs of communities are being met and what could be improved. Service-level changes, adaptations to therapy, engagement of communities, workforce, and staffing are all highlighted as areas to focus on.

Reflective exercise – improving outcomes

Beck et al. (2019) highlight areas for consideration, in order to improve mental health outcomes of racially minoritised populations. Services and practitioners must consider the following, and I would also encourage you to take a moment to consider this for yourself and the context that you work in:

What data is available for the outcomes of populations? What does this show?

What are the needs of individual populations? What are the gaps?

Are professional interpreters being regularly used, as needed?

Are staff competent to work effectively with all populations? Is training available?

Is therapy adapted to consider culture and context? Are adaptations useful?

Can learning be shared amongst the team? Are these conversations prioritised within the team?

How can we better meet the needs of racially minoritised communities? A case example

I will be using a fictional case study of 'Hussain' to demonstrate how flexibility can be used from the point of referral, within assessment, formulation, and intervention. This is only one example, as with every person it is important that an individualised approach is taken considering all aspects of identity (one size does not fit all). The Social GRACES framework (Burnham, 2012) can be kept in mind, as a framework to continually consider domains of identity (e.g. gender, religion, ability, class, ethnicity, and sexuality).

Case study – Hussain (Part 1)

Hussain is a 50-year-old South Asian Bangladeshi Muslim man. Bengali is his first language and English is his second, which he learnt after coming to the UK. His extended family are in Bangladesh, and he lives with his wife Halima and 4 children. His eldest child is 25-year-old daughter Shelina and youngest is ten-year-old Shuhel. He was referred to the service before, but his file was closed. The current referral states he has been out of work as an Uber driver due to a work incident which occurred on the night of September 11 and he is experiencing low mood, with the GP stating that he is 'not psychologically minded' and has prescribed medication.

Point of referral

As you read this information, it will be useful to think about what considerations need to be made and what barriers could exist. Take a moment and note down some of your thoughts before moving on.

- You may consider how the service could be more accessible (e.g. if Hussain prefers to speak in his mother tongue of Bengali): If there are language barriers, consider if an interpreter could be used. If you do not get through to Hussain on the phone, can a letter be sent but also a translated letter in Bengali too? At this point, we do not know if Hussain can read and write in English and/or Bengali. There may be a service protocol; however, can we go that one step further to try and facilitate engagement? For example, an extra phone call, text, or making contact with the GP to see if they could also help encourage contact.
- Hussain was referred to the service before, so we might want to find out what happened previously. Are there any existing notes from this contact? What may have been a barrier during this time?
- The date may be significant of September 11, him being a Muslim man, and this being a date where Muslim people may experience Islamophobia.
- His experience of the GP should also be considered and being prescribed medication, which can also in itself be a barrier. GP's may be more likely to consider medication only for racially minoritised populations, compared to the White population (Memon et al., 2016).
- From my experience, sometimes people may not know what 'psychology' or a 'mental health' service can provide. Can time be taken to explain who you are,

the purpose of the call, and what the service does, without using jargon? What might be some of the thoughts and feelings Hussain is experiencing? What are your own thoughts and feelings of working with Hussain? These are a few considerations, and there may be more that I have not mentioned, at the point of referral.

Top tips – working with interpreters

I have listed some top tips in working with interpreters, from my own practice and from Beverley Costa (2022):

- Always use a professional interpreter (avoid having family members interpret).
- Allow time before the appointment to brief and time after to de-brief.
- Clarify the role of the interpreter is to interpret only exactly what is said.
- Explaining confidentiality also extends to interpreters.
- Allow time for longer sessions.
- Provide feedback to interpreting services.
- Have the client leave the room first and then the interpreter.

Assessment

For assessment, you may follow your usual protocol (e.g. information gathering, questioning, interpersonal skills), with additional considerations. You may check with Hussain if an interpreter is needed, and if so, act accordingly (is there a certain dialect of Bengali that Hussain speaks? Consider the gender of the interpreter and also yourself as the therapist) If your service allows, it will be beneficial to allow time within assessment to build rapport and trust, as I found within my own research, there can be concerns about confidentiality and being misunderstood (Alam, 2023).

- Will Hussain be able to attend the appointment in person? Are there any options of being seen closer to come or in his GP surgery if he feels this could be easier? If he needs support, can an adult family member accompany him? Family members can be supportive in attending appointments but also providing information to aid formulation, with consent.
- You may as a therapist also take that extra step, to call or text Hussain reminders closer to the time of the appointment to aid engagement. As we have seen,

additional barriers exist for racially minoritised communities; therefore, we must take further steps to overcome these.

- As we know, Hussain is Muslim, and we should be curious about his relationship with Islam (e.g. is he devout?) If relevant, further considerations can be if appointments times can avoid clashing with times of prayer and if there are certain religious practices being observed (e.g. some people prefer to attend appointments outside of the holy month of Ramadan).
- Part of your assessment will include a risk assessment, and for some people this may be taboo or seen as sinful in their religion. Therefore, this should be considered and how difficult it may be for someone to discuss thoughts of self-harm or suicide. I have found normalising these thoughts an effective way of asking, explaining our duty of care to keep people safe, and signposting them to support if needed.
- Should there be aspects of someone's culture or religion that you are not sure about, a curious stance is needed to ask about this (e.g. 'I wonder if you could tell me more about that'; 'I am interested to hear more about that and what it means to you'). If appropriate, once rapport has been built after a few sessions, you may ask about any possible experiences of racism once trust has developed (Beck, 2016), for example: 'I am wondering if it is okay for me to ask about whether you experienced racism in that situation?'
- Once rapport has been established, you may name visible differences or similarities, exploring what it might be like for Hussain to see a therapist who is X (e.g. 'how does it feel seeing a therapist who is . . . a man, White?'). This allows for this to be named and to discuss any difficulties or benefits. Gurpinar-Morgan et al. (2014) highlight how therapists should appreciate how a client's ethnic background and culture relate to their presenting difficulties.
- You may consider aspects of Hussain's identity, such as gender within assessment and formulation (e.g. 'what has been your experience of being the only man in your family?'). A genogram is a tool (see Figure 11.1) from systemic therapy that is helpful for mapping out the family system (McGoldrick et al., 2008).

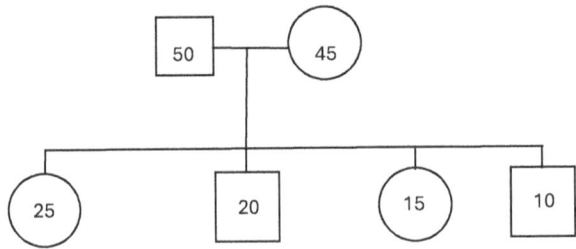

Figure 11.1 Genogram for Hussain

Case study – Hussain (Part 2)

You see Hussain at his GP practice, which is close to home. He attends with his daughter, who waits in the waiting room. He can speak English well, not requiring an interpreter. He worries about someone in the community finding out he is struggling and thinks he should 'just get on with things'. His daughter is due to get married, and he believes that if people find out, they will not want to associate with the family. He does not think he is 'mental' and said someone put black magic on him; he says 'you won't understand'. He thinks he is a failure as 'the man of the house' and as a Muslim.

Hussain said that he feels tired constantly and doesn't want to see anyone. He was quiet and looking down. He used to love going to the Mosque to pray and see friends, going on walks with his wife, taking the kids to football practice, and working. Now he does not have any energy to do things and thinks 'it will happen again' when asking him about when things changed. He has thought 'it would be better if I were not here' but he does not intend to end his life, with religion and family as protective factors.

Formulation

A collaboratively developed formulation provides an opportunity for therapists to ask clients about how this information can be used to gain a better understanding of their presenting problems or where it fits with their current understanding of difficulties (Beck, 2016). From the information that you have, try drawing out what a five areas formulation (Greenberger & Padesky, 1995) might look like for Hussain and practice how you might talk this through with him. Figure 11.2 provides an example from some of the therapists in training I have taught in the past:

Case study – Hussain (Part 3)

In the fourth session, Hussain tells you that this all started on the anniversary of 9/11 after a White male Uber customer called him a 'terrorist', spat at him, and poured alcohol in his car. He felt scared and ashamed to tell anyone. He has experienced Islamophobia before. He was worried that this could happen again and worried for his family as being targets. He did not experience any flashbacks. You explore

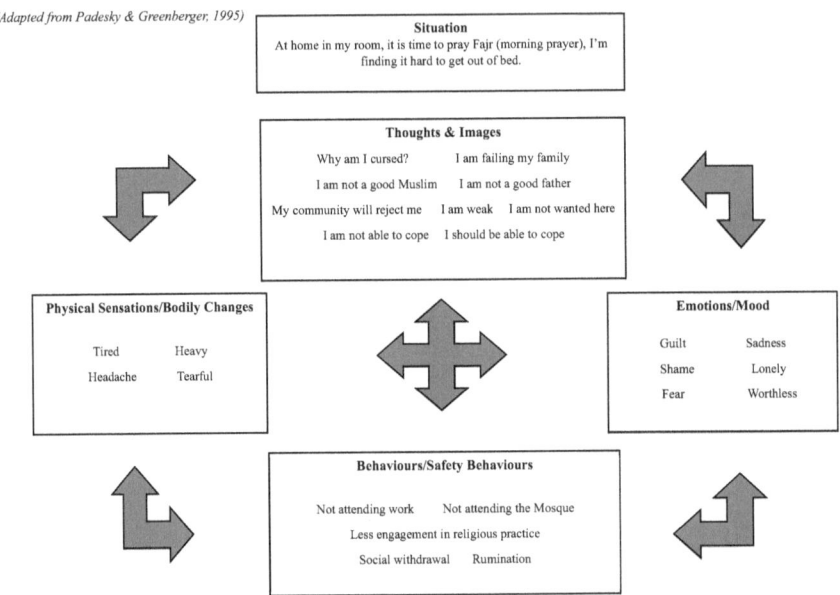

(Adapted from Padesky & Greenberger, 1995)

Situation
At home in my room, it is time to pray Fajr (morning prayer), I'm finding it hard to get out of bed.

Thoughts & Images
Why am I cursed?   I am failing my family
I am not a good Muslim   I am not a good father
My community will reject me   I am weak   I am not wanted here
I am not able to cope   I should be able to cope

Physical Sensations/Bodily Changes
Tired   Heavy
Headache   Tearful

Emotions/Mood
Guilt   Sadness
Shame   Lonely
Fear   Worthless

Behaviours/Safety Behaviours
Not attending work   Not attending the Mosque
Less engagement in religious practice
Social withdrawal   Rumination

Figure 11.2 Five areas formulation for Hussain

Source: Adapted from Greenberger & Padesky (1995)

further Hussain's past, and he said it was tough moving to the UK, leaving his family in Bangladesh and starting a life here. He had to work in hard labour jobs to support his family, and it did not always feel safe.

Hussain grew up in Bangladesh, in a working-class family, being the only son and eldest. His father was 'strong', always working, and Hussain did not see him much.

How might you develop a longitudinal formulation with Hussain? How could you consider his identity, social context, and experiences? Rathod et al. (2015) developed an evidence-based framework to culturally adapt CBT using a longitudinal formulation (Beck et al., 1979). Experiences of racism or discrimination may be a predisposing or precipitating factor for mental health problems (Bhui et al., 2018). Bringing this information into the formulation can give a sense of the client and therapist jointly understanding the wider societal context for someone developing mental health problems. Care should be taken when exploring these ideas not to minimise or discount experiences or concerns about racism. Listening to these stories and helping clients understand their problems in the context of these can be an empowering experience, and it might be part of their recovery process involving politicising their experiences and working towards challenging racism at a wider level in society (Beck, 2016). Williams et al. (2023) provide an evidence-based approach to treating stress and trauma due to racism in the further reading list for more information. See Figure 11.3 for an example and additional considerations of how a longitudinal formulation may look like for Hussain.

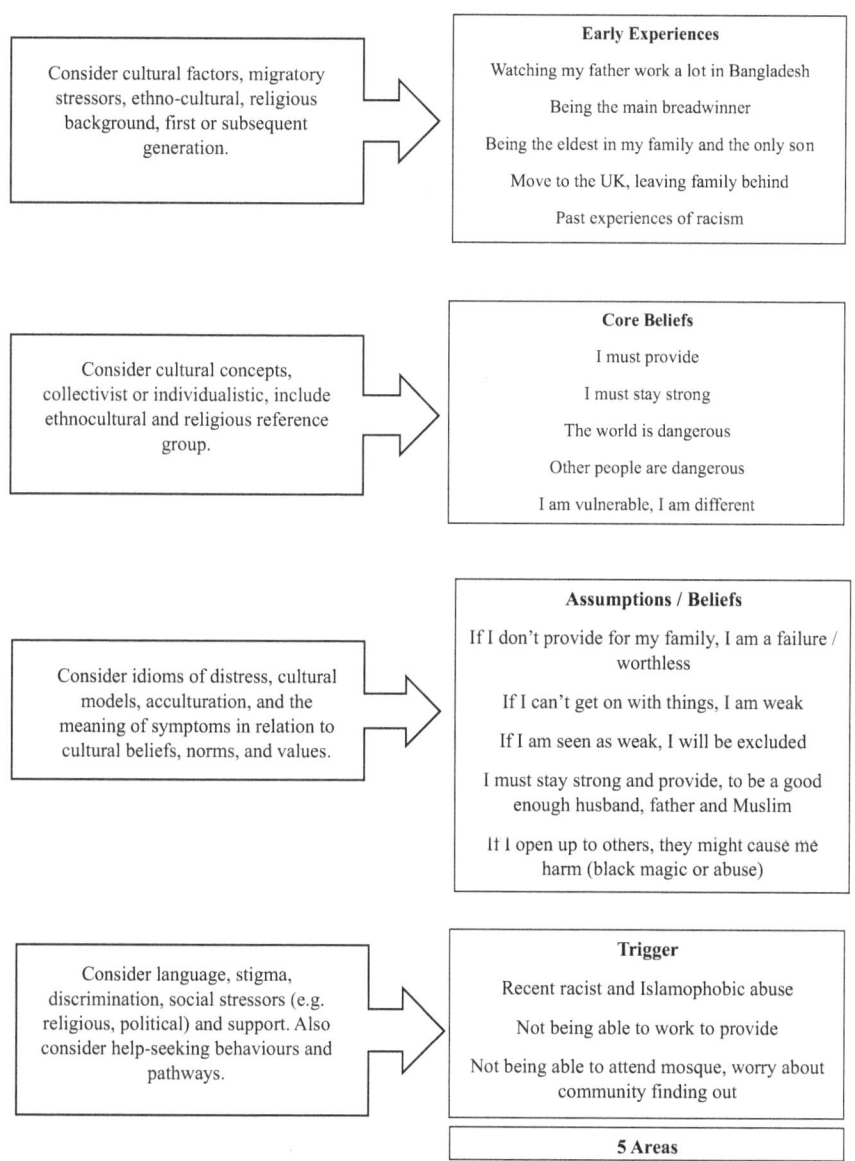

Figure 11.3 Longitudinal formulation for Hussain

Source: Adapted from Rathod et al. (2015)

The view of illness, health, and treatment can vary for people across cultures. Rathod and Kingdon (2009) state how understanding an individual's level of acculturation helps to understand how to engage with them and develop explanations in therapy based on their value systems. For Hussain, you may explore his level of acculturation from Bangladesh to the UK, within his generation and how this has shaped his views. Falicov (1995) also states how other areas to explore with clients could be to understand their own and family migration history, losses and gains from this, roles of family members, and how the family system is organised.

Therapy

Considering information gathered from assessment and collaborative formulation with understanding Hussain's difficulties, you might have your own ideas of what might be useful in therapy for Hussain. Take a moment to reflect on some of your ideas and note them down.

The first point I would like to highlight is how from the point of referral, assessment, and formulation on onwards your interaction with clients will be part of therapy and what may be helpful to them. Building up trust, rapport, and a safe space to talk about experiences, especially those which are painful such as racism and discrimination, will be part of what is therapeutic. For Hussain, he has not had anyone to talk about these experiences with, and this can feel lonely. There are also other roles of a therapist which clients may find helpful, such as writing letters to evidence their engagement in therapy (which Hussain may need for his time off work), linking into community spaces (for Hussain, this may be the Bangladeshi community to help tackle stigma and isolation), and considering if he has reported the incident to the police and if there is any support he needs with this to signpost him or get updates. As therapists, yes, we do offer assessment, formulation, and therapy; however, we can also have other roles which may be more beneficial to the client, using a needs-based approach.

Beck et al. (2019) highlight how services should develop resources or directories of organisations that can offer support and advocacy which will improve engagement in treatment. Services should also consider adapting therapies developed specifically for particular communities, by members of that community where necessary.

- Utilising ideas from narrative therapy may be useful such as using a timeline, having time to explore the losses and gains from migration Hussain experienced, and thinking about his strengths. There may also be systemic ideas, with including family members within the work to facilitate communication, if this is appropriate.
- If a client is religious, we may see where in the community they and us as a therapist could get more guidance on issues. For example, we may see if there are any local Imams (religious leaders) that we could connect Hussain to, or if there are any linked to the service/NHS Trust that we are working in. There may

be a role of a religious leader to help with psychological flexibility and rigid assumptions someone holds, such as having a mental health difficulty and being seen as weak or a bad Muslim.

I did my doctoral research looking at mental health within the Bangladeshi Muslim male community, and a suggestion was for more community work to increase awareness and reduce stigma of mental health difficulties (Alam, 2023). I put together a video with the BBC to highlight how work is being done to link faith with mental health, which could also be used to help encourage people to access support (BBC, 2021a, 2021b). It is important that therapists do not challenge or invalidate someone's beliefs, as this will lead to harmful practice. Clients will also disengage if they believe their spirituality is being pathologised. We need to incorporate this alongside the work we do, such as Hussain's belief that his difficulties may be due to black magic, which may maintain his difficulties. Support from a religious leader or incorporating religious ideas into therapy may aid the process of healing, helping Hussain understand his experiences and consider other explanations to break his vicious cycle.

Mir et al. (2019) highlight how religious coping can help clients. For example, Islamic teachings promote proactive behaviour and can provide hope. This was found through training for staff in a Talking Therapies service in Leeds, where there was an increase in referrals and outcomes for Muslim clients. The training also included therapists to reflect on their own assumptions about religion/Islam, whilst also highlighting the social stigma Muslim people face in the UK. Certain techniques used in CBT such as behavioural activation can be linked with Islamic teachings, emphasising that change begins with the individual. Weak faith could be re-framed in a way in Islam how Muslim people face tests from Allah (SWT) and the idea of 'Sabr' could be brought in, which can translate to patience and persistence despite adversity. There may be other teachings such as 'verily with hardship comes ease' (Quran 94:5) which may help people get through adverse life events. There are other religious teachings that promote wellbeing and prayers that can be recited at times of hardship or for protection. This can be brought into therapy if meaningful to the client. Allah (SWT) is also merciful and forgiving, which may facilitate a compassionate voice for an individual who may be self-critical. For Hussain, we might bring in these aspects of his religion and link this to behavioural activation, such as building a routine, which may coincide with praying five times a day and the process of washing himself before prayer (ablution) as a form of self-care. During my own research, prayer was also described as a way of being present and 'mindful' which may help with a present focus and strengthen a relationship with Allah (SWT) (Alam, 2023).

It is important that we are guided by the client and ask ourselves:

What would be most meaningful for the client?

What are their values?

What goals can be set?

We are not expected to have all the answers, but as therapists, be active in how we can support the client. If there is a need to include religion and spirituality, we must think about how confident we are to explore this and also educate ourselves outside of the therapy room. Adaptations may not always be required, we should try to do this as minimally as possible but be guided by the client and use supervision continually along the way.

Barriers to developing inclusive practice

As we have discussed, there are great benefits to incorporate a client's culture, ethnicity, and religion into therapeutic work. However, this must be done in a genuine way, which makes sense to both the client and therapist. Some clients may not want to discuss these areas, which is up to them, but what is important is that these conversations can be initiated rather than avoided. There are experiences of racism which are difficult to talk about but may be essential in understanding a client's experiences. There can be a great deal that is missed, and a client could be misunderstood if a therapist avoids these conversations, and it feels like 'walking on eggshells'. Time is needed to build up a genuine rapport so that a safe therapeutic space is formed. There may be some of your own blocks and barriers, which are needing to be explored.

Therapists must be aware of their own biases and prejudices, rather than being defensive. Our biases are influenced by our background, cultural environment, and personal experiences (Greenwald & Krieger, 2006). Remember the similarities and differences that exist. With conscious awareness and a sense of curiosity, we can explore a client's experiences and identity. . . . Remember, this is also applicable within supervision!

Supervision

Naz et al. (2019) identified how some ideas from CBT could be used if there are blocks or barriers to conversations regarding identity for a therapist. We might consider what our own 'hot thoughts' are and try using behavioural experiments to step out of our comfort zone. Managers and supervisors must support staff in these conversations and taking action. For example, a therapist might have a thought of 'I might get it wrong, I am not knowledgeable enough about their culture to help them'. This could cause physical changes such as increased heart rate, tension, and emotions of feeling anxious and guilty. They may then avoid these conversations, avoid working with people from different cultures and then continue to feel low in confidence to support different communities. What they could try to do is explore this in supervision and using self-reflection, to try a behavioural experiment. They could tolerate uncertainty, and ask about a client's culture and/or experience of racism in therapy. If you do not feel confident, be kind to yourself, use supervision, and seek training/Continuing Professional Development (CPD) opportunities. Beck (2016) gives an example of how identity and visible difference could be named and spoken about by saying: 'We look very different, you and I, what will it be like for you working with someone like me?' This could lead to developing confidence and an increase in skills/knowledge for the therapist and an improvement in the clients experiences and outcomes.

Clients may be worried about disclosing racism to therapists and may feel high levels of arousal at the prospect of disclosing racist incidents (physical, verbal acts, and microaggressions). Therapists may also feel intense emotions when racism is disclosed to them. Once a good therapeutic relationship has been established, asking about background, family life, migration, and spirituality in a supportive and non-judgemental way can help establish the trust needed to discuss racism. It is important to embody anti-racist practice, by actively valuing and working with equality at the forefront. Therapists must be open to addressing biases and gaps in skills/knowledge. By facing these areas and discomfort, this will aid with aligning to becoming anti-racist practitioners. This should be the case with everyone we work with, that we will not tolerate racism or discrimination from anyone (BABCP, 2020, Anti-racist statement).

Similar to the therapeutic relationship, it is essential that supervision is a safe and supportive space to discuss these issues, where a supervisee can also be vulnerable about their gaps and learning needs. What are the similarities and differences between supervisee and supervisor? What are the visible and invisible differences? Are conversations in these areas currently happening? If not, what are the barriers? How can these be addressed? Can this be made as part of the supervision contract? As a supervisor, we can take forward these principles from therapy and apply them to supervision.

Improving staffing

Services and teams must be representative of the populations that they serve, with a representative workforce. The BME PPG (Beck et al., 2019) identify a cycle of improving staffing where it is essential to recruit a representative workforce, understanding the needs of the workforce, ensuring equality of access to CPD, developing racially minoritised staff into more senior leadership roles, and ensuring fairness in disciplinary issues. There have been issues with psychological professions not being representative, highlighted in an interview I did with the British Psychological Society (BPS), where during my own training I never saw anyone in the profession who represented me (BPS, 2022). Following my own research, Bangladeshi men reported there to be a need to have staff from the same background, with a need for diversity within the workforce (Alam, 2023). However, what is important is that clients have the option to see someone from the same background or a different background, as the systematic review that I completed highlighted how some people prefer to be seen by someone from the same background and some people prefer not to (Alam et al., 2024). It is not necessary for staff to share the same background to be effective if you can demonstrate empathy, have the ability to acknowledge difference, be curious and transparent, whilst taking time to establish trust and build rapport. Think about how similarities and differences can BOTH be discussed and how this impacts therapy.

Top tips

- Use an individual approach, from the point of referral, through assessment, formulation, and intervention.
- Be active in turning towards discomfort and addressing your own blind spots.
- Consider the CBT evidence base but also adapt as necessary.
- Continually use supervision and self-reflection, if you require further CPD, request this to be available for you and your team.
- Consider the changes that can be made at an individual level, team level, service level, and wider. Community work is essential and making links.
- What are the other roles you can have as a therapist to meet the clients' needs? (e.g. advocate)

Conclusion

'Cultural competence' is not a separate requirement that we reach; working with individuals from diverse communities is an integrative and continual process. I have highlighted the need for inclusive practice to better serve racially minoritised communities, with services and individuals needing to do better. A 'one-size-fits-all' approach must be avoided, and we should hold in mind the individual, when assessing, formulating, and using CBT to support communities. Considering the challenges racially minoritised communities face, more must be done to reach out and incorporate all aspects of an individual's identity into therapy.

The case example of Hussain is one example where we can consider flexibility from what may be taught as a 'standard' within assessment, formulation, and intervention. Learning is a continuous process, and practitioners should turn towards discomfort, to address their own blind spots and assumptions, using CBT techniques on themselves and self-reflection to develop. Further research with individual minoritised communities is needed, looking at how to better improve mental health care. Consider your own role as a therapist and what other ways you can bring about change for minoritised communities and really improve access for all.

Acknowledgements

I would like to acknowledge colleagues within the BABCP Anti-Racism SIG who have contributed to the knowledge and learning shared within this chapter. I have learnt a great deal from BABCP president Saiqa Naz, Andrew Beck, Leila Lawton, Rani Griffiths, Daniela Zigova, Afsana Faheem, and Richard Thwaites. I would also like to recognise the trainees who I have taught, who contributed to the formulation of the case example of 'Hussain' and other colleagues who continue to work in improving care for racially minoritised communities.

Further reading

Alam, S., O'Halloran, S., & Fowke, A. (2024). What are the barriers to mental health support for racially-minoritised people within the UK? A systematic review and thematic synthesis. *The Cognitive Behaviour Therapist*, *17*, e10. https://doi.org/10.1017/S1754470X24000084

Special issue of tCBT Journal with cultural adaptations:
www.cambridge.org/core/journals/the-cognitive-behaviour-therapist/volume/56E6BA290
A1C75D68A50E80E70A1FCDA
This link holds a list of research papers looking at working with different racially-minoritized communities.
Special issue of tCBT Journal on being an anti-racist therapist:
www.cambridge.org/core/journals/the-cognitive-behaviour-therapist/special-issues/
being-an-anti-racist-cbt-therapist
This link holds a list of research papers looking at how to become an anti-racist CBT therapist.
Williams, T. M., Holmes, S., Manzar, Z., Haeny, A., & Faber, S. (2023). An evidence-based approach for treating stress and trauma due to racism. *Cognitive and Behavioral Practice*. https://doi.org/10.1016/j.cbpra.2022.07.001

References

Alam, S. (2023). British-Bangladeshi Muslim men: Removing barriers to mental health support and effectively supporting our community. *The Cognitive Behaviour Therapist, 16*, E38. https://doi.org/10.1017/S1754470X2300034X
Alam, S., O'Halloran, S., & Fowke, A. (2024). What are the barriers to mental health support for racially-minoritised people within the UK? A systematic review and thematic synthesis. *The Cognitive Behaviour Therapist, 17*, e10. https://doi.org/10.1017/S1754470X24000084
BABCP. (2020, June 4). *BABCP anti-racism statement*. https://babcp.com/About/News-Press/BABCP-Anti-Racism-Statement
Baker, C. (2018, April 25). *Mental health statistics for England: Prevalence, services and funding*. Briefing paper 6988. House of Commons Library. http://allcatsrgrey.org.uk/wp/download/public_health/mental_health/SN06988-1.pdf
Baker, C. (2020, January 23). *Mental health statistics for England: Prevalence, services and funding*. Briefing paper 6988. House of Commons Library. https://dera.ioe.ac.uk/34934/1/SN06988%20%28redacted%29.pdf
BBC. (2021a, February 19). *Mental health tips for lockdown in Sylheti*. www.bbc.co.uk/news/av/uk-56124256
BBC. (2021b, May 11). *How to get Bangladeshi men talking about mental health*. www.bbc.co.uk/news/av/health-57059479
Beck, A. (2016). *Transcultural cognitive behaviour therapy for anxiety and depression: A practical guide*. Routledge.
Beck, A., Naz, S., Brooks, M., & Jankowska, M. (2019). *IAPT: BAME service user positive practice guide*. BABCP. https://babcp.com/Therapists/BAME-Positive-Practice-Guide-PDF
Beck, A. T., Shaw, B. F., Rush, A. J., & Emery, G. (1979). *Cognitive therapy for depression*. Guildford Press.
Begum, N. (2006). *Doing it for themselves: Participation and Black and minority ethnic service users*. Social Care Institute for Excellence and the Race Equality Unit.
Bhui, K., Halvorsrud, K., & Nazroo, J. (2018). Making a difference: Ethnic inequality and severe mental illness. *The British Journal of Psychiatry, 213*(4), 574–578. https://doi.org/10.1192/bjp.2018.148
Bisby, N., Singam, S., Beattie, A., Ekiko, F., & Cliverd, A. (2003, March). *The mental health needs of the Bangladeshi community in Camden: An action research project*. http://bwhp.co.uk/pdf/reports/mental_health_action_research_report.pdf

BPS. (2022, September 26). *I never saw anyone who liked like me in the profession.* www.
bps.org.uk/psychologist/i-never-saw-anyone-who-looked-me-profession

Burnham, J. (2012). Developments in social GRRRAAACCEEESSS: Visible-invisible and
voiced-unvoiced. In I.-B. Krause (Ed.), *Culture and reflexivity in systemic psychotherapy:
Mutual perspectives* (pp. 139–160). Karnac Books Ltd.

Costa, B. (2022). Interpreter-mediated CBT – a practical implementation guide for working
with spoken language interpreters. *The Cognitive Behaviour Therapist, 15,* E8. https://
doi.org/10.1017/S1754470X2200006X

Faheem, A. (2023). 'It's been quite a poor show' – exploring whether practitioners working
for improving access to psychological therapies (IAPT) services are culturally competent
to deal with the needs of Black, Asian and Minority Ethnic (BAME) communities. *The
Cognitive Behaviour Therapist, 16,* E6. https://doi.org/10.1017/S1754470X22000642

Falicov, C. J. (1995). Training to think culturally: A multidimensional comparative framework. *Family Process, 34,* 373–388. https://doi.org/10.1111/j.1545-5300.1995.00373.x

Fearon, P., Kirkbride, J. B., Morgan, C., Dazzan, P., Morgan, K., Lloyd, T., Hutchinson,
G., Tarrant, J., Fung, W. L., Holloway, J., Mallett, R., Harrison, G., Leff, J., Jones, P. B.,
Murray, R. M., & AESOP Study Group. (2006). Incidence of schizophrenia and other
psychoses in ethnic minority groups: Results from the MRC AESOP study. *Psychological
Medicine, 36*(11), 1541–1550. https://doi.org/10.1017/S0033291706008774

McGoldrick, M., Gerson, R., & Petry, S. (2008). *Genograms: Assessment and intervention*
(3rd ed.). W. W. Norton & Company.

Gibbons, F. X., O'Hara, R. E., Stock, M. L., Gerrard, M., Weng, C. Y., & Wills, T. A. (2012).
The erosive effects of racism: Reduced self-control mediates the relation between perceived racial discrimination and substance use in African American adolescents. *Journal of Personality and Social Psychology, 102*(5), 1089–1104. https://doi.org/10.1037/
a0027404

Greenberger, D., & Padesky, C. (1995). *Mind over mood: Changing how you feel by changing the way you think.* The Guilford Press.

Greenwald, A., & Krieger, L. (2006). Implicit bias: Scientific foundations. *California Law
Review, 94,* 945. https://doi.org/10.2307/20439056

Gurpinar-Morgan, A., Murray, C., & Beck, A. (2014). Ethnicity and the therapeutic relationship: Views of young people accessing cognitive behavioural therapy. *Mental Health,
Religion & Culture, 17*(7), 714–725. https://doi.org/10.1080/13674676.2014.903388

Memon, A., Taylor, K., Mohebati, L. M., Sundin, J., Cooper, M., Scanlon, T., & De Visser,
R. (2016). Perceived barriers to accessing mental health services among black and minority ethnic (BME) communities: A qualitative study in Southeast England. *BMJ Open,
6*(11), e012337. https://doi.org/10.1136/bmjopen-2016-012337

Mir, G., Ghani, R., Meer, S., & Hussain, G. (2019). Delivering a culturally adapted therapy
for Muslim clients with depression. *The Cognitive Behaviour Therapist, 12,* E26. https://
doi.org/10.1017/S1754470X19000059

Naz, S., Gregory, R., & Bahu, M. (2019). Addressing issues of race, ethnicity and culture in
CBT to support therapists and service managers to deliver culturally competent therapy
and reduce inequalities in mental health provision for BAME service users. *The Cognitive
Behaviour Therapist, 12,* E22. https://doi.org/10.1017/S1754470X19000060

NHS Digital. (2020, July 30). *Psychological therapies: Annual report on the use of IAPT
services, England 2019–20.* Community and Mental Health Team. www.digital.nhs.uk/
pubs/psycther1920

NHS England. (2023, October 30). *Patient and carer race equality framework. Making
anti-racism work in all mental health providers.*
www.england.nhs.uk/long-read/patient-and-carer-race-equality-framework/

NHS Race and Health Observatory. (2023). *Ethnic inequalities in improving access to
psychological therapies (IAPT): Full report.* National Collaboration Centre for Mental
Health.

www.nhsrho.org/wp-content/uploads/2023/10/Ethnic-Inequalities-in-Improving-Access-to-Psychological-Therapies-IAPT.Full-report.pdf

Predelli, L. N., Halsaa, B., Thun, C., & Sandu, A. (2012). *Majority-minority relations in contemporary women's movements: Strategic sisterhood.* Palgrave Macmillan.

Raleigh, V., & Holmes, J. (2021, February 17). *The health of people from ethnic minority groups in England.* The Kings Fund. www.kingsfund.org.uk/publications/health-people-ethnic-minority-groups-england#Overall

Rathod, S., & Kingdon, D. (2009). Cognitive behaviour therapy across cultures. *Psychiatry,* *8*(9), 370–371. https://doi.org/10.1016/j.mppsy.2009.06.011

Rathod, S., Pinninti, N., Turkington, D., & Phiri, P. (2015). *Cultural adaptation of CBT for serious mental illness: A guide for training and practice.* Wiley Blackwell. https://doi.org/10.1002/9781118976159

Weich, S., Nazroo, J., Sproston, K., McManus, S., Blanchard, M., Erens, B., Karlsen, S., King, M., Lloyd, K., Stansfeld, S., & Tyrer, P. (2004). Common mental disorders and ethnicity in England: The EMPIRIC study. *Psychological Medicine, 34*(8), 1543–1551. https://doi.org/10.1017/s0033291704002715

Williams, T. M., Holmes, S., Manzar, Z., Haeny, A., & Faber, S. (2023). An evidence-based approach for treating stress and trauma due to racism. *Cognitive and Behavioral Practice.* https://doi.org/10.1016/j.cbpra.2022.07.001

Williamson, E., Walker, A. J., Krishnan, B., Bacon, S., Bates, C., Morton, C. E., Curtis, H. J., Mehrkar, A., Evans, D., Inglesby, P., Cockburn, J., McDonald, H. I., MacKenna, B., Tomlinson, L., Douglas, I. J., Rentsch, C. T., Mathur, R., Wong, A., Grieve, R., . . . Goldacre, B. (2020). OpenSAFELY: Factors associated with COVID-19-related hospital death in the linked electronic health records of 17 million adult NHS patients. *medRxiv* 2020.05.06.20092999. https://doi.org/10.1101/2020.05.06.20092999

Chapter 12

Embedding inclusive principles within your CBT practice

Working with autism, gender identity, and sexual orientation

Allán Laville, Anjali Mehta Chandar, Natalie Meek, and Eleanor Vialls

Introduction

Allán Laville

This chapter provides an overview of Equity, Equality, Diversity, and Inclusion (EEDI) considerations in relation to advancing your clinical practice. As the area of EEDI is vast, we will focus on three protected characteristics from the Equality Act (2010) but also provide a principled approach to all areas of EEDI through the 'appropriate' awareness framework (Laville, 2017). Adopting the 'appropriate' awareness framework addresses previous issues with CBT practice that only focused on the 'here and now' and often did not consider previous experiences of discrimination. This framework views a person holistically, including previous experiences of harassment, bullying, and prejudice that have led to the development of mental health difficulties. By considering previous experiences of discrimination, the therapist can more easily explore core beliefs, particularly those associated with personal identity.

This chapter will focus on the protected characteristics of disability, including neurodiversity, gender reassignment, and sexual orientation. In regard to gender reassignment, we acknowledge that the current legislation is restrictive, so we will use the term 'gender identity' to acknowledge that gender diverse communities also include non-binary individuals. We have chosen to focus on the three areas above due to the intersectional nature of these protected characteristics. The term 'Intersectionality' was coined by Crenshaw (1989) to describe how systems of oppression overlap to create distinct experiences for people with multiple identity categories. As an example, Laville identifies as a White Bi man, who is disabled and neurodivergent. From this, he acknowledges his privilege of being a White man, but also recognises the discrimination and harassment he has faced due to be being Bi, disabled, and neurodivergent. Biphobia and ableism are significant difficulties in today's world and need to be challenged.

DOI: 10.4324/9781003428527-15

Reflective exercise

Reflect on your own protected characteristics and the experiences you have had in relation to them. It is important to note both positive and negative experiences, and how these experiences have informed your own clinical practice.

Following on from the example above, we think it is important to acknowledge our own protected characteristics and the experiences we have had. This starts by acknowledging the various identities we all hold and how all parts of our identity inform our personal and professional life. Laville provides EEDI training to teaching clinicians and includes an activity that scaffolds self-exploration of your own identity and how this informs your clinical and teaching roles. This chapter provides several points to advance your own clinical practice in relation to EEDI. In the following sections, we provide a series a case vignettes to support reflective thinking and development of EEDI clinical practice. We also provide our top tips for working clinically with each community, which will further support the development of your clinical practice.

Training example

Serena (pseudonym) completed the activity of reflecting on each part of their identity as a working-class disabled White female and how different parts of their identity focus more prominently than others. Serena took the learning from this activity to support trainees to discuss their own protected characteristics and how these characteristics may inform their own clinical practice. This provides a good model for trainees in clinical practice, when considering the patient's protected characteristics in relation to life experiences, particularly harassment and discrimination.

It is very encouraging to see that colleagues are now embedding more EEDI activities within their teaching of trainee clinicians.

Working with autism

Anjali Mehta Chandar

Autism, or autistic spectrum condition (ASC), is a neurodevelopmental condition leading to difficulties with social interaction, communication, and restrictive or repetitive behaviours or interests (Pilling et al., 2012). It is considered within the disability-protected characteristic of the Equality Act (2010); however, many neurodiverse people (and indeed those who are not autistic) would argue that autism is not a disability at all. It is merely a difference in neurobiology that means they tend to have particular strengths and challenges.

There is a real need to consider how we can work effectively with autistic people, as we know that they are more likely to experience mental health difficulties. The 'appropriate' awareness framework (Laville, 2017), the case study, and the top tips below suggest how we can do that. We'd also encourage utilising supervision and CPD to enhance your knowledge and confidence further, as recommended by Chandar (2022).

The 'appropriate' awareness framework (Laville, 2017) suggests that we

a) consider the patient's protected characteristic(s);
b) the type of information that the patient is sharing regarding their protected characteristic(s);
c) which treatment intervention and/or signposting options would be most appropriate for that patient.

'Appropriate' awareness avoids assumption-led approaches and supports practitioners to be aware of areas of practice where knowledge could be developed, for example, knowledge of specialist services for particular communities and groups. By utilising good information gathering skills, practitioners should be able to assess whether a patient is interested in engaging in cognitive behavioural therapy and/or specialist signposting options.

Case Study – adapting CBT for autistic clients

Mariah (pseudonym) is a 16-year-old British Asian, autistic cis-female with pronouns she/her. She saw me in private practice for low mood, and in our assessment, I had noticed autistic traits and suggested an autism assessment. Meanwhile, we had 20 sessions following disorder-specific CBT with some additional skills yet progress was limited. She returned post-diagnosis, confused and validated by the diagnosis, and we had six further sessions, spaced one month apart.

This time, the work was more flexible. We had a briefer vicious flower formulation, which guided sessions generally, but we'd largely go with what Mariah required each session,

adding to the formulation if needed. We discussed fitting in at school and how she tiringly 'masked' her differences. Mariah felt unable to drop the mask at school (given an already present lack of belonging for being British Asian in a predominantly White school) but planned to at college. We created identity mind maps and thought about what she liked about her favourite superheroes, and created positive data logs to record how she too has those traits. Mariah wanted some social skills training to help her better manage reciprocal conversations, and we first explored that this was internally motivated (because social skills work can increase suicidality as we might be asking clients to change their authentic selves). Satisfied, we practised tennis ball conversations (remotely, by pretending to throw a ball through the screen) where we could only talk if we had the ball, which Mariah practised with Mum for homework. When Mariah came to a session crying for not being able to manage the sensory overload of her birthday celebrations, we discussed an energy bank, and rated how draining/replenishing different activities are. Homework was to get a balance of energy, and we included Mum in this to reduce demands in the home setting.

Taking a more flexible and affirming approach seemed to benefit Mariah greatly. She was more open, including being able to cry and share all the thoughts she judged herself for. Having a month between sessions also allowed more time for practice. Our therapeutic relationship was also strengthened.

Top tips

- Explore programmes, videos, and podcasts that share autistic people's lived experiences. It is invaluable.
- Authenticity is key. We want neurodiverse people to be able to celebrate and accept their differences and strengths. It can also highlight the need for self-compassion work. Kristin Neff's website has some fantastic exercises.
- Bear in mind the impact of their diagnosis. Some clients relish this and some hate it. Their age at diagnosis can affect this too. Be curious how they feel about it, and don't make assumptions. Use their language for how you refer to it with them, for example, some may not like the word 'autism'.
- Be mindful of intersectionality. How does autism link in with their race, age, marital status, gender, etc. Utilise things like the 'wheel of privilege' to explore this further.
- A formulation driven approach tends to work well, starting with a vicious flower (possibly longitudinal), with interventions to support the various maintenance cycles. However, flexibility to deal with what is happening this week for the client is important. By keeping it routed in a 'what, so what, now what' approach, we can be sure to continue to deliver CBT and change methods, rather than explorative counselling.

- Adaptations to therapy are a small part of the bigger picture. Think more holistically.
- Work alongside parents/partners to help them understand your client, if you have your client's permission. Families may try to mould their loved one into a neurotypical box without realising the damage this can do, particularly by suggesting social skills work. Signposting and psychoeducation can help.
- If your client is a child or young person, consider advocating for the family in the school setting to ensure they get the right support, for example, attend meetings with school and write letters.
- Emotion wheels, comic strip conversations with thought bubbles, and interoceptive exposure are great tools to support clients to access emotions, thoughts, and physical symptoms, respectively.
- The 'figure of 8' reciprocal formulation (Grimmer, 2013) can be an excellent discussion point to help clients make sense of the interaction between theirs and others' thoughts, feelings, and behaviour, aiding difficulties with Theory of Mind.

Working with gender identity

Natalie Meek

Gender is frequently perceived as binary – male or female – but it is best understood as a social construct (Lorber & Farrell, 1991) influencing the expectations, perceptions, and experiences of individuals. The now pervasive view of the gender binary can be traced back to colonialism, and the erasure of gender identities outside of the binary framework within indigenous societies worldwide (O'Sullivan, 2021). Historically, cultural perspectives have existed outside of the gender binary (Fiani & Serpe, 2020). Rather than a stable binary system, gender identity is dynamic, and each person's relationship with their own gender can change across their life (Brady et al., 2022).

The concepts of gender and sex are commonly conflated but refer to separate aspects of identity. Sex is assigned at birth based on biological and anatomical criteria, typically adhering to the male/female binary (Dolan et al., 2020) which fails to recognise the existence and experience of intersex individuals (Ackley et al., 2023). Gender can be static or fluid (Dolan et al., 2020) and is not necessarily congruent with an individual's assigned sex (Coleman et al., 2012). Individuals who identify outside of the gender binary are often described as gender non-conforming, including those who are transgender, non-binary, asexual, gender queer, and gender fluid (although this list is not exhaustive).

Experiences of discrimination

Hate crimes against trans individuals increased by 16% between 2018/2019 and 2019/2020 (Home Office, 2020); however, UK-based charity Stop Hate UK reported that 88% of trans people do not report their experiences of hate crimes (Stop Hate UK, n.d.) which would indicate a higher rate of crimes against gender-non-conforming individuals. People who are gender non-conforming experience health disparities which originate due to systemic bias and discrimination (de Vries et al., 2020) and experience higher levels of mental health diagnoses (Snow et al., 2019). Major barriers to mental health care have been identified for gender non-conforming individuals which include fear of being pathologised, and that practitioners are unknowledgeable, un-nuanced, and unsupportive (Snow et al., 2019).

The Equality Act (2010) identifies gender reassignment as a protected characteristic. Sex is also a protected characteristic, including those identifying as a man or a woman. These narrow definitions of gender identity leave those that identify outside of the gender binary unrepresented.

Case Study – adapting CBT for clients with diverse gender identities

Ben (pseudonym) presented in primary care mental health services with a provisional working diagnosis of social anxiety, accessing CBT face to face. Ben was 19 years old, White British. Assigned female at birth, Ben identifies as male, and uses pronouns he/they. Ben was asexual and was unemployed having recently finished college which he did not enjoy. Ben was diagnosed with autism during their school years, feeling this contributed to his feelings of anxiety in social situations and difficulty maintaining friendships. Treatment goals were developed to find a voluntary job post by the end of treatment, and to socialise in person once a week.

Although I had previously attended training on working with diverse gender identities, I took the time between sessions to refresh my knowledge and understanding. In our first session I introduced myself and my pronouns, I asked directly about their gender, and who in their lives were aware of their identity to make sure I did not 'out' them if family or other healthcare professionals were not aware. When negative thoughts were elicited regarding historic responses to gender identity, I did not move to challenge these thoughts, instead I offered empathy for their previous experiences of being misgendered and deadnamed. We followed a CBT protocol for social anxiety, but adapted this to both their autism and identity, such as not setting experiments to go into spaces where Ben would face discrimination or be at risk. By the end of treatment, Ben was going to a weekly tabletop game session and had found voluntary employment with a charity that was inclusive of all gender identities.

Top tips

- Studies show that discrimination in healthcare settings towards members of the LGBTQIA+ community is often due to a lack of information. Make yourself aware of the language around gender identity; it is not the place of your client to teach you. Attend training on gender identity if necessary.
- It is reported most healthcare workers in the UK would not clarify gender pronouns or ask about gender in mental health settings (Parameshwaran et al., 2017). Make it part of your day-to-day practice to share your pronouns when introducing yourself, as well as asking for the pronouns of each client you work with.
- Ask questions about the client's gender identity and who in their lives is aware of their identity. If your client is not yet fully out, or if being so may cause them to be at risk, make sure you are using the name, pronouns, and gender they wish to be shared in any communication with other services, family, or schools.
- Anti-trans rhetoric is prevalent, and so we may hold implicit bias or have assumptions about people who have diverse gender identities. Use supervision spaces to explore any bias you may hold and work on challenging these biases.
- Misgendering is when someone is addressed using language that does not match their gender identity, which is shown to significantly impact the mental health of transgender people (Dolan et al., 2020). If you misgender a client, name it, correct yourself, apologise, and repair any rupture in the therapeutic relationship.
- Explore any similarities or differences between the gender identity of you and your client. Ask the client how they feel working with someone with a similar/different identity.

Working with sexual orientation

Eleanor Vialls

Sexuality and relationships are a natural part of human diversity (BPS, 2019). Sexual orientation, defined by the Equality Act (2010), is someone's pattern of romantic relationships, including, but not limited to, heterosexuality, gay, lesbian, and bisexual. The provision of this legislation protects people from being discriminated against based on their sexual orientation. The British Psychological Society (BPS, 2019) states a fundamental principle that people with a diverse sexual orientation should have the same rights as a heterosexual individual. It is therefore crucial that psychological therapies address this by ensuring that treatment is adapted to align with patients' beliefs, learning needs, and abilities (NICE equality report, 2021).

We also know from Cocks et al. (2019) that a significant barrier for sexual minority individuals in accessing psychological therapies is the concern that their practitioner will not understand their unique experiences. Therefore, we need to improve visible allyship and improve practitioner's knowledge, understanding, and awareness of sexual diversity considerations in psychotherapeutic care (Laville, 2022).

Case vignette – Part 1 – adapting CBT to be inclusive of client's sexuality and gender identity

When working as a qualified psychological wellbeing practitioner (PWP), I specialised as a perinatal champion. In this role, I supported Sarah (pseudonym), who opted to engage in low-intensity CBT via guided self-help. Sarah was a 33-year-old White British woman, with pronouns of she/her. She identified her sexual orientation as lesbian. At the time of the first session, Sarah was 26-weeks pregnant and seeking support for low mood and negative thoughts about being a good enough parent.

Throughout our treatment sessions, we developed a therapeutic alliance, which was aided by the use of common factor skills (Bennett-Levy et al., 2010) and open and non-assumptive questioning (Laville, 2017). I asked Sarah about her experiences and identity before making any assumptions (Laville, 2017), which was key when developing a therapeutic rapport. To avoid making assumptions, I used inclusive language throughout the treatment sessions. For example, I used terms such as 'parents', as opposed to 'mother and father' and 'partner' as opposed to 'husband or wife'. Sarah also expressed that when the baby was born, she was going to be called 'Mummy' and her partner would be called 'Mumma'. As stated in the guidance for psychologists working with gender, sexuality, and relationship diversity (BPS, 2019), psychological practitioners should use the preferred terms for that individual and how they define their relationship.

This case example is of a client I previously worked with who identified as lesbian and reflected on the elements of treatment that supported her, as well as providing further tips on how to best work with sexual orientation in CBT.

Case vignette – Part 2

Sarah shared that her low mood stemmed from worries about having a baby into a same-sex relationship and worries about being good enough as a parent. I was mindful of unconscious biases that I may have held, and did not want to make any assumptions around Sarah's experiences (Lingras, 2022). Therefore, I asked open questions about Sarah's identity as a lesbian woman and funnelled her worries around having a baby into a same-sex relationship

(Richards & Whyte, 2011). I was able to ascertain that she was comfortable in her sexual orientation as she had identified as a lesbian for most of her adult life, and that she felt equipped to raise a child with her partner. She also felt supported by her community midwife. Therefore, Sarah did not need any signposting to support groups or services at this time. The concern for her was focused more around how they would be perceived by others. Unfortunately, this stemmed from opinions relayed by family members, which perpetuated her low mood. The concern for her was focused around how she would be perceived by others. Unfortunately, this stemmed from opinions relayed by family members, which perpetuated her low mood. Sarah was experiencing internalised stigma (Herek et al., 2009), related to the prejudicial comments made by others. I provided empathy (Richards & Whyte, 2011) to ensure she felt understood, which helped to develop the therapeutic rapport and demonstrate the sessions to be a space where she could share her experiences openly and safely.

I was supervised by a colleague who had previous work experience in a perinatal mental health service (Turpin & Wheeler, 2011). Low-intensity supervision offers space to consider intersectionality and unconscious biases (Lingras, 2022), reflect on the treatment sessions, ensure the treatment fit with the evidence base and adhered to the ethical guidelines (Turpin & Wheeler, 2011; BPS, 2019). Through supervision, I was supported to explore the impact her families discrimination had, utilising the five areas model (Williams, 2001) which also provided a space for Sarah to reflect and problem solve (Richards & Whyte, 2011).

At the time of her treatment sessions, I was also pregnant with my first child. On reflection, this commonality helped me appreciate her experience in more depth, and as a parent to be, I noticed more discrepancies in inclusivity in peri and postnatal services (one example includes mixed-gender parent pictures on pregnancy and birthing guides), which was something to be mindful of. I learnt to hold an open mind, and take a non-assumptive stance when working with Sarah, as well as utilising collaboration to ensure that treatment adhered to Sarah's needs and around her life.

My experience working with Sarah helped me develop my skills to ensure I was working as an inclusive practitioner. I include some best practice tips below for working with sexuality.

Top tips

1) Be mindful of assumptions and offer empathy. It is important that we are open to hearing how our client identifies themselves before assuming this for ourselves (BPS, 2019).

2) Ask questions. Be open to learning about your client's experience, through funnelling and the use of common factor skills (Laville, 2017).
3) Use inclusive language. Keeping language inclusive will ensure that the client and their experiences are not being discounted (BPS, 2019).
4) Seek appropriate supervision. Supervision can allow for space to explore unconscious bias, consider best practice, and reflect on experiences (Turpin & Wheeler, 2011; Cocks et al., 2019).
5) Services should ensure that practitioners are appropriately trained to support diversity (e.g. as stated in the Perinatal Positive Practice Guide, IAPT, 2013).

Further reading

Belcher, H. L. (2022). *Taking off the mask: Practical exercises to help understand and minimise the effects of autistic camouflaging.* Jessica Kingsley.
    This book is written by an autistic psychologist, and provides some fantastic CBT-congruent activities to help clients make sense of, and manage, their masking. I recommend this book to both therapists and clients.
Foy, A., Morris, D. D. A., Fernandes, V., & Rimes, K. A. (2019). LGBQ+ adults' experiences of improving access to psychological therapies and primary care counselling services: Informing clinical practice and service delivery. *The Cognitive Behaviour Therapist, 12*(42), 1–23.
    I recommend this paper to anyone working within psychological services, primary care, or more specifically Improving Access to Psychological Therapies (IAPT) services, to reflect on their practice and delivery of their service. The study presents a thematic analysis that outlines the experiences of the LGBTQ+ community accessing and engaging within mental health services and highlights areas for needed for improvement.
McDowell, M. J., Goldhammer, H., Potter, J. E., & Keuroghlian, A. S. (2020). Strategies to mitigate clinician implicit bias against sexual and gender minority patients. *Psychosomatics, 61*(6), 655–661.
    As clinicians, we are still susceptible to implicit bias, which includes biases towards gender minority patients. This paper explores research on the topic, as well as including some top tips and case studies of what to do, and what not to do. It is a great starting place on your journey to addressing any unconscious bias we may hold.

Conclusion

This chapter has covered key EEDI considerations for clinical practice. Each section has been aligned with the protected characteristics included in the Equality Act (2010). The authors have introduced an effective framework for EEDI considerations and have provided case examples for working with autism, gender identity, and sexual orientation. The authors has also provided a number of top tips for working with each population and key take-home points when considering CBT formulations and treatment plans. Overall, the next steps for clinical practice will be for practitioners, and services, to make sure that EEDI considerations are central on the agenda. It is the responsibility of all of us to ensure that EEDI considerations are effectively embedded within our own clinical practice in order to provide holistic care to our clients.

Key points

1. Avoiding assumption-led approaches by engaging in good information gathering to support the creation of meaningful treatment plans (Laville, 2017).
2. The importance of considering intersectionality and seeing individuals holistically. This was a key factor for Anjali and Natalie when working with their clients.
3. The importance of considering your own protected characteristics and how your own identity informs your clinical practice. This was a key factor for Eleanor when working with her client.
4. The importance of language use and using identity terminology that is congruent with the client's terminology. This is central to developing and maintaining a good therapeutic alliance.
5. The importance of engaging in appropriate EEDI training within training programmes and training provided as CPD. This should then be supported by effective supervision in practice (Chandar, 2022).
6. The importance of authentic practice and visible allyship (Cocks et al., 2019) for minoritised and marginalised communities.

References

Ackley, S. F., Zimmerman, S. C., Flatt, J. D., Riley, A. R., Sevelius, J., & Duchowny, K. A. (2023). Discordance in chromosomal and self-reported sex in the UK Biobank: Implications for transgender-and intersex-inclusive data collection. *Proceedings of the National Academy of Sciences*, *120*(18), e2218700120.

Bennett-Levy, J., Richards, D. A., & Farrand, P. (Eds.). (2010). *Oxford guide to low intensity CBT interventions*. Oxford University Press.

Brady, B., Rosenberg, S., Newman, C. E., Kaladelfos, A., Kenning, G., Duck-Chong, E., & Bennett, J. (2022). Gender is dynamic for all people. *Discover Psychology*, *2*(1), 41.

British Psychological Society. (2019). *Guidelines for psychologists working with gender, sexuality and relationship diversity: For adults and young people (age 18 and over)*. Retrieved June 20, 2023, from https://explore.bps.org.uk/binary/bpsworks/986e577a2e5c686b/dd77909e-434237fe7bd656c718998a266faa1f304fa51648cfd96ff20db3cc0d/rep129_2019.pdf

Chandar, A. M. (2022). Neurodiversity in children and young people. *CBT Today*, *50*(4), 12–13.

Cocks, L., Jonas, K., & Laville, A. (2019). Exploring LGBT mental health and recommendations for clinical practice. *CBT Today*, *47*(3), 10–11.

Coleman, E., Bockting, W., Botzer, M., Cohen-Kettenis, P., DeCuypere, G., Feldman, J., Fraser, L., Green, J., Knudson, G., Meyer, W. J., Monstrey, S., Adler, R. K., Brown, G. R., Devor, A. H., Ehrbar, R., Ettner, R., Eyler, E., Garofalo, R., Karasic, D. H., . . . Zucker, K. (2012). Standards of care for the health of transsexual, transgender, and gender-nonconforming people, version 7. *International Journal of Transgenderism*, *13*(4), 165–232. https://doi.org/10.1080/15532739.2011.700873

Crenshaw, K. (1989). Demarginalizing the intersection of race and sex: A Black feminist critique of antidiscrimination doctrine, feminist theory and antiracist politics. In *University of Chicago legal forum* (Vol. 140, No. 1, pp. 139–167).

de Vries, E., Kathard, H., & Müller, A. (2020). Debate: Why should gender-affirming health care be included in health science curricula?. *BMC Medical Education*, *20*, 1–10.

Dolan, I. J., Strauss, P., Winter, S., & Lin, A. (2020). Misgendering and experiences of stigma in health care settings for transgender people. *Medical Journal of Australia, 212*(4), 150–151.

Fiani, C. N., & Serpe, C. R. (2020). Non-binary identity and the double-edged sword of globalization. In M. Ryan (Ed.), *Trans lives in a globalizing world.* Routledge.

Grimmer, A. G. (2013). *The nine-part model: A tool for sharing dyadic formulations.* Retrieved June 30, 2023, from www.bristolcbt.co.uk/publications/the-nine-part-model-dyadic-formulation

Herek, G. M., Gillis, J. R., & Cogan, J.C. (2009). Internalized stigma among sexual minority adults: Insights from a social psychological perspective. *Journal of Counselling Psychology, 56*, 32–43.

Home Office. (2020). *Hate crime, England and Wales, 2019/2020.* https://assets.publishing.service.gov.uk/government/uploads/system/uploads/attachment_data/file/925968/hate-crime-1920-hosb2920.pdf

IAPT. (2013). *Perinatal positive practice guide.* Retrieved June 20, 2023, from https://kirkleesiapt.co.uk/wp-content/uploads/2018/05/perinatal-positive-practice-guide-2013.pdf

Laville, A. (2017). The importance of data collection, signposting and 'appropriate' awareness in working with sexual orientation. *CBT Today, 45*(4), 14–15.

Laville, A. (2022). LGBT+ history month: The importance of awareness and understanding for LGBT+ considerations within clinical practice. *CBT Today, 50*(1), 14–15.

Lingras, K. A. (2022). Mind the gap(s): Reflective supervision/consultation as a mechanism for addressing implicit bias and reducing our knowledge gaps. *Infant Mental Health Journal, 43*(4), 638–652.

Lorber, J., & Farrell, S. A. (Eds.). (1991). *The social construction of gender* (pp. 309–321). Sage.

NICE. (2021). *Annual equality report.* Retrieved June 20, 2023, from www.nice.org.uk/about/who-we-are/policies-and-procedures/nice-equality-scheme

O'Sullivan, S. (2021). The colonial project of gender (and everything else). *Genealogy, 5*(3), 67.

Parameshwaran, V., Cockbain, B. C., Hillyard, M., & Price, J. R. (2017). Is the lack of specific lesbian, gay, bisexual, transgender and queer/questioning (LGBTQ) health care education in medical school a cause for concern? Evidence from a survey of knowledge and practice among UK medical students. *Journal of Homosexuality, 64*(3), 367–381.

Pilling, S., Baron-Cohen, S., Megnin-Viggars, O., Lee, R., & Taylor, C. (2012). Recognition, referral, diagnosis, and management of adults with autism: Summary of NICE guidance. *Bmj, 344*, e4082.

Richards, D., & Whyte, M. (2011). *Reach out. National programme student materials to support the delivery of training for psychological wellbeing practitioners delivering low intensity interventions* (3rd ed.). Improving Access to Psychological Therapies. Retrieved December 30, 2022, from https://cedar.exeter.ac.uk/media/universityofexeter/school-ofpsychology/cedar/documents/Reach_Out_3rd_edition.pdf

Snow, A., Cerel, J., Loeffler, D. N., & Flaherty, C. (2019). Barriers to mental health care for transgender and gender-nonconforming adults: A systematic literature review. *Health & Social Work, 44*(3), 149–155.

Stop Hate UK. (n.d.). *About hate crime transgender hate.* www.stophateuk.org/about-hate-crime/transgender-hate/

Turpin, G., & Wheeler, S. (2011). *IAPT supervision guidance.* Retrieved June 20, 2023, from www.iapt.nhs.uk/silo/files/iapt-supervision-guidance-revised-march-2011.pdf

Williams, C. J. (2001). *Overcoming depression: A five areas approach.* Arnold.

Chapter 13

Being an effective CBT therapist

What our clients need from us?

Ashley Fulwood and Commentary by Jason Roscoe

Introduction

What makes a person competent in the use of CBT? Providing a concise answer to this question is trickier than it might sound. We might be judged as competent by CBT trainers on account of passing a couple of marked recordings of single therapy sessions seen in isolation, yet if our clients do not feel confident in us or feel unsafe or unheard, they might fail to benefit from the interventions that we seek to provide (Li et al., 2024). Non-specific factors such as the client feeling safe and validated feature time and again in the literature (Flückiger et al., 2018). For example, why is it that two therapists trained to the same standard and using the same interventions can have very different levels of success with their clients? Some people seem to have a knack for putting others at ease or have the charisma to persuade their clients to do the difficult aspects of therapy (e.g. exposure), whereas others struggle. Arguably, 'interpersonal effectiveness' as it is referred to is the hardest skill to develop (Bennett Levy, 2019; Blackburn et al., 2001; Waltman et al., 2017).

Whilst previous chapters have considered how to navigate the training experience, we should not forget the main reason we do this work. Providing compassionate and effective treatment to our clients is paramount, and how they perceive what we do in therapy deserves equal attention. This chapter is written from an Expert by Experience (EbyE) perspective by Ashley, who has accessed CBT treatment for obsessive-compulsive disorder. Hopefully, Ashley's experiences receiving CBT can provide some useful pointers of how to be more effective and engaging as a therapist.

The value of EbyEs

Drawing upon the perspective of EbyEs has become an increasingly popular component of CBT training courses in recent years (BABCP, 2021). EbyE's are individuals who have been through CBT treatment and are in the unique position to offer the perspective of what it is like to receive CBT. Their input on courses can help us to reflect on how the theories and interventions that we learn during our training 'land' with clients. This can also shape the content of teaching and skill

DOI: 10.4324/9781003428527-16

development. The patient perspective allows us to reflect more deeply on the models and methods we are using and how we introduce core aspects of CBT such as agenda setting, homework, and behavioural experiments. After course lecturers and supervisors, EbyE's can be our 'third teacher', offering unique feedback that is only possible when we listen to their experiences of accessing CBT and use this to inform how we translate our classroom learning into patient-friendly therapy.

Ashley's story

Having suffered with obsessive-compulsive disorder for most of my adult life, seeking help for the condition is sadly not a unique experience for me. However, my experiences with therapists I have encountered are varied, and that's become a common theme I have encountered through my work for OCD-UK, a national charity that helps people with OCD. It shouldn't be a mixed bag, but the reality for those of us that reach out for help is that it is. Poor experiences can then lead to reluctance to seek further therapy and even a dismissal of CBT altogether. The good news is that books like this I hope will go some way to ensuring an improved therapeutic journey for those of us that need the help and support of therapists like you. Some of the characteristics to enhance the therapy experience for us patients can be subtle but can actually make or break the trust and understanding between us, so I hope my suggestions will prove helpful in enhancing the therapist/patient experience.

The first meeting

Let's start right at the beginning of the journey with the introductions. As my therapist, I assume you will have already read a little about me from the notes. However, I don't know you; I may have been sent a letter with your name, but as I walk through your door, you are just a therapist to me at this point. By sharing your name straight away, it will offer a sense of familiarity and go some way to creating a therapist/patient trust and connection, which will ultimately allow me to open up about my incredibly personal and often embarrassing situation and problems. It's not unusual for name sharing to be overlooked, but it's a subtle and important first step. If you do share your name, it's so easy for patients to forget a lot of the spoken words in the early parts of therapy, including your name, because we will be sharing vulnerable moments with you, so remember to remind the patient of your name at the start of the second session too.

> **Key point**
>
> Patients want to be safe, understood, and hopeful about change when they first meet you. Your theoretical orientation, whether you are

accredited or how many qualifications you have, is likely to be less important to them. A plethora of research in the field indicates that the therapeutic relationship trumps all, and on this basis, therapists need to be humble about what they can do and take some time to listen to what really matters to the people they are treating.

Helping us to make the most of each session

On the topic of reminders, this also brings me to the second point: encourage your patients to audio record the sessions and to listen back between sessions to make sure no invaluable learning is missed. Some patients may prefer a written transcript of the session rather than audio recording, so although it may take a little time and a very small investment on your part to purchase software such as otter.ai, perhaps if your time resource allows, you can record the session yourself and run the recording through the software to generate a transcription. You could then email the patient at least an overview, if not the full transcript of the session.

Appreciate the nuances of outcome measures

Some assessment forms can lack compassion and will miss the true reflection of the difficult time a person is having because of their ongoing problems. They fail to truly reflect how a person can be left feeling because of their problems and, in my experience, fail to address the collateral damage that OCD causes: for example, the impact on relationships or how some compulsions can impact a person's physical health (e.g. leaving damaged skin from repeated handwashing or breathing difficulties because of all the bleach they use). All because of OCD, but the assessment forms for OCD don't all cover that. They don't take into account the sporadic nature of OCD, how avoidance means some people may not be triggered for several weeks, so a person may score low on a questionnaire but are actually avoiding (a compulsion) to score low.

We are more than a number!

Some therapists, especially those who work within the NHS Talking Therapies Services, will be familiar with the use of the assessment questionnaires/outcome measures such as PHQ-9, GAD-7, and the OCI (Kroenke et al., 2001). Undoubtedly, using these measures can be positive in that it can illustrate a patient's progress through the therapeutic journey. However, it's important to be mindful of the implications of using them to screen people out of services (if they score below a threshold) and why some patients don't like them and may not answer them accurately.

Key point: how to interpret questionnaire scores

My own experience of their use is negative where scoring low was inappropriately used to dictate that I wasn't meeting the clinical threshold for treatment, despite the significant impact of obsessive-compulsive disorder on my life at that same time. The impact of this is that some therapeutic services use such assessment forms to decide if they will offer a patient treatment or not, and I was once rejected for treatment very early in an assessment process (12 minutes) because I measured low on a particular therapeutic measurement score. So they used the assessment form to make a decision before they had started asking me about how the condition truly impacts on me. The assessment form score had already sealed my therapy fate.

Seeing the bigger picture

It's important to be mindful of the fact that the Improving Access to Psychological Therapies (IAPT) Manual advises that a person-centred assessment is a crucial part of the care pathway (National Collaborating Centre for Mental Health, 2019). What the assessment questionnaires fail to address is how much avoidance a person may be practising and the hidden impact on their life that not all patients will be consciously aware of. That's where the skill of the therapist needs to help patients recognise the impact their problems may be having on their lives.

Reflective exercise

Q. What has been your experience of using assessment questionnaires/ outcome measures (e.g. PHQ-9) with clients?

Q. What do you see as their strengths and limitations?

The other factor that's worthy of consideration is that from speaking to other patients, they generally don't like completing the measures. Often, they describe that they are not really accurate or relevant to their problem or how they feel. In other cases, we often hear service users talk about not wanting to upset their therapist by reflecting honestly on how they may feel if their situation has not improved much.

Top tips

- It is imperative that a therapist uses their listening and interviewing skills to provide a person-centred assessment that does not rely on the use of assessment questionnaires/measures to be the sole contributory factor that dictates if a patient is offered treatment or if it's time to discharge a patient.
- Use such forms to guide you, but remember, they can't tell a person's story.

Striking the right balance

Normalising can be a helpful aspect of therapy, such as the type of intrusive thoughts that are experienced by the general population (Purdon & Clark, 1993). This can help reduce shame whilst working on the cognitive aspect of CBT. However, be careful not to fall into the trap of trying to be empathetic but end up trivialising OCD. I have previously felt a therapist was not the right person to help me because they used the words 'we all have a little bit of OCD'. For those of us with OCD, those few words always suggest someone that doesn't understand the condition or our suffering.

Instilling a sense of hope must be an important part of therapy, and if the patient has had poor therapeutic experiences in the past, you will need to work hard to instil hope. It's also important not to torpedo a patient's hope – I once experienced a therapist tell me that I will always have to live with OCD, and in that moment, that therapist had lost me, because I had no confidence in their ability to help me. It also works the other way, and telling me I will be completely OCD free after a dozen sessions is perhaps offering false hope, so ensure you help the patient form realistic and achievable recovery goals for this course of therapy. Having such goals is also good for you as a therapist, in that it can help you measure the patient's progress.

When it comes to helping patients move forward, language is important. Telling a patient to 'stop having those thoughts' or 'stop doing those behaviours' really is unhelpful. I tell our charity service users to answer such suggestions with a one-word response, 'How?' Helping us work out 'how' to think and respond differently in response to our problems is what I am looking for through my therapeutic journey.

Helping a patient make behavioural changes will often involve experiments and exposure exercises, and that will sometimes mean suggesting extreme exercises which are outside of the norms: for example, asking a patient with OCD to place a knife against a loved one's throat or to put their hands inside toilet water. Don't just tell a patient what they have to do, work collaboratively, and where you can, show them by doing the exposure exercise yourself initially. After all, if you're not prepared to do it, why should your patient?

Remember the wise words of Elvis

Finally, whilst it's always important to be friendly and open and have a patient like you, as a patient, I primarily want an effective therapist. Remember, CBT is meant to be a doing therapy not just a talking therapy. For me, the best therapist is one that captures all of that – friendly, understanding, and one that can challenge me and empower me to push myself towards recovery. A useful phrase to remember is 'a little less conversation, a little more action'.

Key points – personalising the CBT that you deliver

- Ashley's preferences mirror some of the 'ideal' characteristics that we look for in trainee CBT therapists (e.g. the capacity to validate how difficult it is to face one's fears yet being *firm enough* to encourage the client to do the tough bits [like exposure]). It also highlights some of the challenges that elements of CBT practice generate for clients and which we might take for granted.
- It's a cliché but first impressions count. How we introduce ourselves, how we explain things – even if we refer to the individual we are working with as a patient or client – can help to create rapport.
- In target-focused cultures such as Talking Therapies for Anxiety and Depression (TTAD), concepts such as 'recovery' and 'caseness' can overshadow our basic therapeutic competences such as empathy. Recognising and reflecting on this often comes down to the micro-skills of how the therapist introduces and interprets things like outcome measures.

Conclusion

Whilst research tells us the types of treatment packages (e.g. CBT for PTSD) and associated interventions (e.g. reliving) that tend to work for most people, what they don't tell us is how it feels to receive these treatments or formulations. Ashley's experiences point to the need to be personable yet professional, guided by evidence-based practices such as routine outcome measures but not a slave to the scores that are generated.

Practising role-plays with another trainee only partly replicates the experience of providing or receiving CBT in the real world. Self-practice of CBT methods and 'real play' where we bring our own material can deepen our understanding of how to personalise our delivery of CBT, yet unless we have accessed therapy or mental health services ourselves, it still doesn't really give us the full picture of what it is truly like to experience CBT as a client. For example, our use of terminology and acronyms that we use with our supervisor in supervision (interoceptive exposure') might confuse or alienate those who we seek to support. Similarly, if we are too focused on demonstrating our competence to clients or providing lengthy explanations of lofty concepts, this can invalidate, bore, or annoy our clients! Finally, the context in which CBT is delivered should not be underestimated. Sitting in a waiting room, in an NHS building brings with it a set of cognitions and emotions that are unlikely to be replicated through simulation alone.

Further reading

Li, E., Kealy, D., Aafjes-van Doorn, K., McCollum, J., Curtis, J. T., Luo, X., & Silberschatz, G. (2024). "It felt like i was being tailored to the treatment rather than the treatment being tailored to me": Patient experiences of helpful and unhelpful psychotherapy. *Psychotherapy Research*, 1–15. https://doi.org/10.1080/10503307.2024.2360448

www.ocduk.org/overcoming-ocd/accessing-ocd-treatment/accessing-ocd-treatment-privately/finding-a-private-therapist/?s=09

This article published on the OCD-UK website contains helpful information for anyone seeing private CBT treatment in the UK with specific tips on what standards to look out for.

Roscoe, J. (2019). Has IAPT become a bit like Frankenstein's monster?. *CBT Today*, *47*(1), 16–17.

References

Bennett-Levy, J. (2019). Why therapists should walk the talk: The theoretical and empirical case for personal practice in therapist training and professional development. *Journal of Behavior Therapy and Experimental Psychiatry*, *62*, 133–145. https://doi.org/10.1016/j.jbtep.2018.08.004

Blackburn, I. M., James, I. A., Milne, D. L., Reichelt, F. K., Garland, A., Baker, C., & Claydon, A. (2001). *Cognitive therapy scale-revised (CTS-R)*. Newcastle Cognitive and Behavioural Therapies Centre.

British Association for Behavioural and Cognitive Psychotherapies. (2021). *Core curriculum reference document*. https://babcp.com/Core-Curriculum

Flückiger, C., Del Re, A. C., Wampold, B. E., & Horvath, A. O. (2018). The alliance in adult psychotherapy: A meta-analytic synthesis. *Psychotherapy*, *55*(4), 316.

Kroenke, K., Spitzer, R. L., & Williams, J. B. (2001). The PHQ-9: Validity of a brief depression severity measure. *Journal of General Internal Medicine*, *16*(9), 606–613.

Li, E., Kealy, D., Aafjes-van Doorn, K., McCollum, J., Curtis, J. T., Luo, X., & Silberschatz, G. (2024). "It felt like i was being tailored to the treatment rather than the treatment being tailored to me": Patient experiences of helpful and unhelpful psychotherapy. *Psychotherapy Research*, 1–15. https://doi.org/10.1080/10503307.2024.2360448

National Collaborating Centre for Mental Health. (2019). *The improving access to psychological therapies manual*. NHS.

Purdon, C., & Clark, D. A. (1993). Obsessive intrusive thoughts in nonclinical subjects. Part I. Content and relation with depressive, anxious and obsessional symptoms. *Behaviour Research and Therapy*, *31*(8), 713–720.

Waltman, S., Hall, B. C., McFarr, L. M., Beck, A. T., & Creed, T. A. (2017). In-session stuck points and pitfalls of community clinicians learning CBT: Qualitative investigation. *Cognitive and Behavioral Practice*, *24*, 256–267.

Chapter 14

First-hand accounts of making it through training

Laura Hamill, Sam Palin, Jessica Palmer, and Commentary by Jason Roscoe

Introduction

For most trainees starting a CBT course, the experience brings about feelings of both excitement and anxiety. Previous chapters have offered perspectives from CBT trainers and supervisors, yet one thing I was always keen to do as a course tutor was to invite back 'survivors' from previous cohorts to meet new starters. Fielding a series of questions from eager yet nervous trainees encouraged them to reflect on what went well in addition to what they might have done differently. It is for this reason that I invited some of the ex-trainees from the University of Cumbria to share their experiences in this chapter.

Jess's story

Previous roles and experience

I completed my undergraduate degree in Counselling and Psychotherapy. It was only in my third year of my undergraduate degree that I realised I much preferred cognitive behavioural therapy having gained a distinction in the CBT module and basing my dissertation on the efficiency of telephone and computerised CBT. Having qualified as a psychological wellbeing practitioner (PWP) and progressing to the role of Senior PWP two years later, I considered myself to be a confident and competent practitioner, with no intention of ever doing CBT training, what else could I possibly learn? That was until a friend and fellow PWP started her training and explained there's more to managing worry than the use of 'worry time'. It piqued my interest and I started to become frustrated by the limitations that came with working as a PWP. I have never been academically gifted so the thought of another year at university terrified me but I was ready for a challenge. In January 2020, I commenced the CBT training course and what a challenge it was!

Adapting from low-intensity to high-intensity work

One of the main struggles I faced when starting the training is that I moved from a role that I felt confident in (e.g. I hit my targets and recovery and if I didn't then

DOI: 10.4324/9781003428527-17

I had the luxury of stepping up) to being in a stage of my career where my confidence soon vanished and was replaced with incessant self-doubt. I found that the CBT training made me aware of a lot of my own core beliefs and experiences that I'd spent a lot of time avoiding and supressing.

Facing my fears – showing videos

When I started the training, my biggest fear was the idea of sharing videos with my peers. On reflection, this was the least of my worries and my advice for anyone considering the training or just starting out is share them, as much and as soon as possible. In my experience no amount of reading or shadowing prepared me for the training but the thing that made the real difference for me was sharing videos. Initially, I found reasons not to, for example, being hit with a global pandemic was a great excuse. I delayed sharing videos for as long as possible and if I could change anything it'd be that. The feedback and guidance from supervision and from my peers made a huge difference to my practice and in me passing the course. Watching videos in supervision allowed me to recognise the transition from my practice as a PWP into that of a CBT therapist, the movement between directed self-help into guided discovery.

The term 'Imposter syndrome' or 'Impostor Phenomenon' was inspired by reports that despite objective evidence of success, some people felt simply 'phony' and that they had managed to fool the people around them into believing they are successful or capable and that they will soon be found out (Topping & Kimmel, 1985). This became a real issue for me, and the first few months felt like I was coasting through and just doing what I needed to pass rather than becoming the therapist I wanted to be. I believed that at some point along the line someone would realise I am not capable.

Being patient with myself

One of the things that stuck with me was being told by our lecturers that for most people, it takes around three years before you start to feel like a fully-fledged CBT therapist. I am now almost two years qualified, and I still believe that to be the case. I do feel more confident as a CBT therapist and (mostly) enjoy the job now.

Overall reflections

In summary, the CBT training is one of the hardest challenges I've faced to date. In my experience, no time would have been a good time for it, although the addition of a global pandemic definitely didn't make it any easier! That said, I wouldn't change a thing as it also remains one of my greatest achievements.

Laura's story

Career path into CBT: joining an improving access to psychological therapies course

Something I noticed that I was good at was working in the care setting. I strive to help others and for them to advocate for themselves. Working as a health care support worker and Occupational therapy assistant enabled me to encourage service users to improve their mental health through therapeutic input. I had a passion to build on my career and therefore studied to have the relevant qualifications to take me through my mental health nursing degree. It came as no surprise that I was interested in therapies during my training and felt the pharmaceutical route alone would not improve overall wellbeing.

High intensity by name and high intensity by nature!

Firstly, I would like to say the journey of being a trainee cognitive behavioural therapist (CBT) is somewhat challenging but also very rewarding. A lie was not told when told by course tutors and previous students on the Improving Access to Psychological Therapies (IAPT) course that it would be an intense year. This made me wonder if I had done the right thing in choosing this path in my career. Nonetheless I pushed through until completing the course with a gap due to having a baby and returning to finish my studies after maternity leave.

The importance of using CBT on yourself

Top tip: know your preferred learning style

One thing that has not changed and has remained the same during the course is that I am a visual learner. Personally, I have never been the 'academic type' that would score highly on assignments and would often compare myself to others. Therefore, the best way to show my skills was through practical ways; showing the dreaded tapes in supervision sessions. I procrastinated to do so at the beginning like many others but learnt that the best way to develop skills was to expose ourselves. Similar to gradual exposure, the fear of showing tapes in supervision became somewhat 'the known' and the dread eased off over time.

It is true to understand CBT as a client; we are to become the client by self-practice SP (Bennett-Levy et al., 2014). Alongside showing tapes, practising some treatments with other students did feel uncomfortable but also really informative. I would advise that the more this is done during the course (and also in clinical practice with supervisors) the more we understand the treatment protocols, increasing our confidence at using these with clients in the process.

Dealing with self-critical automatic thoughts as a therapist

It is important to normalise that we are all in the same boat during our training. Self-critical thoughts pop into our heads; I personally can vouch for that. I remember noticing some clients not improving and often taking these clients to supervision regularly. My own self-critical automatic thoughts included: 'what am I doing wrong', 'why are they not improving', and 'is it me' making me think I was the cause to clients not improving. I then discussed my worries in supervision, and this was evaluated with my clinical supervisor, and a comment from them really stuck in my head. I was asked how I felt after a session with a particular client that I had become stuck with, and I remember describing feeling 'drained'. The next words really hit me, these being 'If you feel that way after a session then you are putting more work in'. I was advised that it appeared the client wasn't engaging in the work during our sessions and to consider having a discussion with the client with some motivational interviewing and reviewing how sessions are going. Stressing the importance of working in collaboration, both the client and therapist work together and not solely the therapist doing the work. Remembering that we are teaching the client the skills to become their own therapist and not doing the work for them. Setting them boundaries earlier on in a tactical, compassionate way that empowers the client. I found becoming aware of my own self-critical thoughts increased my own self-awareness, and using SP would often help my own thinking and improve my clinical practice.

Things that 'stood out' during my training

The usefulness of metaphors

Using metaphors in CBT is common amongst therapists in order to explain a person's situation in a different way in order for the clients to gain understanding. Moreover, they enable new concepts by making connections from metaphors and as such are powerful in therapy with clients (Killick et al., 2016). I found this in my sessions with clients, and particularly the vampire and garlic metaphor helped my clients to understand their problems by making a connection to the story.

Lightbulb moments

During our training, we were told about 'light bulb moments'. There are a few occasions with different clients where something had just clicked. Consequently, these moments often preceded some noticeable progress with treatment.

Lightbulb moment (example)

An example of this in practice was when using the task-interfering cognitions and task-orientated cognitions (TIC/TOC) method in session with a client presenting with recurrent depression (Burns, 1989). When completing this task, the client recognised his unhelpful thinking styles that we had identified in a previous treatment session. The client stated he had a 'lightbulb moment' during the task and was able to make some links from his past and personality traits that led to his difficulties and, as a result, was able to suggest ways to overcome the TIC and replace it with a TOCS. This session led to further work on perfectionism towards the end of therapy based on the light bulb moment the client had.

Don't rush trauma work

Working with trauma is very daunting initially and can ultimately make us feel uneasy taking someone to that uncomfortable place. My advice to others particularly on the course would be not to rush through treatment. Spending those initial sessions on psychoeducation and grounding techniques really helped clients I worked with during my training. I found the use of timelines helpful in cases of complex trauma and giving clients the choice as ultimately it is their choice if and which trauma they choose to work with.

Importance of goals in therapy and referring back to them if stuck

I remember on many occasions where I felt stuck with a client and would often feel like the treatment sessions had somehow become disjointed along the way. One thing that stuck out from supervision was to go back to the client's treatment goals review them and this helps get things back on track again.

Sam's story

Tolerance of uncertainty

As you begin your journey on the course, uncertainty is prevalent, and this remains the norm throughout. You will learn extensively about this concept throughout your training and understand how anxiety is often preceded by uncertainty (Gu et al., 2020). To be able to function effectively on the course, whether that is studying, delivering clinical practice, or having a balanced life outside of the course, it is crucial for you to become aware of this concept and start to work towards becoming more comfortable with the notion of it. Starting to work towards being accepting of the anxiety that comes with uncertain situations will allow you to progressively become accustomed to it. This is typically a very challenging thing to do, largely due to the human mind not being satisfied with the unknown. However, with some targeted study and experiential learning, you can start to work towards becoming tolerant of uncertainty which will not only positively affect your experience of the course but also help you along your path post-training too.

Top tip: setting your own behavioural experiments

A practical step to move towards developing your tolerance to uncertainty may come in the form of a behavioural experiment. I would suggest you focus on situation that you find anxiety provoking. So, an example could be you find parking stressful; therefore, you tend to over plan a trip to investigate where the best parking is and spend time planning where you will park to make things feel safer. The next time this situation arises, tune in to your anxious feelings as you prepare to drive into the place of question but do not engage with the over-planning and go for it! Be mindful of your feelings as you go through the process, without trying to install safety, more often than not from my clinical experience, you will complete the behaviour. What you begin to do is develop or strengthen the belief that you can tolerate uncertainty; thus next time, the anxiety is not as intense.

Competency

Reflecting on my start to the training, I felt worried and anxious about not knowing how to deliver therapy. I was putting pressure on myself to be a competent therapist even when considering I had only had three lectures. It is in the early stages of therapy where you can really feel out of your depth but it is at this stage where you are starting to grow and mould your therapist self, please don't forget this. Despite not knowing all of the theoretical models and treatment plans, you have the most unique characteristic in a therapeutic intervention, your interpersonal skills, do not underestimate the power of this. Research has provided evidence that the patient-therapist relationship is an invaluable component to positive patient outcomes (Llewelyn & Hume, 1979; Murphy et al., 1984; Ryan & Gizynski, 1971; Sloane et al., 1977). These studies consistently reported that patients had found the relationship with their therapist more helpful than the cognitive behavioural techniques that were employed. Now I am not for one second undermining the power of cognitive behavioural therapy (it has enabled me to change the lives of so many in such profound ways and I am only 15 months post-training) but your own idiosyncratic interpersonal abilities hold similar powers.

Taking stock of your strengths and weaknesses

It is extremely important to reflect on your strengths as you progress through the course. Typically, as humans we tend to naturally focus on the negative experiences and outcomes. Becoming aware off your strengths not only helps you to build confidence in the way you can attribute these skills to your therapeutic approach, but also valuably provides clarity on the parts of your interpersonal and academic skills which you can work towards developing on your journey to becoming a CBT therapist.

Reflective exercise

Start of training

Q. What skills do I already possess that will help me at the start of my training?

Mid-course reflection

Q. Which areas am I strongest in and which require more development through reading, role-play, supervision, or clinical contact?

As you proceed on the training course, you will be made aware of the CTS-R (Blackburn et al., 2001) which is the general rubric scoring system for HI CBT trainees. As you become familiar with the components, begin to identify which ones are naturally your stronger areas, for example, interpersonal effectiveness, and then become mindful of the areas potentially you require more time to develop. This can be assisted through clinical supervision but will allow you a firm foundation to continually develop your confidence whilst fine-tuning your areas for improvement.

Supervision and reflection

Watching your clinical recordings in clinical supervision is a crucial part of your development as a therapist during the training. This component of training can be extremely anxiety provoking and at times it is normal for you want to avoid it at all costs. Despite having to tolerate the uncertainty and scrutiny from your peers and supervisor, this part of training is arguably the part of training that hones your interpersonal and clinical skills into the therapist that you are working so hard to become. This occurs through your supervisor providing invaluable observations and critiques that will at first develop your awareness to your behaviour's but then importantly suggest crucial adjustments and additional skills and adaptations to your clinical work. This process is ever evolving but ensuring that you trust the process and are reflecting on your learning as you go will help you to progress through the course. So, please bear in mind when you are starting to experience avoidant thoughts, to challenge them with the understanding that your live recording's will make you a better therapist than you were yesterday. When you begin this process of supervision and reflection, be mindful of your emotional responses to watching the videos and receiving constructive criticism from your supervisor and peers. I found my mind often falling into thinking traps such as 'compare and despair' which is very easy to experience when you are watching your peers videos who will have their own unique way of delivering therapy/techniques. \\

Top tip: mastering your emotions

A helpful reflective tip that I carry with me to this day is to always compare yourself to who you were yesterday, not to who somebody else is today. I also to this day when I show clinical recordings will ensure that during the recording, I am fully focused without any distraction, for example, fidgeting or thinking other thoughts. If you can tune into to your emotional state and your clinical recording, you will start to teach the brain that you are safe, and you do not need to try and escape the uncomfortable feelings you experience. This will allow your brain to see your clinical recordings as an opportunity rather than a threat.

Conclusion

This chapter has provided the accounts of three former 'HIT' trainees, each having shared key aspects of their journeys into CBT, the challenges they faced, and have offered tips on how to overcome common difficulties during training. This final section summarises the key messages that run across all three accounts.

You will learn a lot about yourself

Previous chapters have discussed some of the key challenges that we all face when embarking on a new career. Whether that is moving to a new town, county, or country or letting go of the comfort of being knowledgeable and competent in what you have done before, these experiences will either reactivate old ways of thinking about yourself or generate new worries or doubts. Whilst personal therapy is not a requirement for CBT training, it is highly recommended that trainees engage in self-practice of CBT methods to deepen their understanding of the benefits and difficulties in implementing formulations and interventions.

Try to view supervision as an opportunity rather than a threat

There is arguably no better place to utilise self-practice/self-reflection (SP/SR) than in clinical supervision! Core beliefs that we hold about our worth are likely to be activated for many people when their competence is being examined, and this is often amplified by having to show videos of treatment sessions to a group of peers.

Be patient with yourself

It is human nature to compare yourself to others, and CBT training is often a prime example of where we might view other students as excelling, whilst in our eyes, we are toiling. Our own demanding standards can lead to unnecessary added pressure, and our self-criticism can often leave us feeling inferior. We therefore need to have patience that some skills will develop sooner than others, and this will vary from person to person.

Further reading

Corrie, S., Cockx, A., & Townend, M. (2015). Assessment and case formulation in cognitive behavioural therapy. *Assessment and Case Formulation in Cognitive Behavioural Therapy*.

Nissen-Lie, H. A., Rønnestad, M. H., Høglend, P. A., Havik, O. E., Solbakken, O. A., Stiles, T. C., & Monsen, J. T. (2017). Love yourself as a person, doubt yourself as a therapist?. *Clinical Psychology & Psychotherapy*, *24*(1), 48–60. https://doi.org/10.1002/cpp.1977

Stott, R., Mansell, W., Salkovskis, P., Lavender, A., & Cartwright-Hatton, S. (2010). *Oxford guide to metaphors in CBT: Building cognitive bridges*. Oxford University Press.

References

Bennett-Levy, J., Thwaites, R., Haarhoff, B., & Perry, H. (2014). *Experiencing CBT from the inside out: A self-practice/self-reflection workbook for therapists*. Guilford Publications.

Blackburn, I. M., James, I. A., Milne, D. L., Baker, C., Standart, S., Garland, A., & Reichelt, F. K. (2001). The revised cognitive therapy scale (CTS-R): Psychometric properties. *Behavioural and Cognitive Psychotherapy*, *29*(4), 431–446.

Burns, D. D. (1989). *The feeling good handbook: Using the new mood therapy in everyday life*. William Morrow & Co.

Gu, Y., Gu, S., Lei, Y., & Li, H. (2020). From uncertainty to anxiety: How uncertainty fuels anxiety in a process mediated by intolerance of uncertainty. *Neural Plasticity*, *2020*(1), 8866386.

Killick, S., Curry, V., & Myles, P. (2016). The mighty metaphor: A collection of therapists' favourite metaphors and analogies. *The Cognitive Behaviour Therapist*, *9*, e37.

Llewelyn, S. P., & Hume, W. I. (1979). The patient's view of therapy. *British Journal of Medical Psychology*, *52*, 29–35.

Murphy, P. M., Cramer, D., & Lillie, F. J. (1984). The relationship between curative factors perceived by patients in their psychotherapy and treatment outcome: An exploratory study. *British Journal of Medical Psychology*, *57*, 187–192.

Ryan, V. L., & Gizynski, M. N. (1971). Behavior therapy in retrospect: Patients' feelings about their behavior therapies. *Journal of Consulting and Clinical Psychology*, *37*, 1–9.

Sloane, R. B., Staples, F. R., Whipple, K., & Cristol, A. H. (1977). Patients' attitude toward behaviour therapy and psychotherapy. *American Journal of Psychiatry*, *134*, 134–137.

Topping, M. E., & Kimmel, E. B. (1985). The imposter phenomenon: Feeling phony. *Academic Psychology Bulletin*.

Chapter 15

A week in the life of a qualified CBT therapist

Jessica Baines and Jo Anne Bates

Introduction

This chapter covers a typical week in the life of two recently qualified cognitive behavioural therapists, both working within NHS Talking Therapies Services. We completed our training together, transitioning to working fully remotely three months into the course when the pandemic began. We now both work in NHS Talking Therapies for Anxiety and Depression services (formally Improving Access to Psychological Therapies [IAPT]) and continue to work fully remotely; Jess also has a successful private practice and delivers CBT and ACT to clients face to face.

A typical week for both of us involves

- delivering client sessions;
- screening referrals;
- attending team meetings and clinical administrative tasks (and we attend and/or deliver clinical/safeguarding/peer supervision fortnightly or monthly).

Jo delivers clinical skills supervision to psychological wellbeing practitioners (PWPs) and is currently undertaking training to deliver supervision to HIT CBT therapists whilst Jess provides case management supervision to both PWPs and HIT CBT therapists.

Below is a typical week in our lives as CBT therapists, particularly in respect to working remotely, growing in confidence as our roles develop and what working for a service or within private practice involves day to day.

Monday (Jess – private practice day)

I decided to branch out into private practice six months ago, and for the first three months, I allocated 1 day a week, but I became busier and decided to request a further reduction in hours from my NHS role. Gradually reducing time spent working for NHS Talking Therapies and increasing private practice has allowed time to build referrals and subsequently a caseload, as well as minimise financial risks (Kirk, 2010).

DOI: 10.4324/9781003428527-18

Mondays are a mix of supervision and treatment sessions in clinic, and I really enjoy the variety. I have been asked to provide supervision for trainee PWPs (tPWPs) at a local charity that I previously worked for as a senior PWP. I am also close to completing high-intensity (HI) supervisor training.

In my first supervision session, my supervisee asks for advice with regards to treatment of health anxiety; consequently, we discuss the stepped care model as health anxiety is not a Step 2 appropriate disorder (Department of Health, 2008). I listen to a treatment recording with the next supervisee and provide constructive feedback utilising specific standardised assessment measures (National Curriculum for Psychological Wellbeing Practitioners, 2023). I still have to provide clips as part of my own clinical supervision within my NHS role, though following the rules of exposure (in terms of repeated and prolonged) it doesn't seem to get any easier! A recent study revealed that both supervisors and supervisees were both apprehensive regarding live clips of treatment sessions which may result in colluded to avoid this task (Roscoe et al., 2022b). Nonetheless, observing and receiving feedback from live sessions have many benefits such as ensuring accuracy of case conceptualisation and objective reflection (as opposed to therapist's subjective report) and the opportunity to self-identify learning points and areas for development (Gonsalvez et al., 2016).

Next, I make my way over to the office I rent – luckily, just a short drive away. Currently both my caseloads are health anxiety heavy; anecdotal information from peers, as well as my own experience is that there has been a general increase in health anxiety presentations since the pandemic. The session focus is a review of behavioural experiments conducted thus far and revisiting Theory A/Theory B to assess which theory the outcome of said experiments best fit. I then suggest developing an exposure script specific to the client's main concern – dying of a terminal illness, leaving children behind. Understandably, my suggestion is met with some apprehension, and the client requests time to consider if they are ready to engage in this intervention or to continue work on a hierarchy of avoidance (e.g. conversations about health, hospital visiting, and health-related TV programmes).

Key Point: One of the benefits of working in private practice is flexibility in terms of the number of sessions or treatment 'doses', as opposed to the short-term support in which an NHS Talking Therapies Service operates that can, at times, mean there is a feeling of pressure to move the therapy along.

Tuesday (Jess – NHS Talking Therapies role)

My NHS talking therapy job is a remote role, which is handy as my team are based 190 miles away! All sessions are conducted by video-call, with the occasional telephone sessions for clients who may have barriers in accessing technology.

My first appointment starts at 8.30 am with an OCD client; we are on session 3 and, having previously assessed and formulated using a vicious flower, today's focus is developing Theory A/Theory B. I explain to the client that that our next aim is to generate evidence for Theory B, and this leads into psychoeducation with regards to Exposure and Response Prevention (ERP).

My next session is ten minutes later with a new client, and I note that the PHQ and GAD scores are now below 'caseness' since being on the waiting list. After collection of initial assessment information, it is agreed that completion of the SPIN (Social Phobia Inventory) may be useful. Their subsequent score of this measure confirm that a focus of social anxiety treatment aligns with the clients therapy goals.

After a quick stretch, comfort break, and a glass of water, I am onto the next session which is an long-term condition (LTC) client with a depression presentation. The session is focused around adapted behavioural activation to account for client's pain and fatigue levels.

I completed my HI LTC training around a year following HI training. Having previously completing LTC training at PWP level, I found it very interesting, particularly the lecture we received with regards to ACT (acceptance and commitment therapy). The National Institute for Health Care Excellence (NICE) recommends ACT as a treatment for chronic pain conditions (NICE, 2021), and I have recently gone on to complete an introductory ACT training course. Although I won't be able to integrate ACT into my Talking Therapies role (except for LTC clients), I am hoping to utilise it in my private work.

Before lunch, I catch up on administrative tasks such as adding case notes to our electronic database, booking subsequent sessions, and emailing home tasks and psychoeducation to clients.

After lunch, I provide clinical supervision for a newly qualified therapist. I am required to record all of our supervision sessions currently, in order to provide a clip for the HI Supervisor training course. I am relieved that this is not going to be formally rated but still find it slightly nerve-wracking as it will be peer reviewed.

I prepare for this by reviewing the notes from our previous session and glance over the cases my supervisee has selected for discussion. We create a collaborative agenda, including a wellbeing check in and goal review before moving onto case management. I encourage my supervisee to bring a clip of agenda setting to the next session, as this has been highlighted as an area for development.

My final client of the day cancels at the last minute due to illness, so I utilise the time to clear some emails from my inbox and prepare for my own clinical supervision tomorrow.

The sun is shining, which is an unusual occurrence, so I take the opportunity to finish on time (also a rare occurrence!) and go for a walk after being sedentary for most of the day. Unsurprisingly, a 2020 study found working from home decreased physical activity and increased screen time, with recommendations to employers in encouraging periods of physical activity throughout the working day (McDowell et al., 2020). In my opinion, an important but possibly impractical-to-implement recommendation in most work environments, but particularly an NHS service, due to high caseloads and long waiting times.

Wednesday (Jess – NHS Talking Therapies role)

The day starts with part 2 of in-house diagnostic assessment training – this is mainly aimed at Step 2 practitioners but occasionally HI therapists are required to complete intake assessments to support the wider team. Directly after, I have a client with an OCD presentation. We have previously identified magical thinking within the case conceptualisation, and I raise a Thought Action Fusion (TAF) experiment in which the client writes about a feared catastrophe using myself as the victim, and then exposes themselves daily to the script.

After another treatment session focused on PTSD, I move into clinical supervision during which my supervisor utilises illuminating Socratic questioning, and I become aware that 'compare and despair' thinking style has been activated due to thoughts of being inferior with regards to my newly acquired supervision skills. My supervisor has an extensive history in clinical psychology and has been supervising HI therapist for over five years (I remind myself of this in challenging the thought). One study (Davis et al., 2015) measured personal and professional benefits of self-practice/self-reflection (SP/SR) in which participants were encouraged to identify and challenge a personal and therapist belief to work on, such as 'I am an incompetent therapist'. Over the course of the study, by utilising a variety of CBT methods, there were significant modifications to the original beliefs.

Next, I meet with my line manager, and we review my professional goals such as continuous SP/SR and further time dedicated to reading my vast library of CBT literature, collected since training. After reviewing my current recovery figures and feedback from recently discharged clients, I am asked to consider applying for a team leader vacancy – fortuitously providing further evidence against my previous inferiority-based cognition!

Thursday (Jo)

Today I had telephone treatment sessions all day. Telephone sessions can be slower paced because we describe concepts/models/diagrams more than when working with visuals. We can direct clients to or send resources in advance, but this is not always possible. Learning ways to mitigate a lack of visuals is important, and use of analogies/metaphors to help clients integrate/develop new mental models is known to be effective (Pennebaker, 2000), so I aim to do this where I can.

My first appointment was session 3 with a client who has agoraphobia (interestingly, I have had an increase in agoraphobia cases since the pandemic. As Wegner (2021) writes, crowded spaces were potentially dangerous then, so avoiding them would have been a natural response; I wonder again: 'is the avoidance a heavily invested in new safety-seeking behaviour, or a relapse of historic agoraphobia'?). Session 3 is typically given to developing and sharing the formulation, and I chose the five aspects model (Padesky & Mooney, 1990) to help my client understand the maintenance factors of his difficulties. As my client did not have a visual, I used the analogy of a clock face to help him draw out the model's structure prior to working through it – using numbers to place the model's elements and clock hands for linking these. This analogy has proven useful many times, yet metaphors and analogies can be much more than a strategy for managing a lack of visuals. Stott et al. (2010) describe use of metaphors in CBT as improving cognitive flexibility and being a tool for generating alternative perspectives and understanding of a problem. So researching metaphors/analogies pertinent to CBT, for example, Killick et al. (2016) is useful.

My next client has illness anxiety disorder (IAD). We are also on session 3 – so we were formulating. When using more complex models I send these in advance of a telephone session. I often modify the information within these, for example, I had sent a blank IAD model (Walker & Furer, 2008) in advance of this session but with box descriptors replaced by numbers. Not having the descriptors of model elements included, I find guided discovery is more effective as we work through the model using a lived example, labelling boxes as we go. Today my client was able to gain a good understanding of factors maintaining his anxiety and he felt able to populate the model with other experiences to consolidate his learning as homework.

I'm doing trauma-focused CBT (stabilisation phase) with my next client. My client had not submitted clinical questionnaires nor completed homework, so I needed to explore this with her to determine whether there were practical obstacles to completion or if there was resistance to treatment. We discussed what had prevented her from completing the work, the function of these psychological obstacles, and the unintended consequences of this on the effectiveness of therapy. For me, confidence as a therapist includes having conviction in your clinical judgement and in your role in the therapy dynamic. As CBT therapists, we are not here to just listen; we have an active role in the therapy dynamic of delivering CBT, and sometimes that means challenging resistance and obstacles (Leahy, 2006). Challenging therapy interfering behaviours or cognitions needs to be done sensitively but confidently, and it took me time to gain confidence in this area. CBT therapists gain professional confidence as procedural and declarative knowledge is gained (Maruniakova & Rihacek, 2018). Likewise, as I have gained experience, reflected on previous client resistance and the impact on therapy outcome, I feel more confident having these conversations with clients. I can now more easily use instances of resistance to model CBT techniques (e.g. functional analysis), identify factors pertinent to the formulation (e.g. perfectionism or activation of rules and assumptions), and enable productive conversations; hopefully moving towards meta-competency (Roth & Pilling, 2008). It can be tough to evaluate and challenge our practice, but as our 'therapist self-concept' (our view of ourselves as a therapist, built on our appraisals of ourselves both professionally and personally) influences client change (Nissen-Lie et al., 2017), it is important to update our therapist self-concept through regular reflection and acknowledgement of progress.

I finished the day completing clinical admin (booking appointments, sending out resources and preparing sessions). I finished on time and felt I'd had a successful day – my diary management had been good as I had been busy but not rushed, and I'd had variation in presenting disorders. A full day of the same presentation can be demanding, particularly with PTSD, GAD or depression. Therapist burnout is increasingly recognised (e.g. Baum, 2016; Westwood et al., 2017) so mitigating this where possible is important, for example, distributing presentations that are particularly emotionally or cognitively consuming. However, as we are already trying to marry client availability, our availability, and caseload targets, consistently prioritising variation in presentations for our own wellbeing can be hard. For example, with so many PTSD cases on my caseload at present, it is challenging to put this into practice, but factoring in the stage of treatment can be helpful; for example, stabilisation sessions have a different intensity to reliving sessions, both in content and duration.

Friday (Jo)

I'm working on PTSD with my first client today, focusing on development of a timeline of his experiences. We met via video so I could share my screen whilst documenting our conversation on the timeline. The client found having a visual representation of his experiences was validating to his belief 'I have been through a lot', and there was some shift in his belief 'I've only ever had bad luck' due to seeing the positive experiences, context, and positive post-event appraisals (i.e. 'I showed resilience') we had included. Therefore, this had been an important piece of visual work as a foundation for further processing work.

The more I work remotely, I increasingly use visuals in ways I did not in face-to-face sessions. Morgan et al. found in their 2022 study that therapists working remotely reported their remote working changing over time, moving from an initial crisis response to a new status quo, and this mirrors my own experience and perception that remote methods of delivery are valid and not just a substitute for face-to-face work. Methods I now use include using online street views for virtual 'walks' to do stimulus discrimination work and using online maps to plan routes for behavioural experiments for agoraphobia, and with social phobia, I have moved from telephone to video sessions as exposure and/or an experiment to test alternative cognitions about being on screen/visible.

> **Top tip:** Since the pandemic, there has been an increase in resources regarding remote working (e.g. babcp.com/, oxcadatresources.com/, the cognitive behavioural therapist) and in research of it (e.g. Cromarty et al., 2020). I highly recommend reviewing these to inform your practice – oh and practice using text boxes and arrows in electronic documents!

Since being introduced to the Therapist Belief Scale (McLean et al., 2003), I am mindful of my 'unhelpful' therapy beliefs. I recently read an article on being a credible therapist (Presley, 2023), and the notion of challenging my own standards to model certain behaviours/ideas to clients interested me. I put this into practice today by sending the timeline as it was rather than 'writing it out neatly'; this was particularly pertinent as my client holds himself to high standards, and I wanted to model 'good enough'. Modelling behaviours or thinking styles to our clients can be valuable, and I find there is absolutely space for this in video work, even if it's just modelling that nothing bad happens if we spell something wrong when someone's watching us type!

For my next client, I am still assessing the problem. I was also being shadowed by a trainee CBT therapist (as a recent trainee I remember the benefits of shadowing CBT sessions and so had arranged this despite nerves about being observed!). Afterwards, I reflected that I'd balanced client narrative and therapist questioning, achieving what felt like a productive conversation rather than a Q&A session. This transition from the didactic approach of my previous clinical role to Socratic competency is a skill I consistently work on as it has been a difficult transition – as Roscoe et al. (2022a) found in their study of CBT trainees, we can acquire declarative knowledge of guided discovery by the end of training yet can have difficulty with developing our procedural skills in this area. Acknowledging moments of growing confidence or skill through reflection is important and aids in development of professional confidence (Bennett-Levy & Beedie, 2007; Maruniakova & Rihacek, 2018), so taking time to reflect on this session was beneficial to my therapist self-confidence.

I had my monthly 1:1 clinical supervision today. On qualifying, minimum supervision requirements are reduced (BABCP, 2021), and I certainly felt this reduction, even with my supervisor and team being available for advice ad hoc. I wanted to discuss two formulations today; formulating is what I spend the most time doing outside of appointments – I certainly understand why formulating has been identified as one of the most difficult skills to learn in CBT (Whittington & Grey, 2014) and, as Maruniakova & Rihacek (2018) found, is an area in which 'beginning' CBT therapists demonstrate a strong need for encouragement! The first case I discussed was a client with complex PTSD; I felt I was missing something and after exploring the formulation we identified a gap in the information I had gathered. I felt foolish for having missed this but was assured that complex trauma is exactly that – complex. This is another example of where our therapist beliefs (McLean et al., 2003) can influence us; holding a belief that we should know everything and be proficient in all therapist skills as newly qualified therapists is not realistic – it's OK to need help and encouragement and nothing bad happens if we feel foolish in supervision! After supervision I logged the session on our clinical database and my British Association for Behavioural and Cognitive Psychotherapies (BABCP) supervision log (for accreditation purposes). I noticed my supervision logs show a bias of 'case discussion' as the method of supervision and made a mental note to start submitting more recordings of sessions and to do more role-playing – as Jess has highlighted above, this is a key activity for development as a therapist.

With my final client, today we are working on 'reclaiming life' following successful trauma processing. A barrier to my client prioritising herself was her difficulty saying 'no' to things. The client was having problems identifying the cognitions and emotions linked to saying 'no', so we role-played it, capturing these cognitions and emotions in real time. The more role-plays we did (including swapping roles within them), we successfully captured and challenged barriers to saying 'no', applying learning from previous work to test the accuracy of those cognitions. We also had a giggle, initiated by my client, as the hypothetical situations got more 'abstract'. Studies have found that humour is most therapeutic when it is collaborative, and there is a joint appreciation in the moment (Briggs & Owen, 2022), and this is what happened here. Humour may be a surprising element of psychotherapy, but it can be a useful tool when used appropriately and is included in the cognitive therapy scale-revised (CTS-R; Blackburn et al., 2001) as a skill to develop the therapeutic alliance.

I finished the day completing client admin work and reviewing my diary for Monday to ensure I was prepared. I'm tired, it has been a busy week, but today has been another good day where my love for CBT was confirmed again. Overall this week, I have felt both good about my developing skills and a little foolish and inexperienced, so it presented a realistic and balanced account of my overall experience (which I am assured is 'normal') since qualifying in this role!

Top tips

Keep learning: Read all those books you bought during your training year and have only read sections of for essay or treatment purposes. Organise your lecture notes, you are likely to refer to them in cases of less frequent presentations (e.g. body dysmorphic disorder) or to refresh your memory of a specific intervention.

Pace yourself: Consider other training opportunities carefully; you may want to give yourself some time to consolidate your recent learning and focus on building your case load (or you may jump straight into it as Jess did!).

Know Yourself as a therapist: Keep reviewing your therapist beliefs/ self-concept and clinical skills either with CTSR (Blackburn et al., 2001), shadowing or a self-review of CBT Competencies (Roth & Pilling, 2008).

Working via telephone? Research and create analogies/metaphors for describing diagrams/models over the phone, for example, an analogue clock face for drawing out the five aspects model (Padesky & Mooney, 1990) or Clark Panic Model (Clark, 1986).

Working via video? Be sure to read through the guidance for remote working that has been compiled in recent years such as babcp.com/ and oxcadatresources.com/

Conclusion

We were not expected to know *everything* on completion of our training, and it's important to acknowledge this phase of being a therapist. Just in this one week, our experiences have highlighted the importance of continuing to review our practice (recording sessions and self-reflection), to identify areas of success or for development and to feed into SP/SR (Davis et al., 2015) activities. Additionally, we both utilised clinical supervision: being honest, open to feedback and sharing thoughts that made us feel vulnerable.

This week has highlighted the benefits of our experience and research into remote working as a mode of therapy and we were therefore able to deliver effective therapy. However, we've both experienced some isolation this week too. Remote working and private practice can be lonely. We work to negate this by seeking opportunities to meet/collaborate with others, for example, peer supervision, project work or attending workshops and events. Variation within the clinical role can also be achieved with mentoring, providing supervision/clinical skills development, taking a champion role, or starting private work. This can prevent feelings of isolation, increase job satisfaction and prevent therapist burnout. That said, this week does highlight that these activities do not happen every day – after all, the main purpose of our role is to deliver therapy on a one-to-one basis!

Finally, we feel it's important to enjoy the process of transitioning from a trainee to an experienced CBT therapist, so as we try to, notice those wins and acknowledge the development of skills and acquisition of knowledge!

Further reading

Hughes, G., Moore, L., Maniatopoulos, G., Wherton, J., Wood, G. W., Greenhalgh, T., & Shaw,
S. (2022). Theorising the shift to video consulting in the UK during the COVID-19 pandemic: Analysis of a mixed methods study using practice theory. *Social Science & Medicine, 311*, 115368. https://doi.org/10.1016/j.socscimed.2022.115368
Mueller, M., Kennerley, H., McManus, F., & Westbrook, D. (Eds.). *Oxford guide to surviving as a CBT therapist*. Oxford University Press.
Presley, V. (2023, February 9). Forgoing perfection: The importance of being a credible (not incredible) CBT therapist. *CBT Today, 51*(1), 22.

References

BABCP. (2021). *Supervision guidance for accredited therapists*. https://babcp.com/Accreditation/CBT-Practice-Supervision-CPD/Supervision-Guidance/Supervision-Guidance-for-Accredited-Therapists
Baum, N. (2016). Secondary traumatization in mental health professionals: A systematic review of gender findings. *Trauma, Violence, & Abuse, 17*(2), 221–235. https://doi.org/10.1177/1524838015584357
Bennett-Levy, J., & Beedie, A. (2007). The ups and downs of cognitive therapy training: What happens to trainees' perception of their competence during a cognitive therapy training course? *Behavioural and Cognitive Psychotherapy, 35*(1), 61–75. https://doi.org/10.1017/S1352465806003110

Blackburn, I.-M., James, I. A., Milne, D. L., Baker, C., Standart, S., Garland, A., & Reichelt, F. K. (2001). The revised cognitive therapy scale (CTS-R): Psychometric properties. *Behavioural and Cognitive Psychotherapy, 29*(4), 431–446. https://doi.org/10.1017/S1352465801004040

Briggs, E., & Owen, A. (2022). Funny, right? How do trainee and qualified therapists experience laughter in their practice with clients? *Counselling and Psychotherapy Research, 22*, 827–838. https://doi.org/10.1002/capr.12525

Clark, D. M. (1986). A cognitive approach to panic. *Behaviour Research and Therapy, 24*(4), 461–470.

Cromarty, P., Gallagher, D., & Watson, J. (2020). Remote delivery of CBT training, clinical supervision and services: In times of crisis or business as usual. *The Cognitive Behaviour Therapist, 13*, e33. https://doi.org/10.1017/S1754470X20000343

Davis, M. L., Thwaites, R., Freeston, M. H., & Bennett-Levy, J. (2015). A measurable impact of a self-practice/self-reflection programme on the therapeutic skills of experienced cognitive-behavioural therapists. *Clinical Psychology & Psychotherapy, 22*(2), 176–184.

Department of Health. (2008). *Improving access to psychological therapies implementation plan: National guidelines for regional delivery.*

Gonsalvez, C. J., Brockman, R., & Hill, H. R. (2016). Video feedback in CBT supervision: Review and illustration of two specific techniques. *The Cognitive Behaviour Therapist, 9*, e24.

Killick, S., Curry, V., & Myles, P. (2016). The mighty metaphor: A collection of therapists' favourite metaphors and analogies. *The Cognitive Behaviour Therapist, 9*, e37. https://doi.org/10.1017/S1754470X16000210

Kirk, J. (2010). *Going it alone: Working in private practice.* In M. Mueller, H. Kennerley, F. McManus, & D. Westbrook (Eds.), *Oxford guide to surviving as a CBT therapist* (pp. 275–300). Oxford University Press.

Leahy, R. L. (Ed.). (2006). *Roadblocks in cognitive-behavioral therapy: Transforming challenges into opportunities for change.* Guilford Press.

Maruniakova, L., & Rihacek, T. (2018). How beginning cognitive behavioural therapists develop professional confidence. *The Cognitive Behaviour Therapist, 11*, E5. https://doi.org/10.1017/S1754470X1800003X

McDowell, C. P., Herring, M. P., Lansing, J., Brower, C., & Meyer, J. D. (2020). Working from home and job loss due to the COVID-19 pandemic are associated with greater time in sedentary behaviours. *Frontiers in Public Health, 8*, 597619.

McLean, S., Wade, T. D., & Encel, J. S. (2003). The contribution of therapist beliefs to psychological distress in therapists: An investigation of vicarious traumatization burnout and symptoms of avoidance and intrusion. *Behavioural and Cognitive Psychotherapy, 31*(4), 417–428.

National Curriculum for Psychological Wellbeing Practitioner (PWP). (2023). *Programmes* (4th ed.). Health Education England. www.ucl.ac.uk/pals/sites/pals/files/pwp_review_-_final_report.pdf

National Institute for Health and Care Excellence. (2021). *Chronic pain (primary and secondary) in over 16s: Assessment of all chronic pain and management of chronic primary pain* [NICE Guideline No. 193]. www.nice.org.uk/guidance/ng193/chapter/Recommendations#managing-chronic-primary-pain

Nissen-Lie, H. A., Rønnestad, M. H., Høglend, P. A., Havik, O. E., Solbakken, O. A., Stiles, T. C., & Monsen, J. T. (2017). Love yourself as a person, doubt yourself as a therapist? *Clinical Psychology and Psychotherapy, 24*(1), 48–60. https://doi.org/10.1002/cpp.1977

Padesky, C. A., & Mooney, K. A. (1990). Presenting the cognitive model to clients. *International Cognitive Therapy Newsletter, 6*, 13–14.

Pennebaker, J. W. (2000). Telling stories: The health benefits of narrative. *Literature and Medicine, 19*(1), 3–18. https://doi.org/10.1353/lm.2000.0011

Presley, V. (2023). Forgoing perfection: The importance of being a credible (not incredible) CBT therapist. *CBT Today*, *51*(1), 22.

Roscoe, J., Bates, E., & Blackley, R. (2022a). 'It was like the unicorn of the therapeutic world': CBT trainee experiences of acquiring skills in guided discovery. *The Cognitive Behaviour Therapist*, *15*, E32. https://doi.org/10.1017/S1754470X22000277

Roscoe, J., Taylor, J., Harrington, R., & Wilbraham, S. (2022b). CBT supervision behind closed doors: Supervisor and supervisee reflections on their expectations and use of clinical supervision. *Counselling and Psychotherapy Research*, *22*(4), 1056–1067.

Roth, A. D., & Pilling, S. (2008). The competences required to deliver effective cognitive and behavioural therapy for people with depression and with anxiety disorders. *Behavioural and Cognitive Psychotherapy*, *36*(2), 129.

Stott, R., Mansell, W., Salkovskis, P., Lavendar, A., & Cartwright-Hatton, S. (2010, January 1). *Oxford guide to metaphors in CBT: Building cognitive bridges*. Oxford guides to cognitive behavioural therapy (online ed.). Oxford Academic. (Original work published 2015). https://doi.org/10.1093/med:psych/9780199207497.001.0001

Walker, J., & Furer, P. (2008). Interoceptive exposure in the treatment of health anxiety and hypochondriasis. *Journal of Cognitive Psychotherapy*, *22*(4), 366–378. https://doi.org/10.1891/0889–8391.22.4.366

Wegner, B. (2021). *Agoraphobia: Has COVID fueled this anxiety disorder?* Harvard Health Publishing. www.health.harvard.edu/blog/agoraphobia-has-covid-fueled-this-anxiety-disorder-202103152409

Westwood, S., Morison, L., Allt, J., & Holmes, N. (2017). Predictors of emotional exhaustion, disengagement and burnout among improving access to psychological therapies (IAPT) practitioners. *Journal of Mental Health*, *26*(2), 172–179.

Whittington, A., & Grey, N. (Eds.). (2014). *How to become a more effective CBT therapist. Mastering metacompetence in clinical practice*. John Wiley & sons.

Part III

Fine-tuning and expanding your knowledge and skills

Chapter 16

Get out of your head and into the chair

Bringing CBT to life through chairwork

Mathew Pugh

Introduction

Because cognitive reappraisal and behavioural experiments are seen as hallmarks of CBT, it is often forgotten that it is a fundamentally integrative approach to psychotherapy (Beck, 1991): cognitive behavioural therapists can draw upon a variety of experiential and multi-modal methods to bring about change, including imagery (Hackmann et al., 2011) and chairwork (Pugh, 2019a). But why would we want to be experiential in CBT?

Addressing the levels of meaning associated with distress (e.g. automatic thoughts, dysfunctional assumptions, and core beliefs) usually involves identifying, discussing, and re-evaluating cognitions (Wenzel, 2018). However, even the most skilled CBT therapists sometimes find that these conversations fail to bring about change at a deeper, emotional level. Various factors can contribute to this 'head-heart lag', including implicit, situationally specific, or entrenched beliefs, and parallel information processing streams that are less affected by discussion (e.g. Stott, 2007).

Speaking to the head or heart?

Fortunately, multi-level information processing theories such as Interacting Cognitive Subsystems (ICS; Teasdale & Barnard, 1993) give us some clues about how we can overcome these blocks. Whilst a long discussion isn't possible here (see Pugh, 2019b), the general idea is that changing the deeper meanings underlying distress sometimes relies on experiential modes of information processing. In other words, evocative, multi-sensory, and experiential interventions such as chairwork can help shift deep-rooted (heartfelt) beliefs. At the same time, 'head-level' interventions like Socratic dialogue sometimes restrict emotional processing, which can limit how much change clients experience.

DOI: 10.4324/9781003428527-20

CLINICAL EXAMPLE: *Role-playing the process of cognitive restructuring.*
Ari was stuck. He had spent weeks re-evaluating his negative core belief but still felt worthless. To help shift things, his therapist suggested doing a role-play: she would present the evidence supporting his core belief in one chair, whilst Ari would counter-argue in another chair. 'Acting out' cognitive restructuring was a far more emotional process but helped Ari's 'healthy' perspective feel much more believable.

What is chairwork?

When therapists hear the word 'chairwork', they often think of Gestalt therapy. Whilst Perls (1969) certainly popularised chairwork, it originates from psychodrama: a group-based therapy that uses action and theatre to bring about change (Moreno, 1987). Since then, chairwork has been incorporated in many therapies, including schema therapy (e.g. Van der Wijngaart, 2023), compassion-focused therapy (e.g. Bell et al., 2021a), and CBT (e.g. Pugh, 2019a).

Chairwork seems to be effective (e.g. Pascual-Leone & Baher, 2023; Pugh, 2021a) but it hasn't received as much attention from researchers as other experiential interventions such as imagery. In addition, many CBT therapists initially feel uncomfortable using chairwork, fearing that it might distress, destabilise, or alienate clients (Pugh et al., 2021b). Fortunately, these methods can be broken down into a few basic theoretical ideas and practical applications – the 'pillars' of chairwork (Pugh & Bell, 2020) – which are explored in the next section.

REFLECTIVE EXERCISE: How do you feel about using chairwork? Do you have any doubts or reservations about using these methods? What concerns might your clients have?

Pillar one: the principles of chairwork

Self-multiplicity: The first principle of chairwork is that people have different 'parts', 'selves', or 'I-positions' (Konopka et al., 2019; Lester, 2015). Whether these parts of the self are just metaphors (the 'soft' multiplicity view), fully-fledged subpersonalities (the 'hard' multiplicity view), or fleeting states of mind (the 'modest' multiplicity view) is hotly debated. CBT is most aligned with the third view, referring to these subcomponents of personality as transient 'modes' (Beck, 1996; Beck et al., 2021) or 'minds-in-place' (Teasdale, 1997) that are composed of combinations of affect, behaviour, cognitions, and desires (ABCDs; Revelle & Condon,

2015). Whilst Beck emphasised the importance of modes (Beck et al., 1985; Beck, 1996) and believed they were vital to the evolution of CBT (Beck et al., 2021), many therapists are unfamiliar with this concept and even fewer use it in practice. For the remainder of this chapter, they will be referred to as 'parts' because clients find this term most relatable (Schwartz & Sweezy, 2019).

Information exchange: The second principle of chairwork is that thoughts, feelings, and motivations (collectively, our modes) can be seen as communicative acts that (literally and metaphorically) speak to the self. For instance, CBT has sometimes described negative thoughts as 'self-statements' or 'inner dialogue' (e.g. Meichenbaum, 1977). Accordingly, a key change process in CBT is helping individuals establish internal dialogues that are empirical, compassionate, and decentred (Teasdale, 1997). Chairwork brings these information exchanges to life by acting them out in different chairs.

Transformation: The final principle of chairwork is that parts of the self, their relationships, or a limited oversight of them can contribute to psychopathology (Beck et al., 2021). For instance, depression can arise from a 'depressogenic mind' that gets stuck due to various feedback loops (Teasdale, 1997). Other mood disorders might arise from conflicts between parts (e.g. 'restrictive' vs. 'permissive' modes of eating in bulimia nervosa), mismatches between the activated part and the situation, or limited control over them (Beck, 1996). For this reason, working with parts can be helpful.

TOP TIP: You can bring self-multiplicity into CBT in many ways.

(1) *Listen for parts:* Look out for references to parts in what your clients say. For instance, do they talk about different aspects of themselves (e.g. the 'voice' of their OCD) or ever describe being in 'two minds' about something?

(2) *Float the idea:* See if your clients relate to the idea of having parts. For example, when you draw out a hot cross bun formulation, ask the client to name it (e.g. 'my anxious mode'). What situations bring this part out? What does it say or do? What helps it settle? Crucially, drawing out several hot cross bun formulations will help highlight the client's multiplicity.

(3) *Use metaphors*: For instance, your hand naturally has many fingers and joints (i.e. parts) that give it flexibility, yet they all belong to the same palm (i.e. self) (Villatte et al., 2016).

(4) *Know your parts.* Which parts influence how you deliver CBT? For instance, do you tend to work from your 'logical', 'caring', or 'stick-to-the-manual' part? Would strengthening other parts help you deliver CBT more flexibly or effectively?

Pillar two: the processes of chairwork

The principles of chairwork lead to three complementary processes that guide how chairwork is facilitated:

Separation: Chairwork begins with a collaborative decision about the parts you are going to work with. Once agreed, they are named and placed in different chairs. 'Separating' parts in this way has several therapeutic functions, including making them more distinct, concrete, and supporting decentring (e.g. externalising negative thoughts by putting them on a chair).

Client: *I want to be less self-critical.*
Therapist: *Let's work on that. What shall we call the critical part of you?*
Client: *My inner critic.*
Therapist: *Ok.* [Pulls up a second chair]. *Let's put your critic over here.*

Animation: Once you've identified and separated the parts you are going to address, you need to bring them to life. You can do this in two ways. The first option involves you or the client changing seats and *embodying* the part (e.g. speaking from its perspective in the first-person). Alternatively, the client can *personify* a part by imagining it is held in an empty chair and conveying what is says in the third-person. Embodying a part is usually more immersive and intense, and so tends to be preferred.

Embodiment by the client:

Therapist:*Change seats and be your inner critic. Talk to your empty chair and show me how it puts you down.*

Embodiment by the therapist:

Therapist:*When I change seats, I'm going to play your inner critic and repeat what it says to you.*

Personification:

Therapist:*Imagine your inner critic is sat over there.* [Gestures to the chair]. *What is it saying to you right now?*

> **Top tip:** If a client doesn't like the idea of moving between seats or enacting parts, use personification instead (e.g. *'It's fine if you don't want to change seats and play your inner critic. But let's imagine your inner critic were sat in the chair over there – what does it look like? What is it saying to you? How does that make you feel?'*).

3. **Talk:** Dialogues with or between parts are the engine of chairwork. These dialogues take two forms: 'horizontal dialogues' in which parts interact with one another or the therapist, and 'vertical dialogues' in which the client relates to parts, held in different chairs, from a meta-cognitive or decentred (i.e. standing) position. This second type of chairwork is called 'witnessing' because it's similar to taking an observer perspective.

Client-as-inner-critic: [Speaking to their former chair]. *You're such a loser.*

Therapist:	*Come back to your seat.* [Client moves]. *How do you feel hearing that?*
Client:	*It hurts.*

Client-led horizontal dialogue:

Therapist:	*Do you agree with everything your critic just said?*
Client:	*I'm not a total loser. I do have some positive qualities.*
Therapist:	*Say that back to the critic* [Gestures to the other chair].

Therapist-led horizontal dialogue:

Therapist:	*We've been working strengthening your healthy side in therapy. Can I speak to your critic from that perspective?*
Client:	*OK.*
Therapist:	[Turns to the empty chair]. *That's not true, Jacob isn't a loser. Here's why . . .*

Vertical dialogue:

Therapist:	*Let's stand up and look at you and your inner critic as if we were observers.* [Client and therapist]. *What do you notice about Jacob and his critic from up here?*

Procedures

Psychotherapy books are filled with examples of chairwork. However, these enactments can be distilled into just a handful of key 'dialogues', 'procedures', or 'tasks' (Elliott & Greenberg, 2021; Kellogg & Garcia Torres, 2021; Kipper, 1986; Pugh, 2021b). They include the following:

- *Interviews.* The client changes seats and is interviewed as a part. For example, you could interview a client as a cognitive process ('the part that worries'), an emotion ('the sad part'), behaviours ('the part that binges'), a past or future self ('the version of you that has recovered from anorexia'), or other people ('your best friend'). Interviewing cognitive processes can be particularly helpful way to explore the triggers, content, and motivations of these internal events, much like a functional analysis.

Therapist:	*Change seats and be your inner critic. I'm going to ask that part of you some questions so we can understand it better.* [Client moves to another chair]. *Good to meet you, critic. What do you criticise about Jacob?*
Client-as-inner-critic:	*I hate that he's so lazy.*
Therapist:	*How are you trying to help him by pointing that out?*
Client-as-inner-critic:	*I'm worried he'll get complacent.*

TOP TIP: When you interview a part, try to match its tone and rhythm of speech. This often makes for a more congruent and productive interview.

Dialogues. The client uses two or more chairs to converse with different parts of themselves (including other people). For instance, two-chair dialogue could be set up between the evidence for and evidence against an automatic thought.

Therapist:	*Change seats and be your inner critic.* [Client moves to a new chair]. *Can you show me how it puts you down?*
Client-as-critic:	[Talking to vacated chair]. *You're so lazy. No wonder you're a failure.*
Therapist:	*Change back.* [Client returns to original chair]. *How does that make you feel?*

> **TOP TIP**: If you don't have extra chairs available, you can still facilitate a dialogue by asking the client to move their occupied chair into different spaces.

Dramatisations. Chairs can be used to act out real or hypothetical scenes from the client's life (e.g. Burns, 2020; Kellogg & Garcia Torres, 2021). This includes internal events (e.g. role-playing the process of self-criticism) or external situations (e.g. role-playing a critical interaction with a friend). Unlike dialogues, therapists will play a role on behalf of the client during dramatisations.

Therapist:	*When I change seats, I'll play your inner critic and repeat what it says to you. I'd like you to play the healthy side and defend yourself.*
Client:	*Got it.* [Therapist moves into a new chair].
Therapist-as-critic:	*Jacob, you're so lazy. No wonder you're a failure.*
Client-as-healthy-side:	*That's not true. I've achieved lots in my life.*

> **Top Tip:** I always recommend changing seats when you enact a part on behalf of the client to make it clear that you are playing a role. This is especially important if you are enacting hostile or threatening parts of the self (e.g. the inner critic).

Depictions. In this procedure, empty chairs are used to represent relationships in the client's internal or external world. This can be a useful way to assess, formulate, or measure change.

Therapist:	*Suppose this empty chair represents your inner critic.* [Introduces a seat]. *How near to you was it when we started therapy?*
Client:	*So close.* [Places the chair beside his own].
Therapist:	*And since you've learned how to question your thoughts?*
Client:	*It's much further away.* [Moves the chair several feet away].

Top Tip: You can also create depictions using other objects, like figurines or pillows. If you are working online, try using icons on a shared document or digital whiteboard.

Disclosures. The client uses chairs to explore or develop different self-related 'stories' (i.e. core beliefs). For example, a client might tell the 'same old story' about being worthless in one chair and then build a 'new story' about being worthwhile in a second chair. This can be a useful way to strengthen positive core beliefs and build self-complexity·(Chadwick, 2003). However, unlike dialogues, conversations between these perspectives rarely take place. This is reflected in how the chairs are arranged: both seats face forwards (rather than facing one other), so a dialogue does not take place.

Client:	*I haven't achieved anything this week.*
Therapist:	*Well, that's one perspective. Let's leave this critical point of view here and switch seats.* [Client moves to another chair]. *Speaking from your healthy side in this seat, what have you achieved, no matter how small it seems?*
Client:	*I saw my friends.*
Therapist:	*Well done. What else did you succeed with?*

Witnessing. Whilst the aforementioned procedures capture 'horizontal' forms of chairwork (i.e. interactions with or between parts of the self), witnessing is a 'vertical' chairwork procedure in which the client stands and observes parts/chairs 'from a distance'. This draws on the benefits of self-distancing and third-person perspective taking which can support emotional regulation, wiser reasoning, and 'bigger picture' thinking (Kross & Ayduk, 2017).

Therapist:	*Let's stand and look at this interaction as observers* [Both stand]. *What do you notice about Jacob* [gestures to chair one] *and his critic* [gestures to chair two]?
Client:	*His critic is relentless. It reminds me of how his mother criticised him as a child.*
Therapist:	*What was that like for Jacob?*

Top Tip: To help the client maintain a witnessing perspective during vertical enactments, prompt them to talk about themselves in the third person (e.g. 'As you look at Jacob over there, what do you imagine he is thinking and feeling?').

REFLECTIVE EXERCISE. Now that you're more familiar with chairwork, let's think about you could use it.

1. How could you use chairwork to bring your favourite CBT to technique to life? For instance, if you enjoy cost–benefit analyses, could you set up a two-chair dialogue between the 'advantages' and 'disadvantages' of a thought or behaviour?
2. What reservations might your clients have about chairwork? One objection is that it might seem 'silly'. In this situation, I might interview the part that has these reservations, validating its perspective and negotiating how we can proceed with chairwork.
3. What if you only have one chair? If you need to adapt chairwork, refer back to its underlying principles and processes. So, if all you have is one chair, you can still separate parts by asking the client to move their seat left and right or to stand and sit down as they shift between parts.

Process skills

How therapists facilitate chairwork can affect whether clients agree to do it and how helpful it is (Muntigl et al., 2017). Process skills refer to the moment-by-moment interventions therapists use to ensure that chairwork is as immersive, evocative, and meaningful as possible (Pugh, 2019b). They include the following:

- *Listening in surround sound:* Rather than 'listening in mono' (i.e. viewing the client as being fixed and unitary), listen for expressions of multiplicity (Hartman, 2015). For instance, if a client has 'mixed feelings' about an assignment, you could conceptualise this as two or more parts with conflicting points of view. Once you spot parts, you can work with them using chairwork.

Top Tip: Once you have identified a part, flesh it out using a cross-sectional ('hot cross bun') formulation. For example, what does the client think, feel (emotionally and physically), want to do, and attend to when they are in their 'inner critic mode'?

- *Doubling:* This is an important skill for dialogue procedures and involves offering the client a first-person statement that they repeat or correct (*'If it fits with your experience, try saying this to your critic'*). By saying things on behalf the client, the therapist can gently elicit 'hot' cognitive material, articulate what is unsaid, or clarify what the client is conveying.

> **Top Tip:** Doubling statements are most effective when they are short and to the point. You can also try 'feeding' the client a statement that they complete during a dialogue (e.g. 'Critic, when I hear you say those things to me, I feel so. . . . Can you finish that statement, Jacob?') (Levitsky & Perls, 1969).

- *Imagery:* It's helpful to ask the client to visualise the 'other' in the empty chair before a dialogue begins (Therapist: 'Picture your father in the chair over there – how does he appear?'). Similarly, the therapist might begin a role-play by asking the client to describe the setting (Therapist: 'Before we act out this conversation with your manager, let's imagine we're in her office – what does the room look like?'). This can make enactments more immersive and activate relevant episodic memories.

Conclusion

Chairwork is an exciting way to bring CBT to life, but when should therapists consider using these methods? Evidence for cognitive behavioural chairwork is strongest for skill acquisition (e.g. assertiveness skills training) and re-evaluating core beliefs (e.g. De Oliveira et al., 2012; Lazarus, 1966). Anecdotal evidence suggests that chairwork might be helpful when there is a limited response to standard CBT interventions such as exposure and cognitive restructuring (e.g. Cromarty & Marks, 1995; Newell & Shrubb, 1994). Outside of CBT, research in allied approaches indicates that chairwork can help reduce self-criticism, enhance self-compassion, and support emotional regulation (Bell et al., 2021b; Josek et al., 2023).

Unfortunately, contraindications for chairwork are limited to expert opinions. Therapists should be cautious when using chairwork with people who struggle with emotional dysregulation, aggressiveness, self-harm, or suicidality (Elliott et al., 2004; Pos & Greenberg, 2012). Nonetheless, research indicates that chairwork is still feasible with complex presentations (e.g. Chadwick, 2003). Clearly, training and supervision are important when using these methods.

Finally, if you want to build your confidence using chairwork, my advice would be to 'POP':

- **Practice** (rehearse with a colleague or supervisor);
- **Observe** (watch other therapists doing chairwork so you can learn from them and develop your own style);

- **Participate** (experience it for yourself) – there is nothing like experiencing chairwork from the inside out. Most importantly, be creative and ensure that chairwork is always a collaborative experience for your clients.

Further reading

Pugh, M. (2019a). *Cognitive behavioural chairwork: Distinctive features*. Routledge.
Pugh, M. (2019b). A little less talk, a little more action: A dialogical approach to cognitive therapy. *The Cognitive Behaviour Therapist, 12*, e47. https://doi.org/10.1017/S1754470X19000333
Van Der Wijngaart, R. (2023). *Chairwork: Theory and practice*. Pavilion.

References

Beck, A. T. (1991). Cognitive therapy as the integrative therapy. *Journal of Psychotherapy Integration, 1*, 191–198. https://doi.org/10.1037/h0101233
Beck, A. T. (1996). Beyond belief: A theory of modes, personality, and psychopathology. In P. M. Salkovskis (Ed.), *Frontiers of cognitive therapy* (pp. 1–25). Guildford Press.
Beck, A. T., Emery, G., & Greenberg, R. L. (1985). *Anxiety disorders and phobias: A cognitive perspective*. Basic Books.
Beck, A. T., Finkel, M. R., & Beck, J. S. (2021). The theory of modes: Applications to schizophrenia and other psychological conditions. *Cognitive Therapy and Research, 45*, 391–400. https://doi.org/10.1007/s10608-020-10098-0
Bell, T., Montague, J., Elander, J., & Gilbert, P. (2021a). "Suddenly you are King Solomon": Multiplicity, transformation and integration in compassion focused therapy chairwork. *Journal of Psychotherapy Integration, 31*, 223–237. https://doi.org/10.1037/int0000240
Bell, T., Montague, J., Elander, J., & Gilbert, P. (2021b). Multiple emotions, multiple selves: Compassion focused therapy chairwork. *The Cognitive Behaviour Therapist, 14*, e22. https://doi.org/10.1017/S1754470X21000180
Burns, D. A. (2020). *Feeling great: The revolutionary new treatment for depression and anxiety*. PESI Publishing.
Chadwick, P. (2003). Two chairs, self-schemata and a person based approach to psychosis. *Behavioural and Cognitive Psychotherapy, 31*, 439–449. https://doi.org/10.1017/S1352465803004053
Cromarty, P., & Marks, I. (1995). Does rational role-play enhance the outcome of exposure therapy in dysmorphophobia? A case study. *British Journal of Psychiatry, 167*, 399–402. https://doi.org/10.1192/bjp.167.3.399
De Oliveira, I. R., Powell, V. B., Wenzel, A., Caldas, M., Seixas, C., Almeida, C., Bonfim, T., Grangeon, M. C., Castro, M., Galvao, A., de Oliveira Moraes, R., & Sudak, D. (2012). Efficacy of the trial-based thought record, a new cognitive therapy strategy designed to change core beliefs, in social phobia. *Journal of Clinical Pharmacy and Therapeutics, 37*, 328–334. https://doi.org/10.1111/j.1365–2710.2011.01299.x
Elliott, R., & Greenberg, L. S. (2021). *Emotion-focused counselling in action*. Sage.
Elliott, R., Watson, J. C., Goldman, R. N., & Greenberg, L. S. (2004). *Learning emotion-focused therapy: The process-experiential approach to change*. American Psychological Association.
Hackmann, A., Bennett-Levy, J., & Holmes, E. A. (2011). *Oxford guide to imagery in cognitive therapy*. Oxford University Press.
Hartman, T. (2015). 'Strong multiplicity': An interpretive lens in the analysis of qualitative interview narratives. *Qualitative Research, 15*, 22–38. https://doi.org/10.1177/1468794113509259

Josek, A. K., Schaich, A., Braakmann, D., Assmann, N., Jauch-Chara, K., Arntz, A., Schweiger, U., & Fassbinder, E. (2023). Chairwork in schema therapy for patients with borderline personality disorder: A qualitative study of patients' perceptions. *Frontiers in Psychiatry, 14*, 1180839. https://doi.org/10.3389/fpsyt.2023.1180839

Kellogg, S., & Garcia Torres, A. (2021). Toward a chairwork psychotherapy: Using the four dialogues for healing and transformation. *Practice Innovations, 6*, 171–180. https://doi.org/10.1037/pri0000149

Kipper, D. A. (1986). *Psychotherapy through clinical role playing.* Brunner/Mazel.

Konopka, A., Hermans, H. J. M., & Goncalves, M. M. (2019). The dialogical self as a landscape of mind populated by a society of I-positions. In A. Konopka, H. J. M. Hermans, & M. M. Goncalves (Eds.), *Handbook of dialogical self theory and psychotherapy: Bridging psychotherapeutic and cultural traditions* (pp. 9–23). Routledge.

Kross, E., & Ayduk, O. (2017). Self-distancing: Theory, research, and current directions. *Advances in Experimental Social Psychology, 55*, 81–136. https://doi.org/10.1016/bs.aesp.2016.10.002

Lazarus, A. A. (1966). Behaviour rehearsal vs. non-directive therapy vs. advice in effecting behaviour change. *Behaviour Research and Therapy, 4*, 209–212. https://doi.org/10.1016/0005–7967(66)90068–4

Lester, D. (2015). *On multiple selves.* Transaction Publishers.

Levitsky, A., & Perls, F. (1969). The rules and games of gestalt therapy. In H. M. Ruitenbeek (Ed.), *Group therapy today: Styles, methods, and techniques* (pp. 221–230). Atherton Press.

Meichenbaum, D. (1977). *Cognitive-behavior modification: An integrative approach.* Plenum Press.

Moreno, J. L. (1987). *The essential Moreno: Writings on psychodrama, group method, and spontaneity.* Springer.

Muntigl, P., Chubak, L., & Angus, L. (2017). Entering chair work in psychotherapy: An interactional structure for getting emotion-focused talk underway. *Journal of Pragmatics, 117*, 168–189. https://doi.org/10.1016/j.pragma.2017.06.016

Newell, R., & Shrubb, S. (1994). Attitude change and behaviour therapy in body dysmorphic disorder: Two case reports. *Behavioural and Cognitive Psychotherapy, 22*, 163–169. https://doi.org/10.1017/S1352465800011942

Pascual-Leone, A., & Baher, T. (2023). Chairwork in individual psychotherapy: Meta-analyses of intervention effects. *Psychotherapy, 60*, 370–382. https://doi.org/10.1037/pst0000490

Perls, F. (1969). *Gestalt therapy verbatim.* Gestalt Journal Press.

Pos, A. E., & Greenberg, L. S. (2012). Organizing awareness and increasing emotion regulation: Revising chair work in emotion-focused therapy for borderline personality disorder. *Journal of Personality Disorders, 26*, 84–107. https://doi.org/10.1521/pedi.2012.26.1.84

Pugh, M. (2019a). *Cognitive behavioural chairwork: Distinctive features.* Routledge.

Pugh, M. (2019b). A little less talk, a little more action: A dialogical approach to cognitive therapy. *The Cognitive Behaviour Therapist, 12*, e47. https://doi.org/10.1017/S1754470X19000333

Pugh, M. (2021a). Cognitive behavioural chairwork: Theory, research, and practice. In J. Passmore & S. Leach (Eds.), *Third wave cognitive behavioural coaching: Contextual, behavioural, and neuroscience approaches for evidence based coaches* (pp. 53–77). Pavilion.

Pugh, M. (2021b). Single-session chairwork: Overview and case illustration of brief dialogical psychotherapy. *British Journal of Guidance and Counselling.* https://doi.org/10.1080/03069885.2021.1984395

Pugh, M., & Bell, T. (2020). Process-based chairwork: Applications and innovations in the time of COVID-19. *European Journal of Counselling Theory, Research, and Practice, 4*, 1–8.

Pugh, M., Bell, T., Waller, G., & Petrova, E. (2021b). Attitudes and applications of chair-work amongst CBT therapists: A preliminary survey. *The Cognitive Behaviour Therapist, 14*, e21. https://doi.org/10.1017/S1754470X21000052

Revelle, W., & Condon, D. M. (2015). A model for personality at three levels. *Journal of Research in Personality, 56*, 70–81. https://doi.org/10.1016/j.jrp.2014.12.006

Schwartz, R. C., & Sweezy, M. (2019). *Internal family systems therapy*. Guilford Publications.

Stott, R. (2007). When head and heart do not agree: A theoretical and clinical analysis of rational-emotional dissociation (RED) in cognitive therapy. *Journal of Cognitive Psychotherapy, 21*, 37–50. https://doi.org/10.1891/088983907780493313

Teasdale, J. D. (1997). The relationship between cognition and emotion: The mind-in-place in mood disorders. In D. M. Clark & C. G. Fairburn (Eds.), *The science and practice of cognitive behaviour therapy* (pp. 67–93). Oxford University Press.

Teasdale, J. D., & Barnard, P. J. (1993). *Affect, cognition and change: Re-modelling depressive thought*. Lawrence Erlbaum Associations.

Wenzel, A. (2018). Cognitive reappraisal. In S. C. Hayes & S. G. Hofmann (Eds.), *Process-based CBT: The science and core clinical competencies of cognitive behavioral therapy* (pp. 325–337). Context Press.

Van der Wijngaart, R. (2023). *Chairwork: Theory and practice*. Pavilion.

Villatte, M., Villatte, J. L., & Hayes, S. C. (2016). *Mastering the clinical conversation: Language as intervention*. Guilford.

Chapter 17

'It's not you, it's me'

Addressing therapist schemas during CBT training and beyond

Vickie Presley

Introduction

If you ask therapists to describe their experiences of CBT training, many will be pulled back to the emotional context of their journey. You might hear about the excitement of gaining a training place, the relief of passing a difficult assignment, the joy of helping a client reach recovery, the happiness when connecting with trainee peers, the pride in finally qualifying. But between these milestones, you might also hear about the fear of failure, the anxiety about not being good enough, the embarrassment about getting things wrong, the stress of never-ending deadlines, the confusion about which CBT model to use and when, or the shame of lingering imposter syndrome. Each and every one of these emotional experiences is completely <u>normal</u>: after all, the process of qualifying as a CBT therapist is simultaneously hugely rewarding but also very demanding. As discussed in Chapters 5 and 6, it is not unusual to find that the transition from one professional role to another brings about a feeling of being 'de-skilled' and provokes concerns about personal competence (Lombardo et al., 2009). However, whilst all of these experiences are typical and valid – perhaps even to be expected – they are not simply a by-product of the many training demands. Who we are personally – our own beliefs, values, and past experiences – will undoubtedly interact with how we experience the training year and how we work with our clients. Indeed, there are a number of 'therapist schemas' that are thought to be important to pay attention to during CBT training and beyond (Roscoe & Taylor, 2023). Leahy (2001) describes 15 different types of therapist schema: 'Helplessness' (not knowing what to do), 'Need for Approval' (wanting to be liked), and 'Rejection-Sensitive' (conflict avoidant) are some examples. The focus of this chapter will be 'Demanding Standards' or 'perfectionism', as research tells us that this is a particularly common trainee CBT therapist schema (Haarhoff, 2006).

What is perfectionism?

A number of definitions and models of perfectionism exist in the psychological literature. There isn't space for us to consider all of these here, but you may want

DOI: 10.4324/9781003428527-21

to look at the work of key authors in this area such as Hewitt and Flett (1991) and Shafran et al. (2002). Most definitions and models will emphasise the role of striving to achieve high standards of performance, but many also include other dimensions of the phenomenon thought to be important. Hill et al. (2004) suggested a multidimensional model that includes both helpful and unhelpful dimensions of perfectionism, developing a self-report measure of the construct to reflect this. Trainees may not self-describe as being 'a perfectionist' per se; however, most relate to at least some of these dimensions. Have a look at the sample questionnaire items in Table 17.1 and see if any fit with what you know about yourself. For example, are you the sort of person who worries about getting things wrong? Or who has a tendency for self-criticism? Perhaps the thought of others judging you negatively is anxiety provoking and uncomfortable? Are you the sort of person who likes to have things organised and planned in advance, or who likes to 'do their best'? If this is the case, you may find that the scrutiny of the training programme pulls these things into sharper focus. For example, the academic components may heighten the need to strive for excellence; the direct evaluation of your clinical work may exacerbate concerns about making mistakes; and the building of new relationships with peers, supervisors, and clients may activate a need for approval.

Personal perfectionism: professional context

Before you read any further, it is important to note that I come at this topic from a place of lived experience. My own training year was fraught with anxious feelings of inadequacy, which I promptly attempted to escape from with a plethora of perfectionistic behaviours. Fortunately, I was afforded the opportunities I needed to reflect upon the impact of this on my skills development, my 'therapist self-esteem',

Table 17.1 Dimensions of Perfectionism and Example Questionnaire Items

Dimension of Perfectionism	Example Questionnaire Item
Concern Over Mistakes	'If I mess up on one thing, people might start questioning everything I do'
High Standards for Others	'I get upset when other people don't maintain the same standards I do'
Need for Approval	'I'm concerned with whether or not people approve of my actions'
Organisation	'I think things should be put away in their place'
Perceived Parental Pressure	'My parent(s) are difficult to please'
Planfulness	'I need time to think up a plan before I take action'
Rumination	'I spend a lot of time worrying about things I've done, or things I need to do'
Striving for Excellence	'I can't stand to do something halfway'

Source: From Hill et al.'s (2004) Perfectionism Inventory

and importantly my clients. I can still remember the very moment that I realised that my perfectionist traits were impacting upon not just me but my clients as well.

Personal reflection

I'm working with Pat, a client who is significantly depressed and whose self-worth depends upon the realisation of perfectionistic standards across multiple life domains. It's session 12, and we've competed an effective continuum exercise to help reframe unhelpful dichotomous evaluations of the self. The intervention has gone well, prompting enough cognitive shift for Pat to begin rebuilding a view of themself as something other than a 'failure'. Then, in the very last minute of the session, I suggest that Pat should take the continuum worksheet home and re-write it, because (and I quote) **'mine's a bit messy'**.

I noted the irony of this statement and it's potential to undermine any benefit Pat might have otherwise taken from the intervention immediately, and I chose to use a recording of the session to reflect more closely on my clinical practice. Sadly, this wasn't the only example of the interference of my own schemas in the session. Paradoxically, my need to avoid making mistakes and so escape criticism from both Pat and my clinical supervisor, actually meant that I risked the very things that I was attempting to circumvent.

We all have our own 'perfectionism narrative' that will inevitably be shaped by our personal history, early experiences, cultural heritage, and relationships. I've spent a lot of time reflecting upon the development of my own schemas and how these have the potential to impact upon me personally and professionally, and I hope I've enabled many of the trainees I've worked with over the years to do the same. What I can tell you from these experiences is that perfectionism often serves to conceal, deflect or avoid feelings of shame and anxiety; inevitably self-reflection in this context is not always easy, and might bring about difficult emotions. I therefore encourage you to come to this chapter with gentle curiosity, with a willingness to reflect upon how some of the issues might be relevant to your personal and professional self, but to do so with self-compassion and kindness as part of the process. Remember, there is no judgement here – apart from your own.

The paradox of perfectionism

Perfectionism in the training context

The word I hear most to describe the training year for CBT therapists is 'intense'. There's no denying that the demands placed upon trainees are numerous, and this only intensifies further when these external demands are matched with unhelpfully demanding internal ones. The scrutiny of the training experience is essential for ensuring that therapists are safe, ethical, and competent practitioners when they graduate; however, this can be anxiety provoking for many trainees, and some may find themselves engaging in counter-productive coping strategies. It is very difficult for trainees who expect so much of themselves to lower these expectations and accept that, during training, it is normal to get things wrong, to feel utterly incompetent, and to forget what it's like to know what on earth you're doing. As a result, some trainees might find themselves attempting to avoid any direct observation of their clinical skills through fear of being 'found out' as an imposter, as someone not 'good enough' to be on the training course. These fears might manifest in procrastination over recording clinical sessions for evaluation, or avoiding experiential learning activities such as skills rehearsal as part of teaching sessions. Some trainees will compensate by replacing these active learning opportunities with more passive activities such as over engaging with CBT textbooks or research articles – activities which are 'safe' and free from the risk of judgement and criticism. Such behaviours indicate a degree of experiential avoidance, where there is difficulty remaining in contact with uncomfortable internal experiences (Hayes et al., 1996). Unfortunately, preliminary research tells us that trainees with higher levels of experiential avoidance may struggle more with developing their skills in relation to some key CBT competencies (Presley et al., 2023). This makes sense when we consider this process within a CBT framework (see Figure 17.1). Worries about being incompetent, fears about criticism and failure, concerns about being 'found out' – these self-limiting beliefs cannot be disputed when we avoid any opportunity for disconfirmation, and simultaneously any opportunity to gain the feedback needed to develop our skills.

Perfectionism in the supervisory context

Therapist perfectionism can hamper the supervisory process and limit the learning from this during training. Difficulties with experiential avoidance might also play out here, thwarting opportunities for skills rehearsal or getting feedback on recorded session content. Many trainees might avoid the latter due to feeling exposed and a fear of negative judgement, and some may find this is worse in group supervision (Roscoe et al., 2022). Additionally, trainees might find that they feel reluctant to bring clinical cases where they are struggling, or asking important questions because they might convey incompetence. Other trainees might bounce into supervision presenting all the things that are going well in their practice instead of the things they really need to talk about. Alternatively, trainees might find that they are using supervision to seek reassurance or approval around their decision-making, inadvertently maintaining a lack of confidence in their own clinical judgement. It isn't unusual for trainees to want approval from their clinical supervisor, and they may find themselves compensating for self-doubt by over-preparing, writing copious notes, or armouring themselves with any number of other perfectionistic behaviours. Other trainees might not actually find supervision beneficial but will still avoid disapproval by refraining from asserting their developmental needs with

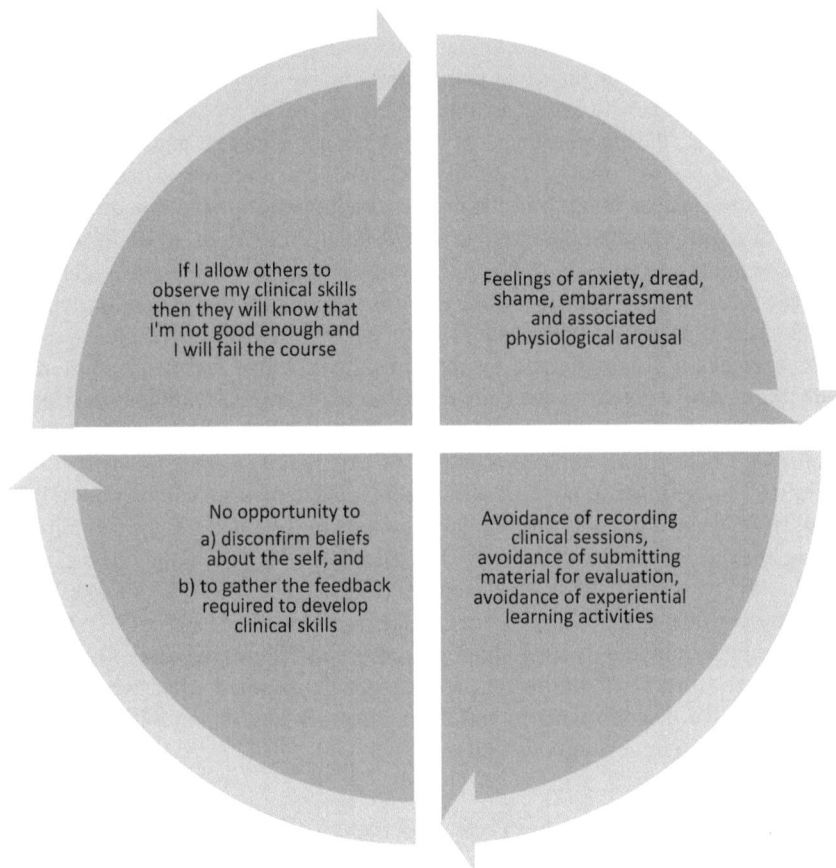

If I allow others to observe my clinical skills then they will know that I'm not good enough and I will fail the course

Feelings of anxiety, dread, shame, embarrassment and associated physiological arousal

No opportunity to
a) disconfirm beliefs about the self, and
b) to gather the feedback required to develop clinical skills

Avoidance of recording clinical sessions, avoidance of submitting material for evaluation, avoidance of experiential learning activities

Figure 17.1 Example maintenance cycle of the consequences of experiential avoidance during training

their supervisor. Of course, it's clear that the different dimensions of perfectionism might impact upon how we engage in supervision in multiple ways – but with the singular outcome that we do not get what we need to develop our clinical competence effectively. When this happens, the lack of progress only serves to reinforce the idea that we are 'not doing well enough', perpetuating the need for perfectionistic safety or avoidance behaviours (and so on). What should be made clear here is that it is absolutely normal to want to escape uncomfortable emotions; that's why as a trainee we might find ourselves doing all sorts of things to deflect from the emotional arousal of feeling de-skilled in a new role which involves lots of competing pressures. However, research tells us that the avoidance of these emotions is unhelpful; in fact, paying attention to emotional experiences and exploring these in supervision are key to maintaining a developmental trajectory, building a supervisory alliance, and protecting wellbeing. Importantly, being able to explore uncomfortable emotions in supervision can provide an insight into the types of beliefs that might be in operation and how these might also play out in a clinical context (Lombardo et al., 2009).

Perfectionism in a clinical context

Perfectionism will very likely shape the clinical interactions we have with our clients. Unfortunately, experience and research tell us that often trying to be a 'perfect' therapist actually has the opposite effect. Leahy (2001) discussed the potential consequences of therapist perfectionism, proposing that such therapists may be impatient and lack empathy, emphasising rationality at the expense of exploring their clients' emotional experiences. Furthermore, he stated they would likely impair the development of an effective therapeutic alliance by setting unrealistic expectations of both themselves and their clients, leaving the client feeling criticised and controlled. Indeed, preliminary research in this area supports the idea that therapist perfectionism might indeed hamper client outcomes (Presley et al., 2017). We found by analysing client outcome data for qualified CBT therapists in relation to their scores on the Perfectionism Inventory, that a number of dimensions of perfectionism were associated with lower outcomes on measures of depression and anxiety. For example, higher therapist scores for 'concern over mistakes' and 'planfulness' were associated with a lesser reduction in anxiety symptoms, and higher scores for 'perceived parental pressure' and 'striving for excellence' were associated with a lesser reduction in depressive symptoms (Presley et al., 2017). There are many reasons why we might have observed some of these patterns in the data. For example, trainees might plan extensively for their sessions, wanting to feel that they are prepared and therefore less likely to get lost in the session, mess up, or let the client down. What we then find is that trainees find it difficult to be spontaneous in the session, their flexibility and creativity is stifled and they can't deviate or collaborate when the client brings something different to their attention. They also model an intolerance of uncertainty which will likely collude with part of the client's own problem formulation. Other trainees might set impossible standards for themselves ('all my client's must reach recovery!') and therefore impossible standards for their clients ('what do you mean you haven't done your homework?!'). Trainees sometimes become aware that they are getting frustrated with their client's lack of progress or engagement and what the impact upon them will likely be; they then criticise themselves for doing so and overcompensate by colluding with client avoidance. This often means they begin working harder than the client, thwarting opportunities for client agency in the change process. Other trainees may focus entirely on executing the technical aspects of CBT practice, seeing this as a marker of their competence. This can result in sessions that are delivered didactically and mechanically, without attention to being present with the client and relating to them empathetically, hampering the therapeutic alliance and progress therein. What is common in each of these scenarios, is that the thera-pist's needs (to feel 'good enough', to be seen as competent, to be liked), play out in a way which detracts from the client's needs. Often this happens outside of the therapist's awareness, and this is why it is so important that as trainee and quali-fied therapists, we commit to monitoring our own emotional arousal and schema activation in our therapeutic work, and take steps to minimise the impact upon the client's therapy journey.

Perfectionism as a barrier to self-care

Whilst there are many trainee coping responses in the multidimensional context of perfectionism that as trainers and supervisors we can see and observe – and hope-fully intervene over – there are other more covert responses that can remain unseen. For many trainees, this comes in the form of excessive self-criticism and self-doubt, often helped along by healthy dollop of 'compare and despair' where everyone else on the training programme appears to be doing so much better than them. This is not a fun place to be. The emotional experiences that accompany these unhelpful thinking styles might vary from sadness or shame to anxiety or frustration – but all are difficult. Many trainees will respond to these thoughts and feelings with a range of compensatory behaviours, and ones that often involve working too hard, working too long, and working on days they shouldn't be. The consequence of this is rarely an emerging sense of accomplishment and triumph. Usually, it means that trainees stop making space for all of the things that nourish them and keep them resilient and steadfast: hobbies or fun activities begin to disappear; connections with loved ones, friends, and family become less frequent; self-care and relaxa-tion becomes something that there's just 'no time for'. In essence, things begin to feel even tougher. Of course, some trainees will find that instead of over-working on course-related activities, they actually begin procrastinating instead. Suddenly, vacuuming the lounge and cleaning out the goldish become far more pressing than completing a case study or self-rating a therapy session recording. As such, trainees can find that they equally get really busy, but not doing the things that they fear they may not do well enough. Again, this response is rarely a helpful one, with procrastination only adding to the list of things that trainees criticise themselves about. All of these things will not happen in a personal silo: trainees are trying to manage the learning journey whilst simultaneously holding a caseload, often in a very busy psychological therapy service. The coming together of these external and internal pressures can be a breeding ground for burnout, and the research supports this relationship. Maladaptive aspects of perfectionism (e.g. self-criticism, rumina-tion, self-imposed demands) have been positively correlated with experiences of burnout (Hill & Curran, 2016); this typically encompasses emotional exhaustion, detachment from others, and a reduced sense of personal competence (Maslach & Jackson, 1981). Once again, the fight to feel 'good enough' has the unintended consequences of the opposite effect.

Conclusion

Reducing perfectionism during training (and beyond)

In conclusion, we know that there are a number of consequences during CBT training when we try too hard to compensate for the inevitable anxieties of role transition. Unfortunately, it's not unusual for perfectionism to become the narrator of the 'not good enough' story, and the more problematic aspects of the phenomenon such as being overly concerned about making mistakes or needing approval from others can lead to uncomfortable emotions and counter-productive behavioural responses.

Jaye has shared his reflections on how he came to understand his own perfectionism through a synthesis of personal and professional factors during the training journey. These insights 'perfectly' encapsulate how we bring our own beliefs, values, and experiences to the training process, and how these then interact with our professional development:

Trainee reflection

Throughout the course, I have identified that my self-worth is associated with achievement and striving for excellence. From my cultural background, this is linked closely to employment and education, and this was ingrained within me from an early age. As such, I have recognised that there is a fear to work with males from the same cultural background – a fear of judgement of whether I would provide a 'good enough' standard of care for them. When ruptures occur in therapy sessions, it activates my schemas of failure. I notice that I offer a lot of reassurance and 'rescuing'. When clients drop out of treatment unexplainably, I notice that I can ruminate about this and must take it to supervision and discuss it with peers several times until I feel satisfied. There have been times when I have catastrophised a client missing a session and thought I may lose my job because I was not 'perfect' in helping all clients gain successful outcomes. Throughout the course, I have had regular thoughts of returning to my previous job role (where I can be 'successful'), yet at the same time, feeling in conflict due to this being a 'back-step'. Moreover, I am very hypervigilant in checking my other peers' progress in comparison to mine.

We should, however, acknowledge that perfectionism is not 'all bad'. If you identify with some of the dimensions of perfectionism listed earlier, it's likely that these will have been helpful or functional for you at various points in your life, and may even be part of the reason for your successes. The final section of this chapter will therefore not advocate for completely erasing any perfectionist traits you might identify with – they are part of who you are. The more helpful stance here is to identify where the various dimensions of perfectionism might be helping or hindering your training journey, and finding ways to do things differently where it is a barrier to your sense of self-efficacy as a budding CBT therapist.

Tips for reflective activities and CBT exercises

1. Which dimensions of perfectionism do you identify with the most? You might consider this question personally and professionally, and see what links there might be. Some of the ideas in this chapter might help you with this question, as might completing a perfectionism measure (e.g. the PI; Hill et al., 2004) or keeping a self-monitoring diary.

2. What sorts of perfectionistic beliefs might be in play within a professional context? You could try to build awareness of this by paying attention to emotional cues within each of the training contexts discussed in this chapter. For example, are you anxious about role-plays? Embarrassed about handing in clinical material for assessment? Frustrated when clients aren't making progress? Stressed about how much there is to do? What beliefs (or expectations) are driving these emotions?

3. How might some of these beliefs manifest behaviourally? What do you do when you feel like this? For example, are there things you are avoiding? Procrastinating over? Worrying or ruminating about? Are you over-working, over-organising, and over-planning? Are you criticising yourself or others?

4. What is the impact of these behavioural manifestations on yourself? And on your clients? How might these behaviours be a) reinforcing some of your beliefs and expectations, b) removing any opportunity to challenge them, and c) eliminating opportunities to receive feedback on your clinical skills?

5. Can you draw out a maintenance cycle of your own perfectionism within the training context? The example in Figure 17.1 might help you with this, as might using the supervisory space to reflect upon these issues further with your supervisor.

6. Can you design a behavioural experiment to begin challenging some of the beliefs that drive your therapist perfectionism cycle? For example, how might you challenge the idea that having a preconceived and detailed plan for every clinical session makes you a better therapist? Or that doing a role-play will result in public humiliation from your peers?

Acknowledgements

Thank you to Jaye for his generosity in allowing me to share his 'Trainee Reflection'.

Further reading

Hill, A. P., & Curran, T. (2016). Multidimensional perfectionism and burnout: A meta-analysis. *Personality and Social Psychology Review, 20*(3), 269–288.

Lombardo, C., Milne, D., & Proctor, R. (2009). Getting to the heart of clinical supervision: A theoretical review of the role of emotions in professional development. *Behavioural and Cognitive Psychotherapy, 37*(2), 207–219.

Presley, V. L., Jones, G., & Marczak, M. (2023). The relationship between therapist experiential avoidance and observed CBT competence during training: A preliminary investigation. *The Cognitive Behaviour Therapist, 16*, e15.

Presley, V. L., Jones, C. A., & Newton, E. K. (2017). Are perfectionist therapists perfect? The relationship between therapist perfectionism and client outcomes in cognitive behavioural therapy. *Behavioural and Cognitive Psychotherapy, 45*(3), 225–237.

References

Haarhoff, B. A. (2006). The importance of identifying therapist schema in cognitive therapy training and supervision. *New Zealand Journal of Psychology, 35*(3), 126–131.

Hayes, S. C., Wilson, K. G., Gifford, E. V., Follette, V. M., & Strosahl, K. (1996). Experiential avoidance and behavioral disorders: A functional dimensional approach to diagnosis and treatment. *Journal of Consulting and Clinical Psychology, 64*(6), 1152–1168. https://doi.org/10.1037/0022-006X.64.6.1152

Hewitt, P. L., & Flett, G. L. (1991). Perfectionism in the self and social contexts: Conceptualization, assessment, and association with psychopathology. *Journal of Personality and Social Psychology, 60*(3), 456–470.

Hill, A. P., & Curran, T. (2016). Multidimensional perfectionism and burnout: A meta-analysis. *Personality and Social Psychology Review, 20*(3), 269–288.

Hill, R. W., Huelsman, T. J., Furr, R. M., Kibler, J., Vicente, B. B., & Kennedy, C. (2004). A new measure of perfectionism: The perfectionism inventory. *Journal of Personality Assessment, 82*(1), 80–91.

Leahy, R. L. (2001). *Overcoming resistance in cognitive therapy.* The Guilford Press.

Lombardo, C., Milne, D., & Proctor, R. (2009). Getting to the heart of clinical supervision: A theoretical review of the role of emotions in professional development. *Behavioural and Cognitive Psychotherapy, 37*(2), 207–219.

Maslach, C., & Jackson, S. (1981). The measurement of experienced burnout. *Journal of Organizational Behavior, 2*(2), 99–113.

Presley, V. L., Jones, G., & Marczak, M. (2023). The relationship between therapist experiential avoidance and observed CBT competence during training: A preliminary investigation. *The Cognitive Behaviour Therapist, 16*, e15.

Presley, V. L., Jones, C. A., & Newton, E. K. (2017). Are perfectionist therapists perfect? The relationship between therapist perfectionism and client outcomes in cognitive behavioural therapy. *Behavioural and Cognitive Psychotherapy, 45*(3), 225–237.

Roscoe, J., & Taylor, J. (2023). Maladaptive therapist schemas in CBT practice, training and supervision: A scoping review. *Clinical Psychology & Psychotherapy, 30*(3), 510–527.

Roscoe, J., Taylor, J., Harrington, R., & Wilbraham, S. (2022). CBT supervision behind closed doors: Supervisor and supervisee reflections on their expectations and use of clinical supervision. *Counselling and Psychotherapy Research, 22*(4), 1056–1067.

Shafran, R., Cooper, Z., & Fairburn, C. G. (2002). Clinical perfectionism: A cognitive-behavioural analysis. *Behaviour Research and Therapy, 40*, 773–791.

Chapter 18

How can we help others if we cannot help ourselves? The importance of self-practice and self-reflection within CBT training

Natalia Barnes

Introduction

Self-practice self-reflection, or SP/SR as it commonly known, is increasingly being recognised as an important aspect if not essential part of becoming a proficient cognitive behavioural therapist (Bennett-Levy, 2019). Engaging in this will provide you with an extra layer of learning according to the declarative procedural reflective (DPR) model (Bennett-Levy, 2006), which I will go on to explain. This chapter will discuss what the DPR model is, with a particular emphasis on the importance of the reflective element made. I have been running a robust SP/SR component of the high-intensity CBT training course at the University of East Anglia since 2021 and have written about how I have done this and the benefits and challenges of this (Barnes, 2022). I am now rolling this out with the fifth cohort to have had this in such a robust way, constantly revising how this is done for trainees to get the best out of this. In this chapter, I am offering an opportunity for trainees to think about how they can do this themselves, regardless of whether this is currently a formal part of your course or not. Good luck on your journey of reflection and in becoming your own therapist. A fictional trainee, Kate, will be used throughout the chapter to highlight key concepts.

> **Key Point:** The key to being a good therapist is to always reflect and adjust, never stay still. By doing your own self-practice and reflections you will learn and grow, by dropping your own safety behaviours you will see a much wider world and open up new opportunities.

What is the DPR model, and how does this relate to SP/SR?

During your training, you will be learning about protocols and skills to treat a variety of disorders; this is known as '*Declarative learning*'. You will then go on to apply this learning to your treatment of client within your clinical work and learn from putting these skills into action, otherwise known as '*Procedural learning*'.

DOI: 10.4324/9781003428527-22

Finally, if you can practice these same skills on yourself, reflect on how that was for you, and then think about what implications this has for you both personally and as a clinician, you will achieve an even higher level of learning; this is the 'Reflective' element, also known as SP/SR.

The DPR model in action

Kate has recently started her training, so far she has been taught:

Declarative information: This is what Kate has learnt from lectures and reading, including some fundamentals of CBT, including cognitive and behavioural theory, and how to complete maintenance cycles and longitudinal formulations with clients.

Procedural: Kate is now trying to put this learning into practice by helping her clients draw their own maintenance cycles and formulations with their own histories, thoughts, and behaviours.

Reflective including SP/SR: Kate reflects on how this is going with her clients but also completes her own formulation. It is only by doing this that she realises that it is quite emotionally difficult to complete a longitudinal formulation, and that it is important to ask questions and be curious by using techniques such as downward arrowing and Socratic questioning to get useful information and make sense of her own problems. She can use this to then understand herself better and also improve her skills as a practitioner.

Why should I do SP/SR?

When I started my career, I trained as a person-centred counsellor. Many therapeutic modalities have either an expectation or strong encouragement to engage in personal therapy, as indeed was I in my training. Why is this important? Think about it like this, as therapists, our job is to enable others to be aware of their own difficulties, how these developed, how these might be maintained, and how clients can overcome these and live a happier and more fulfilling life – all of this, in a safe place providing unconditional positive regard, congruence, and empathy. On top of this, we as humans also have our own backgrounds, difficulties, and challenges we have faced and will continue to face from time to time. We will have our own set of beliefs, ways of seeing ourselves, others, and the future and our own triggers. However, we cannot allow our own beliefs or triggers to interfere with our ability to provide good therapy. We can draw upon the concepts of transference and countertransference to learn more about ourselves and our clients (see Moorey & Byrne, 2019), and having some understanding of their impact on therapy can help us to become more aware of our own feelings and cognitions. We can then use them as an opportunity to learn more about our own contribution to 'stuck points' in therapy

(Prasko et al., 2010). To sum it up, it's not easy. However, it can be incredibly insightful personally and extremely rewarding professionally.

The importance of reflection

The third element of the DPR model, *Reflection*, is increasingly what is being used to maximise therapists learning of skills (Kuyken et al., 2009). The British Association for Behavioural and Cognitive Psychotherapies (BABCP) specifies in their Core Curriculum (2021) that some of the key aspects of therapeutic competence are as follows:

- Reflecting upon and evaluating personal values, clinical competence, and limitations as a CBT practitioner.
- Experiential learning demonstrating how cognitive and behavioural methods can be applied to the self, for example using self-practice/self-reflection.
- Demonstrating an ability to self-care, ensuring fitness to practice and recognising if there is a need for additional support.
- Demonstrating awareness of the self as shaped by individual and cultural diversity.

(BABCP, 2021, page 7)

Example of Kate needing to reflect on her beliefs and behaviours within a therapy session

Kate has now picked up a few clients and is a few weeks into treatment with them. One client with severe depression was not engaging in homework and was telling Kate that they didn't think therapy would be helpful. Kate started to try harder in sessions suggesting activities the client could participate in and trying to guess what thoughts might get in the way. The client was becoming more upset and defensive in session saying that Kate did not understand them and didn't know what she was doing.

Kate was left feeling frustrated and stuck, not looking forward to the sessions with this client and not knowing what else to do.

Can you guess what was going through Kate's mind?

Why do you think this client triggered her to try harder and harder to help?

Why do you think it's important for Kate to pause and think about her own process here?

In order to do SP/SR well, you need to become very aware of your own processes; this is helped by practising CBT interventions on yourself and reflecting on how this went. For example, Kate could ask herself:

- What did I learn about myself? (e.g. awareness of thoughts and functions of certain behaviours)
- What went well and not so well when completing the intervention?
- What are the implications of this for my clinical practice?

Upon using these interventions on yourself, you will be working on your own self-beliefs, otherwise known as your self-schema (*Bennett-Levy, 2006*). This will have many benefits for you, including the following:

1) greater personal awareness;
2) having the tools to work on your own difficulties as a therapist (this is essential in avoiding burnout, increasing self-care, and having more self-compassion);
3) being aware of your limitations and being more attuned to your clients will help you take things less personally, allowing you to take a step back and then do what is best for yourself and the client (rather than making assumptions and jumping in like Kate did and feeling more stuck).
4) finally, greater self-awareness will help us identify when we need to work on our own stuff or identify what might be good to take to supervision and get support with.

This will also benefit your emerging 'therapist self' by

5) improving many aspects of your therapeutic work such as being able to have increased empathy and being able to explain a homework task more clearly;
6) anticipating potential difficulties that can come up and how to adjust our style to overcome these when working with your clients;
7) finally, being more self-aware will help us identify what might be good to take to supervision and get support with.

Key Point: If Kate had worked on her own automatic thoughts and potentially the core beliefs she was being triggered by, she may have been able to identify the client was not looking for answers but needed to think about their own values and take time to do this before generating their own solutions.

Getting started with SP/SR

It is becoming increasingly common for high-intensity CBT courses to have a robust SP/SR element to them (Barnes, 2022), whilst many other courses more informal 'self-practice' exercises throughout such as setting a behavioural experiment or completing a thought record. Others may lack this element altogether, but either way, as a trainee or qualified practitioner, the great thing about SP/SR is you can do this whether guided or on your own (see Bennett-Levy et al., 2014). Research has shown that on the whole, the more trainees engage in SP/SR the more benefits they will get, and the more benefits they get, the more they will engage (Bennett-Levy & Lee, 2014). Despite these benefits, other research has shown that some therapists have strong reservations about its value or the consequences of engaging in SP/SR (Freeston et al., 2019).

Reflective exercise – addressing therapist concerns about SP/SR

What reservations, if any, do you have about engaging in SP/SR whilst doing this course?

Five elements were identified by Bennett-Levy and Lee (2014) as influencing engagement and benefit of SP/SR. These were Course Structure and Requirements, Expectation of Benefit, Feeling of Safety within the Process, Available Personal Resources and Group process. Therefore, I would like you to spend some time reflecting on these elements for yourself prior to commencing on your own SP-SR journey.

Course structure and requirements

Bennett-Levy and Lee (2014) also found that by making SP/SR a course, requirement trainees engaged more. However, before starting the course, you would have likely heard that many trainees find it difficult and fast paced. I would therefore recommend you set yourself some SMART goals (Doran, 1981) for your SP/SR practice, much like you would do with your own clients at the start of therapy. SMART goals are a key principle in CBT (Fenn & Byrne, 2013), and setting these will be a good place to start for you to get maximum benefits (see Table 18.1). You

Table 18.1 SMART Goals

Specific
– How are you going to do this? Where? When? What areas are you wanting to work on?
Measurable
– How many times are you going to do this and for how long? How will you know when you have achieved your goal?
Attainable
– Is this realistic for you to be able to achieve whilst doing the course? Is this sustainable?
Relevant
– Is this relevant to you and your client work? Does this have a value behind it for you and therefore you feel motivated to do this?
Time-related
– Set an initial time frame to give yourself for each task, these can always be modified as you go if needed.

might like to think about much time you can set aside time, which day of the week, the frequency you would like to do this (e.g. daily, weekly, fortnightly), and what interventions you want to prioritise. You could look at your timetable and see what topics are most relevant for you to do a task on yourself and set time aside accordingly to do this.

Examples of SP/SR tasks

Any model or technique that you learn during your training can become a target for SP/SR (e.g. modifying a rule or trying out problem-solving). Here we will focus on completing a formulation and using activity scheduling. One of the tasks I stress as being important to complete is your own formulation. If you are not willing to look at your own difficulties and where these stem from, how these might be maintained and how you can attempt to tackle these, it will be much harder to help a client do this. This process will help you both personally and professionally. If you feel most comfortable you can start with a simple maintenance cycle (e.g. a five areas model or vicious flower) which you will have either already been introduced to, or will be early in your training. I would then advise you complete a longitudinal formulation to get a better understanding of yourself and where your difficulties may stem from.

Let's see how Kate started to draw a longitudinal formulation to help her understand her triggers and behaviours more. Kate asked herself why she often felt triggered in these situations, for example in lectures she often does not want to ask questions in case people think she is stupid. She has also been avoiding playing tapes in supervision other than ones that she thinks are ok and she doesn't want the supervisor and other trainees to think she isn't very good. She sometimes thinks this way in other areas of her life such as thinking she isn't a very good partner or friend. She asked herself questions like 'did I feel like this at any time when I was younger?' and 'What stands out for me in terms of my childhood and adolescence?' Kate also considered 'How did I think about myself when younger and how did I think about others and my environment generally?' Kate came up with the following which mapped out the development of her current difficulties.

Kate's longitudinal formulation

Kates past history

As a child, Kate was bought up by academic parents and two siblings, one was a high achiever at school and the other very good at sport and socialising. Kate felt shy and less competent than her siblings.

When a teenager, Kate struggled to know what she wanted to do at school and just went with what she got best grades at for GCSE. She had one close friend but was pretty shy at school. She got a part-time job but felt anxious and out of her depth whilst her colleagues were quite loud and joked and teased her a bit.

How do you think Kate felt about herself? And others?

As you may have guessed Kate felt, she was inferior to others and that she was not clever. On her worst days, she would call herself stupid and useless. Other people were a bit threatening as they seemed to know more, achieve more and be more confident. Kate also thoughts others were likely to criticise or tease her. She felt the world was just hard work and not that enjoyable.

What rules or assumptions might Kate have?

Kate began to think that unless she tried really hard, people would see she is stupid.

Kate also thought she had to put on a brave face and not show vulnerability or people would tease her and reject her.

So, based on this, what might Kate have been doing in her therapy sessions with the client that was getting worse?

Kate made the assumption that it was her own fault the client was not getting better because she was not a good enough therapist. She therefore thought she needed to try harder to make up for her self-perceived short comings. She avoided supervision based on the assumption her supervisor would also think she was stupid or incompetent and that other trainees may tease her.

Can you see how Kate's difficulties developed and are now being maintained? Because Kate keeps throwing more at the client, the client is actually feeling unheard and frustrated making the situation worse but Kate is not aware why this is and does not seek help hence reinforcing her belief she is incompetent. She is working harder and harder, is not taking a break, and has stopped socialising and self-care because she thinks she just needs to keep studying to get it right.

Based on this information, what techniques can Kate use on herself that might help?

Activity scheduling and time management

One of the main difficulties I hear my trainees come across is time management as you are struggling with the demands of the course, your workplace, your family life and other commitments and also trying to keep up with pleasurable activities.

It would there be beneficial to do some form of activity scheduling to ensure you fit all this in. You will be taught this on your course and can do reading on how best to do this but fundamentally plan out how you would like your week to look in a specific and achievable way and try to stick to this making amendments as you go if it is not working for you, but do not be tempted to skip on a pleasurable activity because you are feeling overwhelmed and stressed for example, as this will often lead to more stress and procrastination rather than releasing stress and then having a clear problem-solving approach. Why don't you use your SMART goals and Values to try to plan in what an average week might look like? You can use a template like below or use your own diary or calendar. You can either put in specific times or leave more generic, everyone works a different way so tailor it to how you best work.

Kate decided to plan her days a little more (see Table 18.2) to ensure she had breaks and times to do more enjoyable activities which would then enable her to have more energy and motivation for study.

Expectation of benefit

Take a moment to reflect on what you would like to get out of SP/SR both on a personally level and as a professional. This is a great opportunity to think about your own difficulties and how you can work on these whilst becoming your own therapist. Professionally, trainees who are able to notice their own NATs, beliefs, and assumptions are more likely to be able to identify when these are being triggered by challenging clients and therefore work on these more effectively. SP/SR

Table 18.2 Activity Scheduling

	Monday
Morning	7:30 am – wake, get ready, and have breakfast whilst reading my fiction book/watching a good sitcom 8:30 am – 30-min walk and listen to music 9.00 am – make a tea and set up computer 9–10:30 am – do some uni work 10:30 am – get up, stretch, walk, or read fiction 10:50 am – make sure notes and tape are ready in the correct place for supervision 11 am–1 pm – supervision
Afternoon	1–1:30 pm – have something healthy to eat and chat to partner or mum 1:30–5 pm – lecture on my break, get up, and stretch, if nice go outside and have a cup of tea
Evening	5–6 pm – make some dinner and eat 6–7 pm – check I am ready for tomorrow; do reading if I am not sure about something 7–10 pm – watch a film with my partner

Table 18.3 Identifying Values

Self-Schema
Have you any particular difficulties that keep cropping up or you are wanting to
   work on now? What skills might be useful for you to use on yourself here?
Family and Friends
Is there anything that you are struggling with that you would benefit having time
   to think about and could use CBT to help you with your friendships or family
   members?
Career
What gets in the way of you making progress or feeling confident on your
   career? Do you need to adjust your work–life balance? Could you benefit
   from problem-solving or goal setting here? Do you need to challenge your
   thoughts?
Hobbies
Are you doing things that make you happy in your spare time? How can you
   make time to prioritise this? Are there things you would like to try out or
   do more of? What is getting in the way and what CBT tools would help you
   achieve this?
Fitness and Health
Are there any ways you can improve your physical health? What might this look
   like in an achievable way? Could you have some SMART goals around this? Or
   incorporate these into an activity schedule?
Client Work
Is there an intervention or skill you are less certain about or struggling with in
   your work with clients? What skill might you benefit from doing more SP-SR
   on so you can improve on this with your clients?
My Therapist Schema
How do see yourself as a therapist? What concerns you the most? Triggers you?
   What do you want to work on and why is this important for you and your
   client work? Can you bring this to supervision or what holds you back from
   this? Could you do some thought challenging about your client work or a
   behavioural experiment for yourself in a session (e.g. using silence, enquiring
   more about a client's anger rather than avoiding it, trying out a technique and
   admitting you are not quite sure and want to have time to think about it and
   come back to it)?

can also help us to create a clear work/life balance Therefore, it is important to
think of what SP/SR activities will be most linked to your own values both personally and as a therapist. I have therefore created a Values worksheet (see Table 18.3)
which I hope will help you work on what you find most important both personally
and professionally.

Feelings of safety within the process

It is important to feel safe whilst using these techniques as you are basically becoming your own therapist and naturally will be thinking about and working on potentially upsetting or anxiety provoking topics. Therefore, it is worth being aware of

what feels achievable to work on by yourself and what you may need support with. Below are some considerations before starting SP/SR.

- Are there any life experiences that feel too distressing to work on by yourself?
- How would you feel sharing certain experiences within an SP/SR group?

Available personal resources

Before commencing on your course, I would recommend you think about what resources you have that you can turn to for support if need be. Think about how you can continue to look after yourself such as spending time talking to your family, partner, close friend, continuing with some form of recreational activity. Also, think about who else you can turn to for support if the SP/SR tasks trigger anything particularly difficult for you such as difficult relationships and traumas. For example, you may need to flag some personal difficulties with a line manager, supervisor, University tutor or advisor, your GP or a therapist depending on what you are needing support with. It may not be easy to work on your own difficulties by any means and therefore having personal support and knowing who to turn to can be essential to ongoing engagement.

Group process

The final factor identified as being beneficial was to make SP/SR a group task to allow people to learn from each other. You may therefore want to share some reflections with peers. Please note, you only have to share the *process* of how you are finding completing the tasks not the *content* if you do not feel safe to do so. For example, you might share what helped you to achieve the task at hand or what got in the way. If you decide to do this, choose who you feel comfortable with and set up an initial meeting with your partner or group to discuss some ground rules to ensure you all feel safe.

Reflective exercise: setting ground rules for SP/SR group work

Is there a group you feel comfortable doing this with? Are you part of an SP/SR group at your university and if not can you create one? Are you part of a group at your workplace and if not can you create one? What ground rules would you like to feel safe in that group setting? What ideas do you have and who do you need to talk to for this to happen?

In addition to the factors above, Farrand et al. (2010) completed some research on the use of blogs to support SP/SR in CBT training. This can help you to remember key learning points, feel supported and build a community feeling. This can also improve supervision because you are actively logging what you are having difficulties implementing on yourself and can make a note to bring this to supervision.

Top tips

- SP/SR offer potential benefits for you personally and professionally.
- There are certain factors you should consider before you start in order to get the best out of this. Spend some time thinking about how to address each factor.
- I would suggest some of the first tasks you do are creating some SMART goals, thinking about your values, completing your own formulation, planning your own activity schedule, and challenging some thoughts.
- Set time to continue to do this regularly, the further you go in your training learning new skills and seeing more clients, the more you will learn if you have time to reflect.
- You may want to create a blogging platform or forum or some kind to note your key learnings for yourself and from others and even have some peer supervision or blog discussions about this learning.
- This could be a journey to a new more fulfilled self; why hold back? Let's start the adventure now.

Conclusion

Although most individuals who engage with SP/SR experience the many benefits of this, some will have adverse reactions (Thwaites et al., 2014). Therefore, it is important to check in with yourself about what might be manageable for you to work on by yourself and when you might need to get specialist help from another therapist. If you feel triggered and unable to cope whilst trying to engage with SP/SR reach out for help from your family, friends, colleagues, GP, or a professional. Think about a safety plan prior to engaging in SP/SR where you think about who you would go to if this becomes too difficult to manage.

Further reading

Gale, C., & Schröder, T. (2014). Experiences of self-practice/self-reflection in cognitive behavioural therapy: A meta-synthesis of qualitative studies. *Psychology and Psychotherapy: Theory, Research and Practice*, 87, 373–392. © 2014 The British Psychological Society.

Laireiter, A.-R., & Willutzki, U. (2003). Self-reflection and self-practice in training of cognitive behaviour therapy: An overview. *Clinical Psychology and Psychotherapy*, 10(1), 19–30.

Thwaites, R., Bennett-Levy, J., Davis, M., & Chaddock, A. (2014). Using self-practice and self-reflection (SP/SR) to enhance CBT competence and metacompetence. In A. Wittington & N. Grey (Eds.), *How to become a more effective CBT therapist: Mastering metacompetence in clinical practice.* Wiley and Sons, Ltd.

References

BABCP. (2021). *Core curriculum reference document.* British Association for Behavioural & Cognitive Psychotherapies.

Barnes, N. (2022). Incorporating SP-SR into a high intensity cognitive behavioural training course within IAPT. *CBT Today.*

Bennett-Levy, J. (2006). Therapist skills: A cognitive model of their acquisition and refinement. *Behavioural and Cognitive Psychotherapy, 34,* 57–78.

Bennett-Levy, J. (2019). Why therapists should walk the talk: The theoretical and empirical case for personal practice in therapist training and professional development. *Journal of Behavior Therapy and Experimental Psychiatry, 62,* 133–145. https://doi.org/10.1016/j.jbtep.2018.08.004

Bennett-Levy, J., & Lee, N. (2014). Self-practice and self-reflection in cognitive behaviour therapy training: What factors influence trainees' engagement and experience of benefit? *Behavioural and Cognitive Psychotherapy, 42,* 48–64.

Bennett-Levy, J., Thwaites, R., Haarhoff, B., & Perry, H. (2014). *Experiencing CBT from the inside out: A self-practice/self-reflection workbook for therapists.* Guilford Publications.

Doran, G. T. (1981). There's a SMART way to write management's goals and objectives. *Management Review, 70*(11), 35–36.

Farrand, P., Perry, J., & Linsley, S. (2010). Enhancing self-practice/self-reflection (SP/SR) approach to cognitive behaviour training through the use of reflective blogs. *Behavioural and Cognitive Psychotherapy, 38,* 473–477. https://doi.org/10.1017/S1352465810000238

Fenn, K., & Byrne, M. (2013). The key principles of cognitive behavioural therapy. *InnovAiT, 6*(9), 579–585. https://doi.org/10.1177/1755738012471029

Freeston, M. H., Thwaites, R., & Bennett-Levy, J. (2019). 'Courses for horses': Designing, adapting and implementing self practice/self-reflection programmes. *The Cognitive Behaviour Therapist, 12,* e28.

Kuyken, W., Padesky, C., & Dudley, R. (2009). *Collaborative case conceptualization.* Guilford Press.

Moorey, S., & Byrne, S. (2019). Interpersonal schemas: Understanding transference and countertransference in CBT. In S. Moorey & A. Lavender (Eds.), *The therapeutic relationship in cognitive behavioural therapy.* Sage. https://doi.org/10.4135/9781526461568.n19

Prasko, J., Diveky, T., Grambal, A., Kamaradova, D., Mozny, P., Sigmundova, Z., Slepecky, M., & Vyskocilova, J. (2010). Transference and countertransference in cognitive behavioral therapy. *Biomedical Papers, 154*(3), 189–197.

Chapter 19

Keeping the shore in sight – how to be flexible in your practice whilst retaining the core principles of CBT?

Jason Roscoe and Denika Campbell-Lee

Introduction

Cognitive behavioural therapy (CBT) has been shown to be an effective therapy for a range of mental health problems (NICE, 2011). Whilst protocols exist for standalone 'disorders', many clients present with comorbidity, often chronic in nature and having failed to benefit from medication or other forms of therapy (Butler et al., 2008; Davidson, 2008). Similarly, the situation/environment surrounding clients may also contribute to their difficulties, making their treatment more complex than 'standard' cases (Moloney & Kelly, 2004). Disorder-specific models and treatment plans can work extremely well for therapists some of the time (Scott, 2018); however, the clinical reality for many CBT practitioners is having to formulate and work with extensive comorbidity and/or chronic difficulties (Roscoe & Wilbraham, 2024) with less frequent supervision than observed in randomised control trials (Roth et al., 2010).

Common challenges

In addition to chronicity and comorbidity, we can often be met with various forms of resistance (Leahy, 2001) from seemingly unmotivated clients or those who experience persistent interpersonal problems that might be described as 'personality disorders' (Davidson, 2008). Alternatively, when working in contexts such as private practice, clients might present with sub-threshold difficulties where they have some, but not all the symptoms of an identifiable disorder or have difficulties where there is no established protocol (e.g. relationship jealousy; Leahy, 2018).

Understandably, novice therapists are prone to wanting to do things 'right' yet in these instances, being too rigid in our application of CBT might alienate and invalidate the client. Alternatively, we might end up applying a treatment to a problem that the client does not have (e.g. CBT for GAD when their worry makes sense given their current stressors). When faced with these dilemmas, it can also be tempting to move away from the model completely, yet being too unstructured or unfocused or having a 'pick and mix' approach to the interventions we use can be problematic and lead us towards 'therapist drift' (Waller, 2009).

DOI: 10.4324/9781003428527-23

Key Point: Working with ambivalent or resistant clients or those who express significant hopelessness about change can become emotionally tiring over a course of therapy and tends to generate strong emotions in therapists such as hopelessness, anger, anxiety, and shame (Ellis et al., 2018). This can lead CBT therapists to assume that if therapy is not proceeding as they expect, it is either due to their incompetence or the inherent failure of CBT as a modality.

One of the key strengths of CBT has been its capacity and willingness to incorporate a broad range of interventions within its umbrella (Beck, 1995). This chapter discusses how to strike the balance between using skills to adapt CBT to fit the needs of individual clients (applying 'meta-competencies') and ensuring that we do not drift too far from the core principles of CBT in the process (Beck, 1995; Roth & Pilling, 2007).

Defining complexity

Complexity can be considered when a client 'presents with a combination of chronic unresponsive problems; comorbidity; psychotic symptoms; enduring difficulties with relationships; and/or pervasive social problems' (Binnie, 2012, p. 480). Furthermore, neurodivergence as well as challenges that clients face due to various forms of discrimination add extra layers of complexity when formulating and planning equitable interventions (Roscoe & Wilbraham, 2024). Additionally, cases can be seen as complex when several factors (e.g. client, therapist, and healthcare factors – limited session numbers) interrelate in a manner that creates obstacles to the therapeutic alliance needed to facilitate effective therapy (Campbell-Lee, 2023).

The 'textbook-clinical reality disparity'

Clients can find themselves falling into the gap between what primary care psychological services can offer and the inclusion criteria for accessing secondary mental health teams. Talking Therapies for Anxiety and Depression (TTAD), formerly known as Improving Access to Psychological Therapies (IAPT) services, have historically taken on many clients who are rejected from Community Mental Health Teams, yet struggle to achieve the same level of recovery rates when treating more complex clients (Moran et al., 2003). For example, Goddard et al. (2015) found that patients who scored higher on a screening tool for personality difficulties had less favourable outcomes in IAPT services.

Is the tail wagging the dog?

Although CBT therapists are employed across a range of services (e.g. Eating Disorders), it is primary care that has been the main provider of CBT in England since the rollout of the IAPT programme in 2008 (National Collaborating Centre for Mental Health, 2019). Furthermore, CBT is recommended by both 'The Matrix' in Scotland (National Health Service Education for Scotland, NES, 2011) and 'Matrics Cymru' in Wales, recommend cognitive behavioural therapy (CBT) as the main evidence-based treatment for several mental health disorders (National Psychological Therapies Management Group & Public Health Wales, 2016). The curriculum content of many UK-based CBT courses is heavily influenced by the disorder-specific models that emerged in the 1980s and 1990s (e.g. Clark, 1986). Each one highlights unique factors thought to be causal in maintaining the problem. For example, the catastrophic misinterpretation of physical sensations in Panic Disorder (Clark., 1986). Prior to this, Beck's generic cognitive model provided a transdiagnostic (and arguably simpler) roadmap to understanding one's individual vulnerability to emotional distress (Beck et al., 1979). For example, core beliefs, rules, and assumptions and their origins help to make sense of several psychological difficulties (e.g. the presence of Major Depressive Disorder and Generalised Anxiety Disorder). Due to their emphasis on maintaining factors, some of the disorder-specific models do not elicit core beliefs or early experiences (e.g. Model for Generalized Anxiety Disorder; Robichaud & Dugas, 2006). The consideration of longitudinal factors might help to explain the understandable emergence of an anxiety disorder in the context of one's formative experiences (Roscoe, 2020), yet some trainees have reported difficulties in their confidence in using longitudinal formulation (Roscoe & Wilbraham, 2024).

Individual differences in how CBT is understood and practised

> **Key Point:** It is possible that too much emphasis is being placed on understanding separate models in CBT training, at the expense of trainees understanding the common themes across disorders (e.g. Clark, 1999).

Rigidity versus flexibility

Where pieces of the formulation jigsaw are missing, it is understandable that novice CBT therapists (who are still acquiring the basic competencies) are especially prone to rigidity. For example, 'the protocol says X so I cannot do Y' or questioning how applicable some formulations and treatment plans (or even CBT per se) are to the populations they serve (Moloney & Kelly, 2004). It has also been found that therapists' can consciously or unconsciously underuse CBT techniques (Hernandez et al., 2021). For example, the unconscious underuse may occur due to factors such as clinicians' anxiety (Deacon & Farrell, 2013; Peters-Scheffer et al., 2013). Therapist rigidity and underutilisation of key 'ingredients' of CBT are threat to the utility of CBT as an effective treatment (Waller, 2009).

Super-shrinks

Okiishi et al. (2003) introduced the idea of 'super-shrinks' (also known as 'meta-competent' therapists), whose clients have substantial levels of reduced symptoms, more frequent higher rates of recovery and show quicker clinical improvements. These meta-competent therapists appear to demonstrate skills which allows them to offer interventions that address individual client needs (Campbell-Lee, 2023). Roth and Pilling (2007) coined the term 'CBT-specific meta-competencies', which relates to the implementation of CBT representing its underlying principles and the application of specific techniques (e.g. capacity to formulate/apply CBT models to the individual clients). This suggests we *can* learn to work flexibly with our clients whilst continuing to adhere to the core structure of CBT. However, despite there being scope for therapist creativity, some practitioners knowingly or unknowingly omit or underemphasise key aspects, such as formulation or active work within sessions (Waller, 2009). This is known as Therapist Drift. The next section introduces the idea of Therapist drift, and its potential influence on therapeutic work.

Therapist drift

Therapist drift is commonly described as CBT therapists' failing to or inadequately delivering treatments they have been trained in, even when they have been provided with the necessary resources to deliver in an acceptable way (Cowdrey & Waller, 2015). For example, the omission or dilution of key ingredients such as exposure in anxiety disorders. The idea of therapist drift appears to be specific to CBT, and is derived from the notion of intervention fidelity, which is arguably applicable to other modalities (e.g. Psychodynamic). Therapists' deviation can result in patients not receiving cognitive behavioural therapy (CBT) described in the evidence-based literature (Waller & Turner, 2016).

Although CBT has the largest evidence base when compared to all other psychotherapeutic treatments (Dobson., 2010), there are aspects of therapy that can be difficult for both patients and therapists. Whilst patients may find it potentially stressful to experience exposure to aversive memories, therapists can also find the implementation of CBT potentially threatening. For both patient and therapist there may be a perceived inability to apply coping resources to perceived stressors (e.g. the difficulties of a therapeutic task). Generally, the main coping resource for therapists has been their clinical skills; however, as a result of this perceived inability, it is has been suggested that many therapists drift away from treatment protocol (Thompson-Brenner & Westen, 2005).

Consequences of drift

According to Cukrowicz et al. (2011), using evidence-based manuals result in better clinical outcomes compared to unstructured approaches. Nevertheless, there are therapists who do not fully adhere to protocols. Research found that therapists treating patients with panic disorder, who do not adhere to treatment protocols, poorer outcomes can be predicted (Huppert et al., 2001). As mentioned previously, lack of treatment adherence can be part of a conscious decision such as some therapists rejecting the use of manuals (Addis & Krasnow, 2000). Therapists may reject manuals because they view it as having a negative impact on the treatment process (e.g. compromising therapist creativity; Henry, 1998). Wiborg et al. (2012) also found that negative attitudes towards manuals can lead to poorer CBT outcomes. On the other hand, some research highlights the benefits and importance of individualised formulation (Kuyken et al., 2009). This approach considers difficulties in a personalised way and can help clients gain a greater understanding of their clinical problems (Redhead et al., 2015). Nonetheless, some therapists may misunderstand this as permission to stray from the model-based formulation.

The challenges in defining therapist drift

Necessary modifications to protocols

Although there is a 'core' conceptualisation of drift in the literature, 'moving away from traditional protocol', some authors use different terminology relating to this definition (Campbell-Lee, 2023). After commenting on the discrepancies within literature relating to drift, Toomey et al. (2020) recommended clarifying how fidelity (or drift) is defined and understood. Much of the research focuses on therapist factors (e.g. therapist attitudes; Levita et al., 2016) to provide explanations for why therapists drift in CBT. However, this can be seen as problematic, as it remains unclear exactly what does and does not constitute drift; is it drift, or is it individualisation/adaptation? For example, Marques et al. (2019) discovered that some components can be modified to better suit the client. They suggest it is important for therapists to understand and discern which components can be altered, and which should be maintained. Furthering this, recent research describes the importance of cultural adaptations in CBT (Hanchard, 2019) as the therapy has been noted to conflict with cultural values at times (e.g. Kingdon et al., 2015). In more recent years, research has begun demonstrating that CBT can be successfully applied, even when the therapist has drifted from the traditional model.

Differential focus in protocols

Whilst avoidance and safety-seeking behaviours appear to obviously dilute the potential effects of CBT, other clinical adaptions require further consideration. For example, the term 'exposure' is used interchangeably with 'behavioural experiments' within CBT, yet historically the former term refers to the use of a habituation-based approach to the treatment of anxiety disorders. In the UK, many training courses are influenced by Cognitive Therapy where clients are encouraged to face feared objects or situations but rather than 'exposing' them to the point of habituation, the idea is that they stay in the situation long enough for belief change to occur (Bennett-Levy et al., 2004). In this respect, the underutilisation of exposure by cognitive therapists would not equate to drift as they are merely adopt-ing a different stance towards CBT treatment as would be the case of how reliving is used in Ehlers and Clark (2000) PTSD protocol.

Shining a light on factors that contribute to drift

For the purpose of this chapter, we will focus on the two most commonly cited rea-sons for drift; – skills deficits (Wisniewski et al., 2018) and dysfunctional therapist beliefs (Roscoe & Taylor, 2023). Skills deficits often improve as one progresses through training but occasionally, they persist and need additional targeting in supervision. Therapist beliefs are not always explicitly identified by trainees or their supervisors (see Haarhoff, 2006) and may need to be specifically targeted through self-practice/self-reflection (SP/SR) exercises (Barnes, 2022).

Spotting drift in practice

We shall now look to explain the difference between drift (actual omissions) and the use of meta-competencies, which helps therapy to remain faithful to the core principles of CBT yet flexible enough to take account of the individual client (Roth & Pilling, 2007). The case study below illustrates a more 'clear-cut' case of drift in that the clinician (David) fails to deliver the active ingredients of the GAD protocol with his client Becky due to his passivity in sessions. David is a fictional therapist as is his client Becky, yet they are representative of many cases that Jason has helped to supervise.

Case study 1: Drift

David worked in a primary care CBT service and was providing sessions via an online platform. He had been a person-centred counsellor prior to CBT training.

David found it difficult to contain and focus his client Becky who he was supposed to be treating for Generalised Anxiety Disorder (GAD). Each session she would attend as highly anxious about a new situation that she worried about that week.

David would let Becky talk about this at length and hoped that he would find an 'opening' in the conversation to set an agenda, but it never came. Often it would be 15 minutes into the session before David felt he could speak.

David brought this case to supervision after seven sessions stating that no progress had been made. He had yet to create a formulation and had not delivered any model-specific interventions. This was also reflected in the absence of changes to Becky's minimum data set scores.

Understanding the beliefs and contexts that can perpetuate drift

Having read David's story, you might find yourself identifying with this clinical scenario. There are several questions to consider that might help to understand how drift arose. Examples are as follows:

- Was online the only medium for working with this client? Would face to face have changed the dynamic?
- Why was David able to see this client for seven sessions without supervision?
- Was role transition from counselling to CBT addressed within supervision?
- Was Becky informed of what CBT would entail at the point of entry to the service?

A recent literature review (Campbell-Lee, 2023) revealed some common reasons for therapist drift (e.g. therapist personalities) (Waller et al., 2016), which centralises the therapists' role in causing drift. This can be seen as unbalanced, and some studies recommended that causes should be measured individually at therapist level, client level, and service delivery setting. It has been demonstrated that the strength of the therapeutic relationship and therapeutic change can be related (Waller & Turner, 2016), indicating that both therapist and client can have an impact on how therapy is delivered. The manner in which therapy is implemented is not solely dependent on the therapist, but can also depend on the capacity of the service and client factors. Further to this, many services have introduced remote therapy (e.g. via telephone), which can also increase the risk of therapist drift (Faija et al., 2020).

The activation of maladaptive therapist schemas

From a therapist schema perspective, David might fear upsetting or angering Becky (Leahy, 2001), or he may lack the skills to effectively pause and refocus clients due to insufficient 'declarative knowledge' (e.g. missed teaching days on specific topics) or lack of 'procedural' knowledge' from sufficient hours building skills in this area (Bennett-Levy, 2006).

These assumptions tend to share the same themes – intolerance of uncertainty and fear of upsetting clients. The above is not an exhaustive list but research suggests these are common and tend to be associated with maladaptive therapist schemas such as rejection-sensitivity (Leahy, 2001; Roscoe & Taylor, 2023).

Negative beliefs about aspects of CBT formulation or treatment

The third reason relates to negative beliefs that CBT therapists hold about CBT formulations or interventions. Rather than a fear of the outcome, these beliefs are more related to the values that some therapists hold about client care or what a therapist is there to do (see Lee et al., 2013).

Common therapist assumptions associated with drift

Focusing the client

If I interrupt the client whilst they are talking then it means I am rude and invalidating.

If I focus the client with an agenda, I might miss important details that are relevant to the formulation.

Utilising specific CBT methods

If I make the client relive their traumatic experiences, I will retraumatize them.

Handling high levels of affect

If the client becomes distressed during exposure, I should back off and soothe them instead.

Plugging gaps in 'wave two' protocols

Therapists can feel that disorder-specific protocols overlook key aspects of a client's problems (e.g. emotional regulation), and drawing on third-wave or integrative approaches (e.g. DBT) can be seen to 'plug' these gaps (Kennedy & Pearson, 2020). For example, Roscoe (2020) carried out a straw poll via a CBT practitioner forum on social media, and 94 out of 109 respondents (86%) endorsed the statement 'I blend techniques from EMDR/CFT/ACT into CBT treatment'.

Keeping the shore in sight

It is likely that most CBT therapists will identify with at least one of the reasons given for drifting. If we assume that drift is both common and at times necessary, we need a simple way of gauging when this is happening. One way of helping this 'stick' in our mind is the use of a metaphor. Here we propose viewing the evidence-based models and related interventions like an island.

Rowing in the same direction

As therapists, it is like we are in a rowing boat, holding an oar, and we are often in choppy waters. The sea conditions might represent either the clinical context in which we are working (e.g. limited session numbers) or the session-by-session mood state of the client we are treating. The current of the ocean at times, might move us further away from the island. What has not been mentioned yet is that the client is also in the boat with us and has an oar too. The client might want to row in the opposite direction to the shore and at times, we can find ourselves in a battle of strength to see who 'wins'. This can often be referred to as an 'unspoken tug of war' as was the case with David and Becky. We are trying to pull the client towards an agenda and a focused conversation whilst the client is trying to pull us into a supportive chat or to act as a sounding board for their most recent concern.

Losing sight of the shore

No matter how experienced we are as therapists, we cannot stop the weather conditions and we cannot make the client row with us. What we can do is keep an eye on where the shore of the island is, at any given time. Examples are as follows:

- Have we got closer to the shore as the sessions have gone on?
- Are we very far away, so far that it is almost out of sight?

Gauging this requires the skill of 'reflection in action' (Schon, 1987) and helping the client to see this too often involves 'meta-communication' (Katzow & Safran, 2007). These are incredibly hard competencies to master and being that attuned to every client, week in week out is nigh on impossible. Due to human limitations, we might have to accept that some 'drift' is inevitable, especially as some studies do outline the inevitability of drift (e.g. Hanchard, 2019). Recent research by Campbell-Lee et al. (2024) found evidence of therapists using a putative meta-competency (reflection), which may encourage them to individualise therapy, and move away from standardised protocol to work with complexity. Consequently, reflection can also help therapists adhere to a protocol (*how do I deliver it in this particular situation?*), which gives more reason for researchers to examine the effects of drift, exploring whether it can have positive implications, and whether factors such as complexity makes drift more inevitable. Furthermore, in the service of developing a 'good enough' rapport with the client, allowing some drift from shore in early sessions to row closer later in treatment might be warranted.

Accepting short-term drift for rowing towards the shore 'together' in the long term

Weck et al. (2015) discovered that when alliance facilitated competence, it was associated with treatment outcome, which supports Waller's (2009) claim that as well as needing to apply CBT appropriately, it is also vital for there to be an effective working relationship. This arguably indicates that drift can be influenced by therapeutic alliance. For example, the client might have a history of feeling invalidated and trying to row to shore too soon might reinforce this and trigger a rupture (Leahy, 2001). Consequently, the therapist drifts from protocol in the short term to maintain the rapport in order to collaboratively row to shore in the long term.

Using meta-competencies to manage complexity

Arguably, the impact of clinical complexity has been under-emphasised in current competence measures (e.g. CTS-R), perhaps due to these scales being developed for core competencies with assumed standard cases (Blackburn et al., 2001). In an attempt to address this, Roth and Pilling (2007) included 'meta-competencies' (generic; necessary for therapists of any theoretical orientation; and CBT specific; capacity to formulate/apply CBT models to the individual clients) in their list of competencies which are to be used in the competent delivery of CBT treatments.

Levels of competence

Figure 19.1 illustrates the framework developed by Campbell-Lee et al. (2024) that offers an alternative way to consider differing levels of therapist skill: Level 1 – therapist skills for *particular* problems (e.g. reassurance seeking recognition in Heath Anxiety); Level 2 – skills demonstrating the delivery of core aspects in a competent and replicable way for all disorders (e.g. reviewing homework); and Level 3 – skills which facilitate the decision of which core aspects should be prioritised, considering the client's presentation and stage of treatment (e.g. formulation over goal setting). Level 3 skills also optimise therapy delivery in regard to client needs with particular problems (e.g. clients with highly recurrent difficulties requiring additional time and encouragement to collaborate with decision-making).

All skill levels are of equal importance; therefore, Level 3 skills do not replace Level 1 and 2 skills. The difference is that meta skills at Level 3 co-ordinate and organise the other skills which helps therapists understand how to apply CBT to the specific needs of the client. Level 3 is where more experienced therapists are expected to operate, given that complex client presentations tend to require a higher level of decision-making for therapists.

> **Key Point:** It is the *co-ordination* of all three levels that leads to therapy being skilfully applied and appropriately personalised.

It is hypothesised that as therapists move towards proficient and expert levels (Dreyfus., 2011), they are more likely to develop and demonstrate meta-competencies, incorporating Level 3 into their practice. For example, an experienced therapist with meta skills, may prioritise building the therapeutic relationship over agenda setting in a therapy session. Another example is, when it is unclear which aspect of a co-morbid presentation to prioritise, these therapists would implement procedural and declarative knowledge which is required of competent therapists, but these skills would also be regulated by reflection (a meta-competency) to effectively consider client need (Bennett-Levy., 2006). This is where 'rowing away from the shore' temporarily helps to keep therapy viable in the long run. It is hypothesised that Arguably, meta-competent therapists are likely

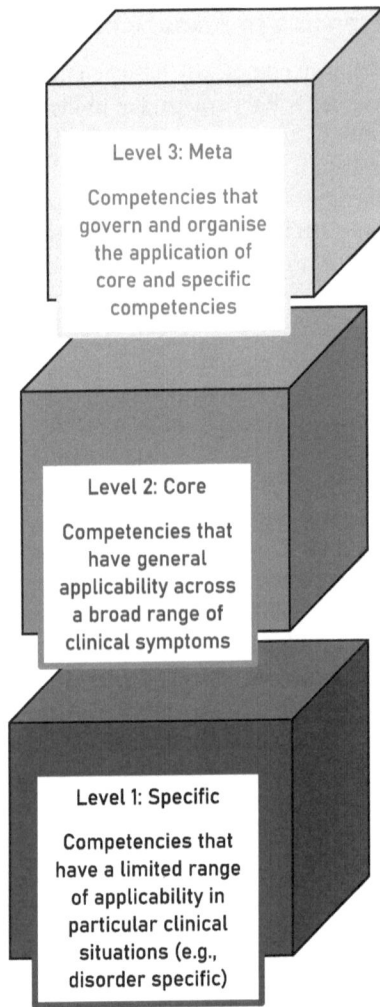

Figure 19.1 CBT competency blocks

to prioritise the application of particular skills. However, this is not to say that therapists in training trainee do not have meta skills, just that they have had less opportunity for their meta-competencies to develop.

Key Point: The capacity to individualise and prioritise is the function that meta-competencies support and is therefore highly likely to be needed in complex, difficult-to-treat, and/or atypical cases.

The importance of adequate reflection

Campbell-Lee et al. (2024) found evidence consistent with the capacity to reflect being a meta-competence. Differences between more experienced and trainee therapists were discovered in their capacity to reflect on complex scenarios. As therapists are required to attune their skills to work with complexity, this evidence suggests that reflective capacity increases over time, especially as therapists are likely to be exposed to more complex cases over their careers. Furthermore, reflection is deemed more necessary when working with complex cases, due to protocols requiring therapists to be flexible, possess adequate problem-solving abilities, and have the capability to respond to unexpected circumstances working with a range of presenting clients (Milne et al., 2001) to differences in client presentation and unexpected circumstances.

Case study 2: Flexible use of CBT drawing upon meta-competences

Nicola had been working with her client John for three sessions and had found it difficult to contain him as he would come into sessions and launch into a ruminative monologue about a range of situations in his life that felt unjust.

Looking at her formulation that she had managed to develop to this point, Nicola recognised that John had been resistant to low-intensity CBT that he had received previously as he felt it was dismissive of his feelings. Nicola validated John's feelings by summarising what he was saying but then directed the conversation back to their agreed goals. Nicola put this on the agenda for discussion and John agreed to do a functional analysis on this behaviour.

John realised that his rumination was 'eating into' time to work on managing his depression and they agreed that John would have a five minute 'check in' at the very start to 'feel heard' and after that point Nicola would set the agenda.

Utilising a defusion method from acceptance and commitment therapy (ACT), they also agreed that if John got 'hooked' on any ruminative thoughts later in the session that they would both try to spot this and find a way to refocus on the agreed session items.

Meta-competencies versus drift

What the two vignettes of David and Nicola have in common are the adaptation of a manualised approach to treatment in response to the individual client. In the first one, David is not using meta-competencies, he is failing to take charge of the session, perhaps due to a maladaptive assumption about what it means to interrupt a client. He is not providing the client with an evidence-based treatment, and after the 12 sessions are up, the client is likely to leave having learned very little about how to manage her GAD. In other words, the shore was nowhere in sight.

If this session had been recorded, it would have failed on several criterion of the CTS-R (Blackburn et al., 2001). For example, agenda setting, pacing, collaboration, and conceptual integration were all seriously impeded by David's inability to focus Becky on the goals of treatment.

In contrast, Nicola does use her meta-competencies. Firstly, she accepts that to engage David in treatment, she needs to allow a small amount of the session to be unfocused. However, Nicola 'keeps the shore in sight' by agreeing that they will time the unfocused element with a stopwatch, and after five minutes, they will set the agenda. Secondly, Nicola uses some skills that she has learned from an ACT workshop to help David to 'unhook' from thoughts that he becomes highly 'fused' with at times (Harris, 2013). The use of the 'Press Pause' technique allowed Nicola to keep therapy focused and did not push their rowing boat further out to sea. Whilst Press Pause does not feature in any of the disorder-specific literature, it can be utilised without compromising the core principles of CBT practice (Beck, 1995).

Key points

- Most therapists will drift in certain contexts, whether that is at the start of their CBT career or many years in. For example, therapists might fail to impose structure with some problems (e.g. depression) whilst being too rigid with others (e.g. GAD).
- Drift may also arise through a desire to plug perceived gaps in existing CBT protocols, or it may relate to dysfunctional therapist assumptions (e.g. fears of upsetting the client; resistance towards the structure or style of CBT).
- Conscious efforts to develop reflection (meta-competency) will help therapists to justify their drift based on the needs of the client, and consideration of the complexity of the case.
- Self-practice of CBT (e.g. SP/SR) and good-quality supervision can enhance self-reflective skills and help identify and work through drift as and when it arises.

Top tips

- Before deviating from an established formulation or intervention, pause and ask yourself 'why am I doing this?'. Is the change justified by certain obstacles in treatment (e.g. emotional dysregulation) or is it due to personal preference (e.g. for third-wave approaches) or a dislike for the structure of CBT/aspects of a specific model?

- Consider if you have the requisite skills to deliver an ancillary intervention from another modality (e.g. you have been trained to use compassion-focused methods). It is also advisable to check what additional modalities your supervisor is trained in.
- If you are a supervisor reading this chapter, then try to normalise drift with your supervisees and the need to adapt protocols to meet the needs of clients. Consider sharing some of your own experiences of meta-competence practice, drift, and the lessons you have learned from this.

Conclusion

A significant proportion of trainee CBT therapists worry about 'getting it right' which can result in rigidity or avoidance due to fear of failure. The good news for them is that moving 'away from the shore' temporarily does not constitute drift, but rather a treatment plan that takes account of the client's formulation and presentation, session by session whilst retaining the core principles of CBT. Although the difference might appear subtle, this is not the same as changing focus every session whereby no progress is made on the agreed goals for therapy. When thinking about client complexity, it could be that therapists moving away from traditional protocol are using meta-competencies, to manage multiple complexities (there are many other examples that could be provided where specific techniques from 'third-wave' and integrative therapies can augment standard CBT, or examples where traditional CBT is adapted, without compromising the core principles).

Further reading

Campbell-Lee, D., Barton, S., & Armstrong, P. (2024). Higher-order CBT skills: Are there differences in meta-competence between trainee and experienced therapists? *The Cognitive Behavioural Therapist*, *17*(7), 1–3. https://doi.org/10.1017/S1754470X24000047

Roscoe, J. (2020). Rethinking therapist drift: Incompetence or ingenuity? *CBT Today*, *48*(1), 10–11.

Waller, G., & Turner, H. (2016). Therapist drift redux: Why well-meaning clinicians fail to deliver evidence-based therapy, and how to get back on track. *Behaviour Research and Therapy*, *77*, 129–137. https://doi.org/10.1016/j.brat.2015.12.005

References

Addis, M. E., & Krasnow, A. D. (2000). A national survey of practicing psychologists' attitudes toward psychotherapy treatment manuals. *Journal of Consulting and Clinical Psychology*, *68*(2), 331–339. https://doi.org/10.1037/0022-006X.68.2.331

Barnes, N. (2022). Incorporating SP-SR into a high intensity cognitive behavioural training course within IAPT. *CBT Today*.

Beck, J. S. (1995). *Cognitive therapy: Basics and beyond* (1st ed.). Guilford Press.

Beck, A. T., Rush, A. J., Shaw, B. F., & Emery, G. (1979). *Cognitive therapy of depression.* Guilford Press.

Bennett-Levy, J. (2006). Therapist skills: A cognitive model of their acquisition and refinement. *Behavioural and Cognitive Psychotherapy, 34*(1), 57–78. https://doi.org/10.1017/S1352465805002420

Bennett-Levy, J., Westbrook, D., Fennell, M., Cooper, M., Rouf, K., & Hackmann, A. (2004). Behavioural experiments: Historical and conceptual underpinnings. In Bennett-Levy, J, Butler, G, Fennell, M, Hackman, A, Mueller, M & Westbrook, D (Eds.), *Oxford guide to behavioural experiments in cognitive therapy* (pp. 1–20). Oxford University Press.

Binnie, J. (2012). Using cognitive behavioural therapy with complex cases: Using the therapeutic relationship to change core beliefs. *Issues in Mental Health Nursing, 33*(7), 480–485.

Blackburn, I. M., James, I. A., Milne, D. L., Reichelt, F. K., Garland, A., Baker, C., & Claydon, A. (2001). *Cognitive therapy scale-revised (CTS-R).* Newcastle Cognitive and Behavioural Therapies Centre.

Butler, G., Fennell, M., & Hackman, A. (2008). *Cognitive behavioural therapy for anxiety disorders.* The Guilford Press.

Campbell-Lee, D. (2023). *A doctoral thesis examining the field of therapist drift in cognitive behavioural therapy, and the exploration of meta-competence in cognitive behavioural therapy* [Doctoral thesis, Newcastle University].

Campbell-Lee, D., Barton, S., & Armstrong, P. (2024). Higher-order CBT skills: Are there differences in meta-competence between trainee and experienced therapists? *The Cognitive Behavioural Therapist, 17*(7), 1–3. https://doi.org/10.1017/S1754470X24000047

Clark, D. M. (1986). A cognitive approach to panic. *Behaviour Research and Therapy, 24*(4), 461–470.

Clark, D. M. (1999). Anxiety disorders: Why they persist and how to treat them. *Behaviour Research and Therapy, 37*(1), S5.

Cowdrey, N. D., & Waller, G. (2015). Are we really delivering evidence-based treatments for eating disorders? How eating-disordered patients describe their experience of cognitive behavioural therapy. *Behaviour Research and Therapy, 75*, 72–77. https://doi.org/10.1016/j.brat.2015.10.009

Cukrowicz, K. C., Timmons, K. A., Sawyer, K., Caron, K. M., Gummelt, H. D., & Joiner, T. E., Jr. (2011). Improved treatment outcome associated with the shift to empirically supported treatments in an outpatient clinic is maintained over a ten-year period. *Professional Psychology: Research and Practice, 42*, 145–152. https://doi.org/10.1037/a0021937

Davidson, K. (2008). *Cognitive therapy for personality disorders: A guide for clinicians.* Routledge.

Deacon, B. J., & Farrell, N. R. (2013). Therapist barriers to the dissemination of exposure therapy. In E. A. Storch & D. McKay (Eds.), *Handbook of treating variants and complications in anxiety disorders* (pp. 363–373). Springer Science + Business Media. https://doi.org/10.1007/978-1-4614-6458-7_23

Dobson, K. (2010). *Handbook of cognitive behavioural therapies.* Guildford Press.

Dreyfus, S. (2011). The five-stage model of adult skill acquisition. *Bulletin of Science Technology & Society, 24*(3), 177. https://doi.org/10.1177/0270467604264992

Ehlers, A., & Clark, D. M. (2000). A cognitive model of posttraumatic stress disorder. *Behaviour Research and Therapy, 38*, 319–345.

Ellis, T. E., Schwartz, J. A., & Rufino, K. A. (2018). Negative reactions of therapists working with suicidal patients: A CBT/mindfulness perspective on "countertransference". *International Journal of Cognitive Therapy, 11*, 80–99.

Faija, C. L., Connell, J., Welsh, C., Ardern, K., Hopkin, E., Gellatly, J., Rushton, K., Fraser, C., Irvine, A., Armitage, C. J., Wilson, P., Bower, P., Lovell, K., & Bee, P. (2020). What influences practitioners' readiness to deliver psychological interventions by telephone?

A qualitative study of behaviour change using the theoretical domains framework. *BMC Psychiatry, 20*(371). https://doi.org/10.1186/s12888-020-02761-3

Goddard, E., Wingrove, J., & Moran, P. (2015). The impact of comorbid personality difficulties on response to IAPT treatment for depression and anxiety. *Behaviour Research and Therapy, 73,* 1–7.

Haarhoff, B. A. (2006). The importance of identifying and understanding therapist schema in cognitive therapy training and supervision. *New Zealand Journal of Psychology, 35,* 126–131.

Harris, R. (2013). *Getting unstuck in ACT: A clinician's guide to overcoming common obstacles in acceptance and commitment therapy.* New Harbinger Publications.

Hanchard, J. (2019). *A deeper look at how therapists experience working with Black clients in clinical practice using cognitive behaviour therapy: A grounded theory* [Unpublished Doctorate Dissertation]. City, University of London.

Henry, W. P. (1998). Science, politics and the politics of science. *Psychotherapy Research, 8*(2), 126–140. https://doi.org/10.1093/ptr/8.2.126

Hernandez, M. E., & Waller, G. (2021). Are we on the same page? A comparison of patients' and clinicians' opinions about the importance of CBT techniques. *Cognitive Behavioural Therapy, 50*(6), 439–451. https://doi.org/10.1080/16506073.2020.1862292

Huppert, J. D., Bufka, L. F., Barlow, D. H., Gorman, J. M., & Shear, M. K. (2001). Therapists, therapist variables, and cognitive-behavioural therapy outcome in a multicentre trial for panic disorder. *Journal of Consulting and Clinical Psychology, 69*(5), 747–755. https://doi.org/10.1037/0022-006X.69.5.747

Katzow, A. W., & Safran, J. D. (2007). Recognizing and resolving ruptures in the therapeutic alliance. In P. Gilbert & R. Leahy (Eds.), *The therapeutic relationship in the cognitivebehavioral psychotherapies* (pp. 90–105). Routledge.

Kennedy, F., & Pearson, D. (2020). *Integrating CBT and third wave therapies: Distinctive features.* Routledge.

Kingdon, D., Rathod, S., Phiri, P., & Pinninti, N. (2015). *Cultural adaptation of cognitive behavioural therapy.* Wiley.

Kuyken, W., Padesky, C. A., & Dudley, R. (2009). *Collaborative case conceptualization: Working effectively with clients in cognitive-behavioural therapy.* Guilford Press.

Leahy, R. (2001). *Overcoming resistance in cognitive therapy.* Guilford Press.

Leahy, R. L. (2018). *The jealousy cure: Learn to trust, overcome possessiveness, and save your relationship.* New Harbinger Publications.

Lee, J. A., Neimeyer, G. J., & Rice, K. G. (2013). The relationship between therapist epistemology, therapy style, working alliance, and interventions use. *American Journal of Psychotherapy, 67*(4), 323–345.

Levita, L., Duhne, P. G. S., Girling, C., & Waller, G. (2016). Facets of clinicians' anxiety and the delivery of cognitive behavioral therapy. *Behaviour Research Therapy, 77,* 157–161. https://doi.org/10.1016/j.brat.2015.12.015

Marques, L., Valentine, S. E., Kaysen, D., Mackintosh, M.-A., Dixon De Silva, L. E., Ahles, E. M., Youn, S. J., Shtasel, D. L., Simon, N. M., & Wiltsey-Stirman, S. (2019). Provider fidelity and modifications to cognitive processing therapy in a diverse community health clinic: Associations with clinical change. *Journal of Consulting and Clinical Psychology, 87*(4), 357–369. https://doi.org/10.1037/ccp0000384

Milne, D. L., Claydon, T., Blackburn, I.-M., James, I. A., & Sheikh, A. (2001). Rationale for a new measure of competence in therapy. *Behavioural and Cognitive Psychotherapy, 29*(1), 21–33. https://doi.org/10.1017/S1352465801001047

Moloney, P., & Kelly, P. (2004). Beck never lived in Birmingham: Why CBT may be a less useful treatment for psychological distress than is often supposed. *Clinical Psychology, 4*–10.

Moran, P., Leese, M., Lee, T., Walters, P., Thornicroft, G., & Mann, A. (2003). Standardised assessment of personality – abbreviated scale (SAPAS): Preliminary validation of a brief screen for personality disorder. *British Journal of Psychiatry*, *183*(3), 228–232. https://doi.org/10.1192/bjp.183.3.228

National Collaborating Centre for Mental Health. (2019). *The improving access to psychological therapies manual*. NHS.

National Health Service Education for Scotland (NES). (2011). *The Matrix. Mental health in Scotland: A guide to delivering evidence-based psychological therapies in Scotland*. Retrieved from http://www.nes.scot.nhs.uk/media/20137/Psychology%20Matrix%20 2013.pdf (accessed April 15, 2017).

National Institute for Health and Clinical Excellence (NICE). (2011). Common mental health disorders. The NICE guideline on identification and pathway to care. *The British Psychological Society and The Royal College of Psychiatrists*, *123*, 222–227.

National Psychological Therapies Management Group and Public Health Wales. (2016). *Matrics Cymru: The Welsh Matrix. A guide to delivering evidence-based psychological therapy in Wales*. Retrieved from http://www.1000livesplus. wales.nhs.uk/ matrics-cymru-draft-consultation (accessed February 15, 2017).

Okiishi, J. C., Lambert, M. J., Nielsen, S. L., & Olgles, B. M. (2003). Waiting for supershrink: An empirical analysis of therapist effects. *Clinical Psychology & Psychotherapy*, *10*(6), 361–373. https://doi.org/10.1002/cpp.383

Peters-Scheffer, N., Didden, R., Korzilius, H., & Sturmey, P. (2013). Therapist characteristics predict discrete trial teaching procedural fidelity. *Intellectual and Developmental Disabilities*, *51*(4), 263–272. https://doi.org/10.1352/1934-9556-51.4.263

Redhead, S., Johnstone, L., & Nightingale, J. (2015). Clients' experiences of formulation in cognitive behaviour therapy. *Psychology and Psychotherapy: Theory, Research and Practice*, *88*(4), 453–467. https://doi.org/10.1111/papt.12054

Robichaud, M., & Dugas, M. J. (2006). A cognitive-behavioral treatment targeting intolerance of uncertainty. In Davey, G.C & Wells. A. (Eds.), *Worry and its psychological disorders: Theory, assessment and treatment* (pp. 289–304). John Wiley & Sons Ltd.

Roscoe, J. (2020). Rethinking therapist drift: Incompetence or ingenuity? *CBT Today*, *48*(1), 10–11.

Roscoe, J., & Taylor, J. (2023). Maladaptive therapist schemas in CBT practice, training and supervision: A scoping review. *Clinical Psychology & Psychotherapy*, 1–18. https://doi.org/10.1002/cpp.2802

Roscoe, J., & Wilbraham, S. (2024). 'When it goes well, it works fantastically': Motivations to train and their impact on the practice of CBT. *The Cognitive Behaviour Therapist*, *17*, e6.

Roth, A. D., & Pilling, S. (2007). *The competences required to deliver effective cognitive and behavioural therapy for people with depression and with anxiety disorders*. HMSO, Department of Health.

Roth, A. D., Pilling, S., & Turner, J. (2010). Therapist training and supervision in clinical trials: Implications for clinical practice. *Behavioural and Cognitive Psychotherapy*, *38*(3), 291–302.

Schon, D. A. (1987). *Educating the reflective practitioner: Toward a new design for teaching and learning in the professions*. Jossey-Bass.

Scott, M. J. (2018). IAPT: The need for radical reform. *The Journal of Health Psychology*, *23*, 1136–1147.

Thompson-Brenner, H., & Westen, D. (2005). Personality subtypes in eating disorders: Validation of a classification in a naturalistic sample. *British Journal of Psychiatry*, *186*(6), 516–524. https://doi.org/10.1192/bjp.186.6.516

Toomey, E., Hardeman, W., Hankonen, N., McSharry, J., Matvienko-Sikar, K., & Lorencatto, F. (2020). Focusing on fidelity: Narrative review and recommendations for improving intervention fidelity within trials of health behaviour change interventions. *Health*

Psychology Behavioural Medicine, 8(1), 132–151. https://doi.org/10.1080/21642850.20 20.1738935

Waller, G. (2009). Evidence-based treatment and therapist drift. *Behaviour Research and Therapy, 47*, 119–127. https://doi.org/10.1016/j.brat.2008.10.018

Waller, G., & Turner, H. (2016). Therapist drift redux: Why well-meaning clinicians fail to deliver evidence-based therapy, and how to get back on track. *Behaviour Research and Therapy, 77*, 129–137. https://doi.org/10.1016/j.brat.2015.12.005

Weck, F., Richtberg, S., Jakob, M., Neng, J. M. B., & Hofling, V. (2015). Therapist competence and therapeutic alliance are important in the treatment of health anxiety (hypochondriasis). *Psychiatry Research, 228*(1), 53–58. https://doi.org/10.1016/j.psychres.2015.03.042

Wiborg, J. F., Knoop, H., Wensing, M., & Bleijenburg, G. (2012). Therapist effects and the dissemination of cognitive behaviour therapy for chronic fatigue syndrome in community-based mental health care. *Behaviour Research and Therapy, 50*(6), 393–396. https://doi.org/10.1016/j.brat.2012.03.002

Wisniewski, L., Hernandez, E., & Waller, G. (2018). Therapists' self-reported drift from dialectical behaviour therapy techniques for eating disorders. *Eating Behaviours, 28*, 20–24. https://doi.org/10.1016/j.eatbeh.2017.12.001

Chapter 20

Working in specialist services

Andrew Haley, Rebecca Light, Cassie-Ann Simmonds, and Commentary by Jason Roscoe

Introduction

The launch of England's flagship mental health initiative, Improving Access to Psychological Therapies (IAPT) in 2008, saw a considerable expansion of CBT therapist posts and with it, training places on the adult pathway (National Collaborating Centre for Mental Health, 2019). A large workforce has developed over this time and career opportunities have broadened for CBT therapists meaning that some train directly in or move on to work in, specialist services such as Child and Adolescent Mental Health Services (CAMHS), Eating Disorders, Community Mental Health Teams (CMHT), Early Intervention and more bespoke services such as 'step 3.5' teams (HEE, 2019). This chapter provides the reader with an overview of what it is like to work in some of these specialist services, ranging from the perceived benefits through to the personal challenges that each therapist has experienced. The first section discusses what it is like to applying CBT within a Step 3 plus service.

Working in a step 3.5 service

Andrew's story

In 2006, I completed the postgraduate diploma training in cognitive therapy. Prior to this I had worked as a senior occupational therapist in a variety of mental health settings. After qualifying as a cognitive therapist, I gained my first post at one of the IAPT demonstration sites, before moving on to work in a Psychological Therapy service in order to work closer to home. I quickly recognised that the clients who accessed this service had more complex and challenging difficulties than those who accessed IAPT. I was faced with a steep, but enjoyable learning curve as I developed my skills and knowledge in a service that would become what is now known as a step 3.5 service (or step 3+ as some are called). I continue to work in an NHS Step 3+ service and find my work enjoyable and rewarding.

DOI: 10.4324/9781003428527-24

Initial attraction

As I began to work with clients who had a variety of complex problems, I found that the skills, knowledge, and experience I had from working in previous mental health settings assisted me in relating to the difficult and distressing situations clients experienced. Having the opportunity to formulate from core principles and combine my general mental health experience alongside developing my skills as a cognitive behavioural therapist in a creative manner excited me. I was also part of a team who worked from different modalities and there was an open culture, which facilitated supportive clinical discussions. This enabled me to access a multitude of knowledge and experience when dealing with challenging situations, such as risk issues or ruptures.

Typical presentations

Clients who access Step 3.5 range from 16 years onwards and often have a lengthy history of engaging with mental health services. Comorbidity is common and they may have a diagnosis or features of personality disorder, but their presenting problems are linked to a common mental health difficulty. Clients may also present with neurodiversity such as Attention Deficit Hyperactivity Disorder (ADHD) or autistic spectrum condition (ASC) and interpersonal or relational problems that can lead to issues with trust. Most clients have experienced some adverse conditions and/or trauma during childhood.

In addition, the following difficulties can be prevalent within this client group:

- issues linked to substance and alcohol misuse/addiction;
- the use of self-injurious behaviour as a means of coping and a history of para-suicide;
- difficulties with emotional regulation and impulse control;
- antisocial, reckless, and promiscuous behaviours that may place them at risk;
- ambiguity about change, due to secondary gain, loss, or fear.

Specific challenges

The immediate challenge I faced when working with Step 3.5 clients was that their difficulties did not always fit with a single, disorder-specific model. I had to develop the skill of collaboratively developing a transdiagnostic, idiosyncratic formulation. Although idiosyncratic, these formulations adhere to key cognitive behavioural principles and are informed by the evidence base, consisting of core cognitive and behavioural processes that are common across a range of different disorders (Grant et al., 2010).

I found that the following assisted me in developing transdiagnostic formulations:

- having a good understanding of the disorder-specific cognitive models;
- having a clear understanding of the core principles of cognitive therapy;

- having knowledge and experience of working with a wide range of mental health difficulties in different settings;
- being open to new learning and actively seeking learning opportunities;
- being open to working creatively and adaptively whilst maintaining model compliance;
- being committed to and investing in supervision and CPD.

When working with complexity there is an implicit invitation to continue expanding knowledge and skill, which I find to be rewarding, interesting, and fulfilling. The process of ongoing development continues to increase my understanding of how wider theoretical concepts inform the process of formulation and the understanding of human experience. Developing my understanding of how relational trauma and deprivation impacts on child development has been invaluable. Combined with this, understanding multi-level theories such as the Interacting Cognitive Subsystems (Teasdale & Barnard, 1993) has been invaluable, when attempting to establish how an emotional or a behavioural response may manifest in a situation without any identifiable cognitions or external triggers.

> **Reflective exercise**
>
> Would working in a Step 3.5 service appeal to you?
> What might you enjoy about working with complexity?
> How would you find the process of creatively developing a transdiagnostic formulation?
> What aspects of this client group might be familiar to you?

Personal challenges

Step 3.5 clients who have experienced relational trauma can have difficulty engaging in a collaborative therapeutic relationship. They may have minimal and fixed, dichotomous beliefs about themselves and others and from the offset they may be demanding, critical, and rejecting of therapy and the therapist. When I initially encountered these moments in session, I could feel anxious, and I could be diverted from the task of therapy and become complicit with avoidance. Supervision has helped me to hold and understand what is happening in these moments, what beliefs, feelings, and responses are being activated in me and the client. This reflection has helped to inform the process of formulation, which in turn has assisted in developing a shared awareness of the interpersonal processes that are arising and how to work with them. Reviewing the work of Safran and Segal (1990), Leahy (2008) and Moorey and Lavender (2019) has assisted me in this. I have also engaged in further training in psychotherapeutic approaches which work with a cognitive understanding of concepts such as transference and countertransference. I continue to learn from these interpersonal moments when they arise, and

I value the benefit of having a team to support me in these moments. I respect and acknowledge the wisdom of maintaining my own wellbeing as working with rupture and moments of crisis can place extra demand on clinicians, especially when carrying a full case load.

Key points

- Often Cognitive Therapists who work in Step 3.5 have worked at Step 3 to gain the experience and skills required to work with complexity.
- Further training and skills in cognitive models and approaches that work with complexity can be advantageous such as schema therapy, and CBT for personality disorders.
- Therapeutic change with this client group can be minimal, it takes time and may not be recognised with disorder-specific measures.
- On occasions working with Step 3.5 clients can be challenging on a clinical and interpersonal level. Therefore, it is essential to be a reflective practitioner who is open to seeking out and accepting supervision and guidance and who can acknowledge and prioritise their wellbeing needs.

Further reading

Moorey, S., & Lavender, A. (Eds.). (2019). *The therapeutic relationship in cognitive behavioural therapy*. Sage.

Whittington, A., & Grey, N. (Eds.). (2014). *How to become a more effective CBT therapist, mastering metacompetence in clinical practice*. John Wiley & Sons Ltd.

Working with children and young people (CYP)

Rebecca's story

Initial attraction

For many therapists working within children and young people services, there is a sense that children represent the future, and through supporting them with their mental health, we can have a positive impact on both their future and the next generations. When working with adults, it is often seen that the experiences of our formative years contribute largely to the development of belief systems and increase our vulnerability to developing mental health problems.

Children and young people have a remarkable ability to learn, change, and adapt, with the distinct advantage of still having neural plasticity as their brains develop. For this reason, applying CBT with children and young people is often highly rewarding as the dramatic shifts created can be more pronounced than with adults where belief systems can be more fixed and harder to challenge.

Similarities and differences from applying CBT with adults

Whilst it is important to consider what differences exist, there are key similarities in what CBT interventions look like across the ages. CBT within settings such as Child and Adolescent Mental Health Services (CAMHS) settings retain the following principles and processes:

1. **Focused on the connections between thoughts, feelings, and behaviours.**
   Interventions offered to children may have a more behavioural focus, depending on the cognitive and verbal abilities of the child and may also be facilitated through changes made by the parent. Whichever way CBT is facilitated, the therapist will need to use a formulation which takes account of the key principles of how interacting thoughts, feelings, and behaviours serve to maintain problems, even if they do not appear to be explicitly the focus for a change method.
2. **Uses a structured and goal-based approach.**
   The therapist still takes an active role in providing psychoeducation and facilitates progress towards goals through the delivery of sessions with clear agendas, and between session practice of skills or activities.
3. **Is dependent on a collaborative approach with a positive therapeutic relationship.**
   Whilst this may appear an obvious similarity, consideration needs to be given to with whom the therapeutic relationship needs to be built and maintained. Children need to be collaboratively involved in therapy for it to be successful.

Case Example: Sophie (15-year-old girl). *Presenting Problems:* features of low mood (namely withdrawal, self-critical thinking and fatigue), perfectionism, and associated procrastination.

Treatment Plan: Through individual CBT, Sophie developed a better understanding of how behavioural activation worked, and how she could use this to overcome her procrastination behaviours, focusing on tasks she was most likely to engage with and successfully complete first, and also setting small goals to initiate activity.

Systemic factors: Sophie had a very challenging relationship with her mother which lead to her wanting to exclude her mother from the details of her therapy (driven by a need for control and fear of further criticism). In so doing, her mother didn't understand the maintenance cycle of her low mood, poor motivation and procrastination and as a result resorted to more criticism and pushing her to do more of the thing she was least motivated to do (with an underlying belief of challenging laziness). This reinforced the self-critical thinking Sophie experienced, undermining the success of the intervention.

Involving parents in treatment: To get Sophie's therapy tasks back on track, it was essential for her mother to have an understanding of the formulation and therapy goals. Sophie was reluctant to involve mum in the sessions which she held as a safe place just for her and was reluctant to allow me to share details without her present for fear that mum would misinterpret what was said or talk about her in a negative way she could not defend.

Augmented formulation: This case required the systemic maintenance factors to be explicitly built into the formulation and treatment to be collaboratively developed with both parent and child.

Key differences working with children and young people

There are some very specific considerations and training needs which are particular to this demographic. Of particular note, the power imbalance between adult therapist and child cannot be ignored. Often, the therapeutic relationship with the parent is equally important. Navigating the path to tread between these areas can be challenging. There is a growing research base on the importance of bringing systemic practice more explicitly into the CBT provided to children and young people (see Dummett, 2018).

The way in which therapy is delivered will depend on their individual cognitive and verbal abilities, their developmental stage, and their attachment experience

Communicating and sharing understanding with children and young people requires a very specific set of skills which need to be developed through a sound understanding of child development, adapted communication styles and the legal frameworks relevant to children.

Developmentally, children gain the necessary skills to engage in meaningful cognitive and behavioural work at very different rates. It is essential to have the theoretical underpinnings to assess these stages before an appropriate treatment plan can be made.

Key Point: If your CBT training, and your previous experience in mental health has been focused on adults there are some key texts which may support the theory base in relation to child development (Gerhardt, 2003; Maddox, 2018) but experience of working with children, alongside close supervision from an experienced, child-focused practitioner is essential beyond theoretical understanding.

In addition, many children presenting with mental health difficulties may do so in the context of other developmental challenges (e.g. query ASD and ADHD), as well as with difficult attachment relationships that they are still living within, which all impact on how best to engage them with therapeutic work.

There are different legal frameworks and systems to understand when applying CBT with children and young people

It is important that anyone working directly with children is aware of and trained within the necessary frameworks for safeguarding, understanding confidentiality and legislation, specifically the Mental Capacity Act (2005) and the Mental Health Act (1983). Additionally, an understanding of the education system, health care and social care systems specific to children are important considerations. Also, the matter of informed consent can be more complex, and therapists should be knowledgeable regarding Gillick competency to assess a child's ability to consent to treatment.

Reflective exercise

Would working in CYP service appeal to you?

What might you enjoy about working with children and young people?

How might the experiences of your parents or being a parent yourself impact on how you work with this demographic?

What areas do you feel you would need additional training, experience or supervision for in order to offer effective and safe practice?

Intervention may not always involve working directly with the child; work is often through a parent or care-giver or with the wider system

Working with parents can occur in a range of ways; from simply reducing the extent to which they maintain problems through psychoeducation, through to employing them in the role of lay or co-therapist. This brings with it a specific set of skills as a therapist. In these cases, the therapist has to simultaneously understand the cognitive and emotional needs of the parent (which often brings a high likelihood of self-blame and sensitivity to criticism) alongside the child's developmental needs, and hold these in mind whilst supporting the parent to learn the skills required to elicit behavioural changes (for the parent and the child).

Further reading

Creswell, C., & Willetts, L. (2010). *Overcoming your child's fears and worries.* Constable Robinson.

Fuggle, P., Dunsmuir, S., & Curry, V. (2013). *CBT with children, young people and their families.* Sage.

Stallard, P. (2005). *A clinicians guide to think good feel good: Using CBT with children and young people.* John Wiley.

Stallard, P., Myles, P., & Branson, A. (2014). The cognitive behaviour therapy scale for children and young people (CBTS-CYP): Development and psychometric properties. *Behavioural and Cognitive Psychotherapy*, 269–282.

Working with severe and enduring mental illness

Cassie-Ann's story

This section explores my personal experience as a CBT therapist working within a community mental health team. It also discusses how my career as a CBT therapist began, what led to my specialism and includes reflections on the rewards and challenges of my role.

I started my career as a registered mental health nurse in 2017 and have always worked within secondary care services supporting individuals with severe and enduring mental illnesses. In 2019/2020, I returned to university to study a master's in cognitive behavioural and psychotherapy. In 2021, I was coming towards the end of my second year when I applied for my first CBT post, which was at the Psychosis and Bipolar Psychological Care Network (PBPCN) within my NHS service. However, as I still had some training hours to complete, I was provided with an opportunity to finish my training and work as a trainee CBT therapist.

The PBPCN provides psychological therapy to individuals who have a diagnosis of either psychosis or bipolar and are under the care of the community mental health team. The service offers a range of psychological interventions in accordance with NICE guidelines, one of them being CBT.

To work within this area, a core profession of either nursing, social work or occupational therapy, alongside CBT training is required. A core profession is required within this area because there is a requirement within the role to act as the main professional, which involves co-ordinating an individual's care whilst providing therapy.

I was thrilled to obtain the role, but nervous to work with such complexity with minimal CBT experience. However, I received weekly supervision and attended in-house training on CBT for psychosis and bipolar and found that CBT for psychosis and bipolar was not much different to the generic CBT models.

One of my concerns specialising within this area was that I would lose my skills to deliver the generic models of CBT; however, that was not the case. Many people with psychosis and bipolar experience comorbidities, and although the PBPCN is a diagnosis-led service, the treatment is service user led and based on their presenting problem. Therefore, I have worked with a range of comorbidities and utilised most if not all the CBT models in my current practice. Despite being in this role for over two years, I continue to find the role of a CBT therapist within secondary care challenging, but enjoyable and rewarding at the same time.

Reflective exercise

What might attract you to delivering CBT in secondary care?
What might feel scary about that for you?

Rewards

When completing assessments, people tell me they do not know much about their illness, the symptoms they are experiencing, and why they may have it. In my experience, the patient's diagnosis and symptoms are explained during a busy multidisciplinary team meeting, where the patient is usually feeling a world wind of different emotions due to a recent relapse or being diagnosed with a new illness. I often hear that what they were told has been forgotten which is understandable under the circumstances. During CBT therapy for psychosis and bipolar, the first few sessions are focused on normalising and psychoeducation. I believe this is the most important part of the therapy, as many people I speak to believe, they are strange, feel alone, confused, embarrassed, and worry about their diagnosis or symptomology, as severe mental illnesses are rarely talked about.

Whether I am facilitating a group therapy programme or delivering 1:1 CBT, helping the person to see how common their symptoms are, providing them with the opportunity to see or hear from others with similar experiences helps to build hope. When individuals hear that anyone under the right set of circumstances can experience psychosis or bipolar and that they are not 'crazy' or 'abnormal' that really seems to help people feel less alone and hopeful that things may improve for them.

Challenges

One of the many challenges I come across within my role is complexity; individuals tend to have multiple diagnoses, and their presenting problems fall between two treatment pathways and often overlap. In my experience, complexity can make treatment tricky; however, it is important for the individual to understand that one problem is treated at a time and that the treatment structure is outlined during the assessment.

> **Top tip:** I often find individuals feel overwhelmed with their symptoms and can bring a lot to the session to discuss each week. Therefore, it is important to remind yourself and the individual of the agenda, the treatment goals, and problem list; having a copy of these laid out during each session can be helpful.

The most common differential diagnoses I have experienced within secondary care are Emotionally Unstable Personality Disorder (EUPD) in the backdrop of bipolar, psychosis with EUPD or Post-Traumatic Stress Disorder (PSTD) with psychosis alongside a type of anxiety and/or depression. This is where my assessment skills, knowledge of severe and enduring mental illnesses and my knowledge of services available within secondary care become helpful.

Managing complexity

I would assess the primary concern, focusing my assessment on what the individual wants and if their current presenting problems were more in line with EUPD for example. I would have this discussion with the individual and explain how they have two diagnoses that fit within two different treatment pathways. Advising that one service may offer more suitable treatment for their presenting problem than the other. I would then discuss my assessment with the referrer and a practitioner who works within the personality disorder management clinical network (PDMCN), and generally, an assessment under the PDMCN is offered, providing the individual with a choice of which treatment they would prefer.

> **Reflective exercise**
>
> What would you find challenging working with complexity?
> How would you overcome these challenges?

Top tips

- Always have a clinical rationale for the decisions you have made, and document this clearly within the clinical records.
- You and the patient are a team, the individual is the expert in their symptoms, and you are the expert in delivering the therapy.

In conclusion, working with severe and enduring mental illness is not as challenging as it sounds, and secondary care services within the NHS provide many opportunities for therapists with a core profession to develop a specialism. Although within secondary care therapists face many challenges in terms of complexity, the complexity is what makes the role so rewarding.

Further reading

The British Psychological Society. (2011). *Good practice guidelines on the use of psychological formulation.*

Freeman, D. (2016). Persecutory delusions: A cognitive perspective on understanding and treatment. *The Lancet Psychiatry, 3*(7), 685–692. https://doi.org/10.1016/S2215-0366(16)00066

Mansell, W., Morrison, A., Reid, G., Lowens, I., & Tai, S. (2007). The interpretation of, and responses to, changes in internal states: An integrative cognitive model of mood swings and bipolar disorders. *Behavioural and Cognitive Psychotherapy, 35*(5), 515–539. https://doi.org/10.1017/S1352465807003827

Morrison, A. (2017). A manualised treatment protocol to guide delivery of evidence-based cognitive therapy for people with distressing psychosis: Learning from clinical trials. *Psychosis, 9*(3), 271–281. https://doi.org/10.1080/17522439.2017.129509

Conclusion

In this chapter, three clinicians have described their experiences of delivering CBT to specialist populations. Some CBT therapists will train within adult primary care settings before making the transition to other services. Conversely, there are now specialist CBT curriculums in England where practitioners are recruited from core professions such as nursing to train directly in one of these specialist roles (see HEE, 2019). There are of course other services that CBT therapists go on to specialise in which are not covered in this chapter. One example is therapy that is delivered fully remotely, via computerised CBT or in some cases, by text message. It is hoped that these accounts of practising CBT across various contexts has given you a 'flavour' of how they differ from working with anxiety disorders and depression.

References

Dummett, N. (2018). Cognitive – behavioural therapy with children, young people and families: From individual to systemic therapy. *Advances in Psychiatric Treatment*, 23–36.

Gerhardt, S. (2003). *Why love matters: How affection shapes a baby's brain.* Taylor & Francis.

Grant, A., Townend, M., Mulhern, R., & Short, N. (Eds.). (2010). *Cognitive behavioural therapy in mental health care.* Sage.

Health Education England. (2019). *National curriculum for cognitive behavioural therapy for severe mental health problems.*

Leahy, R. L. (2008). The therapeutic relationship in cognitive-behavioural therapy. *Behavioural and Cognitive Psychotherapy*, 769–777.

Maddox, L. (2018). *Blueprint: How our childhood makes us who we are.* Little Brown.

Moorey, S., & Lavender, A. (Eds.). (2019). *The therapeutic relationship in cognitive behavioural therapy.* Sage.

National Collaborating Centre for Mental Health. (2019). *The improving access to psychological therapies manual.* NHS.

Safran, J. D., & Segal, Z. (1990). *Interpersonal processes in cognitive therapy.* Guildford Press.

Teasdale, J. D., & Barnard, P. J. (1993). *Affect, cognition and change.* Lawrence Erlbaum Associates Ltd.

Chapter 21

Training in third-wave and integrative approaches

Jim Lucas, Tobyn Bell, Heather Howard Thompson, and Commentary by Jason Roscoe

Introduction

There is no singular path to 'thriving' as a CBT therapist although some find that other modalities compliment or supersede how they work with certain clinical presentations. Whilst CBT can be effective for many people, it is not a panacea, nor is any therapy for that matter and many psychotherapists choose to train in more than one therapeutic modality, even those who hold strong allegiances towards CBT. This chapter offers perspectives from CBT therapists who have chosen to do additional training in third-wave or integrative approaches and who now adopt this as one of their preferred methods of working with clients. There are many other modalities that CBT therapists will train in that are not covered in this chapter (e.g. DBT, CAT, IPT, couples); however, it is not feasible to discuss them all within the confines of a short chapter.

The 'third-wave', integrative therapies and approaches that can be integrated with CBT

CBT training curriculums are largely influenced by 'second-wave' models where the content of thinking and the concept of 'safety behaviours' were seen to be important considerations that 'first wave' behavioural approaches could not always explain, particularly when clients failed to improve through approaches such as repeated exposure alone (Salkovskis, 1991). The development of acceptance and commitment therapy or ACT (pronounced ACT rather than A.C.T) where focus shifted from *content* of thoughts to *context* and function, signalled the rise of a 'third wave' in CBT (Hoffman, 2018). Some people consider compassion-focused therapy (CFT) as belonging to this category; however, whilst it shares some features with ACT (e.g. use of mindfulness; changing relationship with thoughts), CFT is ostensibly an integrative therapy (Bell, personal communication), drawing heavily on evolutionary science and attachment theory (Gilbert & Simos, 2022). In this respect, it has more in common with Schema Therapy, another integrative therapy which draws upon elements of CBT but is also influenced by psychodynamic and attachment theory and object relations (Young et al., 2006).

DOI: 10.4324/9781003428527-25

We then have approaches such as Eye Movement Desensitisation and Reprocessing (EMDR) which can be integrated within CBT, ACT, or CFT (e.g. Beer, 2018). The key aim of this chapter is to demonstrate how approaches that have similar features to CBT (e.g. agenda setting, imagery, focus on behavioural change) may compliment or 'speak to' an individual therapist's 'epistemic style' or world view' and help them manage clinical challenges more effectively (Kennedy & Pearson, 2020; Neimeyer & Morton, 1997).

Why are CBT therapists drawn/attracted towards ACT/third-wave therapies?

Jim Lucas

Overview

After completing their training, many CBT practitioners train in third-wave approaches, including ACT. CBT therapists may choose ACT as their default approach due to its simplicity, scope, precision, and depth. The author will briefly describe the ACT approach in this chapter, noting the similarities and differences from traditional CBT. Drawing on his personal experience, he describes the benefits of learning ACT and why some CBT practitioners prefer to use ACT as their primary therapeutic framework. Finally, he recommends further reading for those interested in learning more about ACT.

What is ACT? How is it similar and different from traditional CBT?

ACT is a psychotherapeutic approach developed over three decades (the 1970s to 1990s) by Hayes et al. (1999). It is based on a scientific philosophy called *Functional Contextualism*, which is fundamentally different from *Elemental Realism* that underpins traditional Cognitive Therapy (Hughes, 2018). Simply put, ACT focuses on increasing *psychological flexibility* by targeting specific behavioural processes. Whilst distinct, these six processes are interrelated and target different dimensions, including emotion, cognition, attention, self, motivation, and overt behaviour (Hayes et al., 2022). ACT therapists explore your relationship patterns with these dimensions and seek to influence them away from suffering and towards better health and wellbeing (Hayes et al., 2012).

Key Point: Functional contextualism represents a progressive paradigm that explores how culture and evolution influence a person's experience and difficulties. Rather than reducing suffering to problematic cognitions, ACT focuses on how a person's learning history, setting, and habits affect their experience.

An ACT therapist does <u>not</u> seek to identify and change the *form* of faulty thoughts or physiology. Nor do they aim to eradicate or reduce unwanted emotions frequently referred to in traditional CBT as *symptoms*. ACT emphasises how your experience and habits *make sense* because of how your learning history has shaped you. Through a functional contextual lens, everything you do can be explained by the context in which you have and continue to move.

Many clinicians are attracted to this scientific and philosophical shift. ACT represents a departure from the traditional dualism of 'normal versus abnormal' psychological states. It would be inconsistent for an ACT practitioner to refer to suffering as a disease, syndrome or disorder. Despite the tendency to entangle ourselves with beliefs that one is 'broken' or 'defective', we can observe each other as *complete humans* (Walser, 2019*)*. Whilst we may want to change our habits, pursue goals, and invest in personal growth, we are fundamentally acceptable, wonderful, and capable.

Such a perspective on human beings is not only practical, but it also carries hope. We are capable of extraordinary change regardless of past events or current circumstances. We have a choice, and no matter how dire your situation is, there is always the possibility that you can take your life in a new direction.

Reflective exercise

Consider someone you love. Imagine they come to you describing their distress. What would they need to change about themselves to make them acceptable to you?

Probably, your answer is 'nothing'. You may not appreciate all of their behaviour, but you recognise you love them for who they are.

What would it be like to see your clients as complete and capable?

What are the benefits of learning ACT?

Research shows that when people are psychologically inflexible, their mental health and wellbeing worsen (Kashdan & Rottenberg, 2010). Conversely, psychological flexibility accounts for 45% of everything we know about why therapy works (Hayes et al., 2022).

Although there are many paths to change, a therapist who regularly utilises acceptance, mindfulness, and behaviour change tools in their clinical work will likely outperform practitioners who rely on counselling skills, cognitive restructuring or increasing self-esteem (Lucas, 2023)

Clinicians report many reasons for wanting to learn and apply ACT to help clients reduce suffering. Many people encounter life-changing injuries and chronic illnesses. They find little comfort or transformation in challenging the accuracy of their thinking. Instead, they find hope and vitality connecting with the values that bring fulfilment. Values exploration is a central process in the ACT model, which many practitioners and clients appreciate. Rather than merely focusing on 'symptom reduction', you can focus on meaning and purpose. For example, it may no longer be possible for a person who has Multiple Sclerosis to play football with their child. However, you can engage in similar possible activities by exploring the values underpinning your desire to do this activity. The qualities of *connecting*, *playing*, and *teaching* may be what makes these interactions so precious, allowing you to explore alternative possibilities once you can see those more significant motivations.

My journey into ACT

As well as values, many clinicians are drawn to the acceptance process within ACT. I first discovered ACT in a journal article about the well-known 'tug of war' exercise. A colleague and I agreed to include it in our NHS service in a CBT for long-term anxiety sufferers group programme.

In the tug-of-war exercise, you and your client hold opposite ends of a rope. You play your client's 'anxiety monster', pulling on the rope whilst they pull back. After pulling back and forth, you notice the struggle with your experience. You go nowhere, feeling tenser and getting sore arms. On this occasion, and after a few minutes of tugging, it occurred to my client they could let go of the rope. I asked them what they noticed then, and their response changed my professional life. Their eyes filled with water, and we both felt a strange sadness. Before they said anything, this feeling enveloped me, and then they spoke: 'I've wasted years of my life fighting with the anxiety when all I needed to do was stop'.

At that moment, I witnessed something I'd never seen before. There was a heartfelt moment between us. Inside it, there was pain, and there was a beauty. They connected with something that hurt and shared that moment with me. Something changed that day for both of us. For them, it was the realisation that control would never work. For me, it was the discovery that transformations happen experientially.

Why do some CBT therapists ultimately prefer to use them as their default method?

Many CBT therapists begin their ACT journey by integrating tools and techniques into their current working methods. For example, they incorporate values into fear exposure interventions and cognitive defusion into behavioural activation. Others go on to adopt ACT as their primary therapeutic model. I am one of those people, but I haven't disregarded everything I learned from my CBT training. If anything, I have evolved my framework, staying close to scientifically sound behavioural principles and drawing on powerful behaviour change methods commonly used in traditional CBT.

There are four reasons why I think some clinicians ultimately prefer to use ACT as their default method. They are

1. simplicity;
2. scope;
3. precision;
4. depth.

Simplicity

ACT is one model, so you needn't learn and retain multiple formulation templates and procedures. One might say ACT is transdiagnostic but given that it's a model of the human condition, that wouldn't quite fit. Instead, you and your client learn a straightforward way to understand their distress and develop specific skills to help their life.

Scope

Ongoing functional analysis and experiential methods are the driving forces of ACT interventions. Your task is to examine what people do, how their history and environment influence them, and how those actions get reinforced. In other words, you can use ACT with anyone and any presenting psychological problem.

> **Top tip:** Sometimes, we may feel thrown by what we see and hear. Set your confusion and self-doubt aside and pick up your tools. When you lean into the ACT model's principles and processes, they'll show you the way.

Precision

One could argue that many CBT protocolised treatments are over-packaged. Whilst randomised control trials point to their degree of effectiveness, they don't tell us which bits work and which bits are unnecessary. ACT practitioners focus on behavioural processes, seeking to build flexibility. They are free to observe and respond to the unique, unhelpful patterns repeated by an individual as they occur in the therapy room. By intervening in what happens here and now, you can work more directly on how clients unintentionally perpetuate their suffering. You can work with greater creativity, selecting interventions that fit the context.

Depth

ACT operates within an evolving scientific programme based on a post-Skinnerian account of human language and behaviour (Hayes et al., 2001). Functional contextualism, relational frame theory, and evolutionary science inform and guide its research programme. It is far from perfect, and the data broadly shows it is no more effective than CBT (A-Tjak et al., 2015; Gloster et al., 2020; Ost, 2014).

I once heard Steve Hayes say, '*We know ACT is wrong. We just don't know where it is wrong*'. When I witnessed that statement from its founder, I was struck by his boldness, authenticity, and humility. It's far too familiar for our leaders in psychology to claim superiority in their favoured therapeutic model. Such certainty limits progress, and like many others, I feel at home in a community that wants to evolve its processes and methods in line with scientific advancements.

Summary

Many therapists who train in CBT go on to learn third-wave approaches, including acceptance and commitment therapy. Initially, they may be attracted to its focus on values construction and acceptance interventions, which they don't learn in traditional CBT. After taking their first steps with ACT, they often discover the flexibility and creativity that comes from focusing on processes before procedures.

Although counter to evolutionary instincts and cultural messages, the willingness to be open can be transformational, it often opens up the possibility of change, bringing hope and sparking agency to take small steps forward. Rather than fighting with yourself, you learn to accept yourself, warts, and all! Acceptance is an experiential process of curiosity and making room for your emotions. It's not about putting up with bad behaviour or unwanted situations. It is the act of choosing to receive and carry your feelings instead of trying to avoid, control, or problem solve them.

Top tips

CBT practitioners can integrate ACT interventions with relative ease. However, they should be aware of the philosophical differences and guiding behavioural principles that may be less explicit in traditional CBT training programmes.

To get a better working knowledge of acceptance and commitment therapy, explore different learning formats. Read a book, listen to a podcast, or attend a training course.

Self-practice/self-reflection will help you develop your skills from the inside out, giving you the capacity to operate from an embodied stance, which is critical to effective ACT practice.

Further reading

Harris, R. (2006). Embracing your demons: An overview of acceptance and commitment therapy. *Psychotherapy in Australia*, *12*(4).

Hayes, S. C., Barnes-Holmes, D., & Wilson, K. G. (2012). Contextual behavioral science: Creating a science more adequate to the challenge of the human condition. *Journal of Contextual Behavioral Science*, *1*, 1–16.

Wilson, K. G., & Sandoz, E. K. (2008). Mindfulness, values and therapeutic relationship in acceptance and commitment therapy. In S. Hick & T. Bein (Eds.), *Mindfulness and the therapeutic relationship*. Guilford Press.

Why train in compassion-focused therapy?

Tobyn Bell

'I understand the logic that I'm not a failure, but I still feel like one.'
'I know I'm not to blame for the abuse, but I feel it's my fault.'

Overview

Most cognitive therapists will recall clients sharing sentiments similar to those above: where hard-won insights fail to be reassuring and the heart lags some way behind the head. During the 1980s, Paul Gilbert, the originator of compassion-focused therapy (CFT), became curious about these very issues in his practice of cognitive therapy (Gilbert, 2009). Gilbert observed that clients prone to shame and self-criticism would often report such 'rational-emotional dissociation' (Stott, 2007) despite having become skilled at cognitive restructuring. The alternative, more balanced and data-based thoughts they'd generated were often experienced with an emotional tone of coldness or harshness, and they had difficulties in experiencing feelings of safeness, contentment, or warmth in their relationship with themselves and with others. These observations prompted Gilbert to develop an approach to therapy that trained clients in compassion, helping them to *feel* the benefit of such care and bridge the head-heart divide.

What is CFT? How is it similar and different from traditional CBT?

CFT is a model grounded in motivational processing and explores the drives that existed millions of years before the elaboration of higher cognition. These basic motives shape and organise the mind in distinctive and powerful ways, and whilst the human mind can very well be dominated by competitive, conflictual, and attainment-focused motives, it is also demonstrably capable of compassion and care. CFT focuses on activating, engaging, and cultivating care-based motives as a way to change the relationships we have with others and ourselves, particularly our struggles and difficult emotional experiences. One major benefit of changing motives- rather than cognitive content alone- are the shifts this can create across our entire mindset: impacting our thinking and reasoning, our focus of attention, our behavioural impulses, our feeling states, and style of relating. CFT seeks to stimulate this whole-system change (recruiting and co-ordinating a range of bio-psycho-social processes) by engaging basic motives focused on the giving and receiving of care (Gilbert, 2010).

The 'tricky brain'

CFT discusses motivational psychology within an evolutionary framework, and this context provides clinicians with a means to de-pathologise, de-personalise, and de-shame common factors of the human experience that can underlie so much of our suffering and struggle. In discussing human experience in this broader evolutionary perspective, clients can be supported to understand the core functions of their behaviours and emotions, and how they flow from the evolved drives that sit behind them (e.g. for attachment or harm-avoidance). Complex and contradictory drives and reactions are well explained through an evolutionary lens, and CFT practitioners are keen to highlight the inherently 'tricky' way the human brain has developed.

> **Key Point:** Clients can be helped to make sense of their desire to stay attached to an abusive family member or understand their feelings of rage and envy towards a best friend.

The motivational psychology of CFT also provides a bridge for CBT therapists to discuss developmental needs and stages and to de-pathologise the difficulties that occur when they are thwarted. Refreshingly, CFT is a model of human functioning rather than disorder, and the approach encourages clinicians to take the broadest of perspectives to understand why the mind is so difficult to manage.

To develop the soothing system and to experience the regulating effect of care, CFT involves a multitude of experiential and body-based interventions. CBT therapists will find much to deepen and extend their repertoire of experiential practices and will notice an increased focus on body-related processes. Gilbert's (2020) adage to 'use the body to support the mind' highlights the way that CFT works from a 'bottom-up' – rather than 'head first' – principle whereby clients are supported to use various soothing and grounding practices (such as slowing the pace of breathing and changing posture and facial expression) before engaging cognition. CFT also includes a variety of experiential practices to build and enact the client's compassionate self (a version of themselves that embodies various compassionate qualities). Such practices include the use of mental imagery, acting techniques, sensory-focusing, chairwork, and letter-writing. The client can then be supported to embody their compassionate self to help them face the difficulties that brought them to therapy.

What are the benefits of learning CFT?

CFT offers therapists a model for exploring and balancing emotions. In CFT, emotions are clustered according to their evolved function (Gilbert, 2009). Certain emotions (such as anger and anxiety) form part of our *threat-protection system*, alerting us to physical and social danger and priming us for protective action. Other emotions (such as excitement and joy) form part of our *drive-acquisition system* and function to motivate, orientate, and reinforce our actions to achieve and consume. Whilst a CBT therapist, utilising disorder-specific models, might be accustomed to working with such emotions (e.g. stimulating the drive system in behavioural activation; or targeting threat-based reactions in social anxiety experiments), they may not routinely target the cultivation of parasympathetic feeling states associated with the *soothing-safeness system*. Within CFT, clients are encouraged to access, elaborate, and tolerate emotions associated with safeness and contentment that, in mammals, have evolved to support care, affiliation, and attachment.

> **Key Point:** CFT differs from CBT in the emphasis on explicitly building access to the soothing system, as a means to balance and regulate problematic threat and drive-based experiences.

Multiple selves

In the last decades, cognitive therapists have emphasised the importance of building new self-representations and ways of being rather than dismantling negative maintenance cycles and structure of belief (Mooney & Padesky, 2000; Korrelboom et al., 2012). It raises the question as to what type of 'self' would be most beneficial to cultivate. Is it a self-representation based on drive and achievement to bolster self-esteem? Or might it include a compassionate self that helps us to flourish whilst also supporting us through life's inevitable difficulties? When compared to self-esteem, self-compassion creates a more stable sense of self-worth (Neff & Vonk, 2009) and provides more of a buffer against problems such as depression (Petrocchi et al., 2019). CFT focuses on building the compassionate self as a counter to self-criticism or contingent self-worth, but also focuses compassion on the very threats and fears that drive these experiences.

Validating fears, blocks, and resistance

For the CBT therapist, CFT offers a means to integrate a relational focus. The approach is grounded in attachment theory and focuses on how relationships and community have key roles in influencing our maturation and wellbeing. To demonstrate the difference in emphasis, negative core beliefs in CFT are understood as indicative of distressing emotional memories (e.g. the belief 'I am bad' might signify 'I have emotional memories of being treated as bad and unacceptable') (Gilbert, 2010). Much of the therapeutic work of CFT is working with fears, blocks, and resistances to compassion. Rather than cognitively challenging these reactions or treating them as therapy interfering behaviours, they are validated and understood as previously adaptive responses to interpersonal trauma or ruptures in attachment (Steindl et al., 2023). The social mentality model that underpins CFT highlights how our internal world and self-to-self relating is intrinsically coloured by our external relationships, making the model contextually sensitive and trauma focused.

> **Top tip:** When beginning with CFT, it can be disconcerting to find clients reacting to compassion exercises with anxiety, sadness, or any number of threat-based reactions.
>
> It can be very easy to think you've done something wrong in your delivery and to focus on yourself. Whilst there is always scope to reflect on our own practice as clinicians, focusing on your clients' responses will often give you key insights into their fears, blocks, or resistances (FBRs) to compassion and care.
>
> This is where the therapy really begins. FBRs are often linked to early experiences of care and can offer a window into our client's attachment relationships and injuries. As such, FBRs need to be treated with respect and sensitivity, but they also take you directly to the places where care is most needed. To paraphrase the proverb: 'the obstacles are the path'.
>
> Such FBRs can take you into the client's prior experiences of receiving care (e.g. to attachment experiences of neglect). The FBRs now become our therapeutic focus. They can validate, understand, and target the ways.

Another compelling reason to consider training in CFT is the rapidly growing body of science supporting its effectiveness. The most recent reviews by Craig et al. (2020) and Millard et al. (2023) have found that CFT does indeed increase compassion-based outcomes whilst reducing clinical symptomatology. CFT has a developing evidence base across multiple presentations, including eating disorders, psychosis, depression, and anxiety disorders (see Basran et al., 2022, for overview). Research also suggests that the effectiveness of evidence-based treatments, such as CBT, is reduced in clients with high levels of shame and self-criticism (Marshall et al., 2008) and it is exactly these experiences that CFT targets. Research suggests the best way to work with self-criticism is not to focus on reduction, but on cultivating its antidote in compassion (Wakelin et al., 2022). The science also shows that compassion can be trained (Kirby, 2017) and CFT provides a clear and systematic way in which to do so. A course of CFT typically involves working on competencies and attributes (such as empathy and distress-tolerance) linked to the development and application of compassion. True to its spirit, CFT is integrative in nature and works well in completing and facilitating other evidence-based treatment: for example, in a phased-based approach to PTSD (Lawrence & Lee, 2014).

Reflective exercise

Compassion can be misperceived as a 'soft' or 'easy' option but consider the following situation.

A child you know is anxious about attending a party with their friends. The child had been excited all week but, on the day, they are too frightened to go.

Ask yourself, what is the compassionate thing to do in this scenario and how would you show care to this child? Compassion involves engaging with suffering, with sensitivity, rather than avoiding it. What would that look like here? Compassion also involves a motivation to be helpful in alleviating suffering and working with its causes. What would that look like in this example?

Summary

CFT is not a soft option. It isn't about pampering oneself or soothing away difficulties, letting yourself off the hook, or accepting the unacceptable. It is about caring for yourself and others, and listening deeply to what hurts so that you can provide or access what is needed. This takes courage and often requires us to connect to the 'shadow' sides of our character: the parts of ourselves we may be inclined to disown, hide, or project onto others. It also takes commitment, practice, and the strength to be vulnerable with others. None of this is easy. CFT also asks us not to focus solely on 'self-compassion', but to consider compassion as a series of flows: self-to-self, other-to-self, and self-to-others. It isn't a navel-gazing exercise but rather a fundamental call to embrace what it is to be interconnected and human, using both your head and your heart.

Further reading

Gilbert, P., & Simos, G. (Eds.). (2022). *Compassion focused therapy: Clinical practice and applications*. Routledge.
Kolts, R. L., Bell, T., Bennett-Levy, J., & Irons, C. (2018). *Experiencing compassion-focused therapy from the inside out: A self-practice/self-reflection workbook for therapists*. Guilford Publications.

EMDR and how it can aid and develop your clinical practice?

Heather Howard Thompson

Overview

Developed in the late 1980s by psychologist Dr Francine Shapiro, Eye Movement Desensitisation and Reprocessing (EMDR), has transformed the treatment of trauma and related mental health conditions (Shapiro, 2018). In the first part of this section, I will briefly describe what EMDR is and how it differs from CBT. I will then discuss my own journey as a psychotherapist and why I am such an advocate for EMDR. I will then move on to explore the unique benefits and outcomes that differentiate it from CBT. This includes my reasons why EMDR therapy can be helpful in cases where I have found CBT to have limited effectiveness. Finally, I will explore how EMDR can help expand your clinical skills and CBT practice.

What is EMDR? How is it similar and different from traditional CBT?

EMDR therapy is a therapeutic approach that helps individuals process and heal from traumatic experiences. It is guided by the Adaptive Information Processing (AIP) model (Shapiro, 2007), which suggests that psychological difficulties arise when traumatic memories are not adequately processed and are stored or stuck in the brain's neural network. EMDR aims to facilitate AIP through the reprocessing of these memories, using bilateral stimulation (e.g. rapid eye movement, taps or sounds). This helps to alleviate distressing emotions and associated physiological symptoms, shifting the brain into memory processing mode similar to that of REM sleep.

The evidence base for EMDR therapy continues to grow (see Wilson et al., 2018). Data from this narrative review examined the evidence of the efficacy of EMDR therapy as a treatment for Post-Traumatic Stress Disorder (PTSD). A meta-analysis found EMDR therapy improved PTSD diagnosis, reduced PTSD symptoms, and reduced other trauma-related symptoms. Furthermore, Chen et al. (2014) looked at 26 scientific studies and concluded that EMDR therapy significantly reduces PTSD symptoms, including depression and anxiety and is especially effective at reducing patients' distress. Research has shown positive outcomes for EMDR therapy across different populations, including veterans, chronic pain, low self-esteem, OCD, depression, and complex PTSD (Carletto et al., 2021; de Jongh et al., 2019; Griffioen et al., 2017; Marsden et al., 2018; Silver et al., 2008). Finally, the National Institute for Health and Care Excellence (NICE), which provides guidelines for healthcare practices in the UK, has recognised EMDR as an effective treatment for PTSD (NICE, 2018).

Why use EMDR therapy with clients?

Chen et al. (2015) examined 11 scientific studies to find out whether EMDR or CBT was more effective in treating PTSD. They found that EMDR was more effective overall. There are of course, contradictory studies and more research continues to be carried out. As you will see in my vignette, I continue to use CBT, DBT skills, and EMDR in my clinical work with clients. Let's now explore how EMDR can be an effective treatment of choice for clients, based on my experiences of using a range of therapies effectively in my private practice.

Client preference

The choice as to which therapy to use with a client may depend on individual client preferences. In my experience, it is useful to be able to offer different approaches, based on the client's (e.g. history of previous therapy and their willingness to complete intersession work). Some people may find EMDR's approach helpful in processing traumatic memories, whilst others may prefer the cognitive and behavioural strategies in CBT. It is important to note that therapy effectiveness can vary from person to person, and the therapeutic relationship between the client and the therapist also plays a crucial role. Ultimately, the decision between which therapeutic approach you use should be made collaboratively, based on the individual's specific needs, preferences, and the nature of the presenting concerns.

Targeting underlying trauma

EMDR recognises that many mental health conditions including negative beliefs about ourselves, and unhelpful behaviours are rooted in unresolved trauma. By using EMDR, we aim to identify and address the traumatic memories that may contribute to an individual's current symptoms. By targeting the underlying trauma directly, EMDR therapy can result in profound and lasting changes.

Resolving negative beliefs

EMDR specifically targets negative beliefs that have developed as a result of traumatic experiences. For example, a client may have been told at primary school that they will never achieve anything in life if they struggle with academic work. This could lead to them believing 'I'm not good enough'. By reprocessing this negative belief at a deep emotional level, EMDR therapy helps individuals develop more adaptive beliefs about themselves and their experiences. Bilateral stimulation appears to assist in processing memories, and through the phases of 'desensitisation' and 'installation', this negative belief can be changed to a more adaptive belief (e.g. 'I am good enough'). This can have a significant positive impact on their current low self-esteem or enable them to try new things that they may have previously avoided.

Addressing complex trauma

Life can be challenging for most people, and we often go through multiple traumas (which can be anything that at the time, has a an intensely negative emotional impact). We may not even recognise the effect that these incidents can have on our wellbeing. Research shows that clients with Complex PTSD benefit from trauma-focused therapies for PTSD, specifically trauma-focused CBT and EMDR (NICE, 2018). Whilst both approaches have demonstrated efficacy in treating PTSD, some studies indicate that EMDR's unique way of focusing on processing traumatic memories may be particularly beneficial for those with complex trauma histories (Korn, 2009).

EMDR's bilateral stimulation and attention to sensory components during memory processing may facilitate the integration of fragmented and overwhelming traumatic experiences in a way that aligns with the challenges posed by complex trauma. Other evidence-based interventions can also be used during the preparation phase of the EMDR process, such as the Flash Technique (Manfield et al., 2017). This can help the client process extremely distressing memories in a way which helps them to tolerate the distress more effectively resulting in significant improvements in overall wellbeing.

EMDR can also be applied to 'small t' traumas such as experiences of bullying or social humiliation. For example, a client who presents with anxiety in social situations might be able to identify a past memory of being shamed by a parent in front of a group of friends age 7. You then have a choice of using CBT for social anxiety disorder or taking an AIP-focused approach with EMDR. In summary, being trained in EMDR gives you the added option for clients and expands your range of techniques that you can offer.

Promoting emotional regulation

Emotional dysregulation is a common symptom in various mental health conditions. EMDR helps individuals develop effective emotional regulation strategies by integrating distressing emotions associated with traumatic memories. Through the reprocessing of these emotions, clients can experience a greater sense of emotional stability and resilience. Phase two of the standard EMDR protocol (Shapiro, 2018) is the preparation phase, where it is vitally important that you work on resource building and teaching clients how to practise regulating their emotions to enable them to process traumatic memories. I use the 'Window of Tolerance' exercise (Siegel, 2020) before starting EMDR preparation as this is a fantastic tool with clients. Siegel proposes that everyone has a range (or zone of 'optimum arousal'; Ogden et al., 2006) which they can comfortably experience, process, and integrate emotional experience.

The window of tolerance acts as a safety zone, ensuring that the client remains regulated during therapy sessions. This preparation phase allows individuals to build resilience, strengthen their capacity for emotional regulation, and enhance their ability to cope with distressing emotions that may arise during and between therapy sessions. This helps to enhance the effectiveness of EMDR therapy and improves overall outcomes for clients.

Vignette – My CBT and EMDR journey

I started out in the field of mental health as a student mental health nurse in 1994. After qualifying I worked on an acute psychiatric ward and then moved into a community mental health team, working with clients experiencing severe and enduring mental health problems. I become interested in people's histories and extensive traumas that led to or exacerbated their mental health struggles.

I then moved to an NHS Occupational Health department and helped develop their Health and Wellbeing Team. It was during this time that I realised that I lacked the skills needed to help with the trauma that staff members presented with. I was going through a particularly difficult time in my own life having experienced numerous personal traumas, so therefore chose to access private therapy. This was my first introduction to EMDR, and it totally changed my life! My negative beliefs about myself and intrusive images stopped within a matter of weeks. I was hooked and that started my EMDR journey on a professional level.

In 2012 I started to train in EMDR and practised the skills learned with clients attending Occupational Health, along with continuing to use CBT skills which I learned on a short-term CBT course at The University of York in 2008/09. In 2013, I finally started my Postgraduate Diploma in CBT and qualified in 2015. After a brief stint in prison (working as a Primary Care Mental Health Team Manager!), I left the NHS in 2015 and started working full time in private practice. Using CBT, EMDR, and elements of Dialectical Behaviour Therapy, I've found that I increasingly work with clients that have accessed therapy in the past who are still struggling, or they present as 'complex'.

EMDR has become the mainstay of my practice and has proven to help clients with long-term difficulties where other therapies have previously failed. I continue to use CBT and DBT skills where appropriate, but find EMDR with the right preparation, is transformative, particularly for clients presenting with Complex PTSD.

How EMDR can help expand your clinical skills and CBT practice

In my own practice, I have found EMDR to be extremely effective in treating not only PTSD but also a range of mental health problems and current symptoms (including emotions, physical sensations, behaviours, and negative thoughts) that ultimately stem from traumatic experiences.

Reflective exercise – Could EMDR help 'complex' clients?

Paper and pen to the ready!

Consider any clients that have struggled to engage with CBT; have had CBT in the past and are still struggling with symptoms, didn't complete homework or that you found difficult to work with (e.g. they seemed 'too complex').

Do they have a history of traumatic memories that could have led to their current difficulties? Think about how their past experiences could have led to their negative thoughts, emotional experiences, and unhelpful behaviours.

Key points

- By adding EMDR to your toolbox as a psychotherapist, you can provide individualised care for clients, expanding your expertise and client base. This helps you build in confidence as a practitioner, knowing that you have more skills to help a wider range of clients.
- With lots of preparation, emotional regulation strategies and a strong therapeutic relationship, EMDR can help heal the most complex of trauma histories.
- If you incorporate EMDR into your practice, you offer an additional evidence-based treatment option for clients. If you are in private practice, this can attract new clients who are specifically requesting EMDR or those who have not responded well to traditional CBT methods.

When might you use EMDR instead of other therapies?

- Consider an individual's specific needs and preferences.
- If the client struggles to complete homework tasks.
- If a client has tried other therapies but hasn't found a resolution.
- Clients who have trouble talking about traumatic events because they're too painful to discuss.
- Clients who can tolerate some distress.

Summary

The purpose of this section was to introduce you to EMDR and provide an insight into how it might help expand your skills, especially for traumatised client who struggle to 'get on' with CBT. Personally, I am glad that I trained in multiple therapies, and I hope this gives you some ideas as to how you can develop and flourish in your career path. With time and practice, you will start to see how you can use CBT, EMDR, and other therapeutic interventions, formulating with the clients to determine their main areas of distress and deciding on which area to work, in which order and with which therapy. This allows flexibility, using evidence-based treatment that suits the needs of the client and gets to the root of the problem.

Top tips

- Find a Clinical Supervisor that is also EMDR trained and preferably accredited (see https://emdrassociation.org.uk/find-a-therapist/)
- EMDR works with distressing memories, not only PTSD.
- The Window of Tolerance is a useful tool for explaining the impact of trauma to clients.

Be creative when it comes to resource building and spend time in the preparation phase (you can use CBT skills to do this).

Further reading

De Jongh, A., Bicanic, I., Matthijissen, S., Amann, B.-L., Hofmann, A., Farrell, D., Lee, C.-L., & Maxfield, L. (2019). The current status of EMDR therapy involving the treatment of complex posttraumatic stress disorder. *Journal of EMDR Practice and Research, 13*(4), 284–290.

Shapiro, F. (2018). *Eye movement desensitization and reprocessing (EMDR): Basic principles, protocols and procedures* (3rd ed.). The Guilford Press.

Conclusion

In this chapter, we have looked at three therapeutic modalities that CBT therapists often train in post-qualification. Three highly experienced clinicians have given accounts of what has drawn them to that modality and how this has helped to shape how they work therapeutically. A common theme is encountering certain limitations in the application of 'second-wave' or standard CBT models and interventions (Hofmann, 2018).

A few words of caution

Whilst you may find yourself drawn to some of the theories or interventions associated with the approaches discussed in this chapter, it is important to reflect upon one's reasons for this.

Reflective exercise

Am I drawn to any of the approaches discussed in this chapter? If so, which one?

What are the main reasons for this?

Could any of my reasons be due to misconceptions about aspects of CBT? (Things I didn't grasp fully during my training, negative beliefs/fears about aspects of CBT)

We should not rule out the possibility that some therapists hold misconceptions about CBT formulations or treatment plans leading to applying them incompetently or in an unnecessarily rigid manner (e.g. Parker & Waller, 2017). For example, if one believes that CBT is restrictive or invalidating, then it is easy to see why they might look to other therapies that they deem to fill these gaps. Whilst one or more of the approaches described in this chapter may have struck a chord with you, it might be worth spending some time answering the questions in the reflective exercise before dashing off to add more strings to your bow.

A brief word on supervision

Practising multiple modalities automatically generates questions about who will supervise your work, how much time you will need to allow for this and if you are in private practice, how much this will cost you. Paying different supervisors for different modality specific supervision is likely to be expensive but might ensure subject specialism. Alternatively, many CBT therapists in private practice will pick a supervisor who is trained in both CBT and EMDR for example. The obvious advantage is that it is likely to be less expensive than the first option, but it is worth asking if the supervisor can offer high-quality supervision in two modalities.

Key points

- Some CBT therapists 'thrive' once qualified by augmenting their practice with skills from third-wave and integrative approaches.
- Not all CBT therapists will feel the need to augment their work with third-wave or integrative approaches. However, some CBT therapists may find that they are naturally more aligned with another therapy (e.g. ACT) and adopt this as their primary modality.
- Training in additional modalities brings challenges in addition to the perceived benefits (e.g. trying to reconcile competing theories)

Reflect on your reasons for wanting to train in a different modality.

References

A-Tjak, J. G. L, Davis, M. L., Morina, N., Powers, M. B., Smits, J. A. J., & Emmelkamp, P. M. G. (2015). A meta-analysis of the efficacy of acceptance and commitment therapy for clinically relevant mental and physical health problems. *Psychotherapy Psychosomatics, 84*(1), 30–36. https://doi.org/10.1159/000365764

Basran, J., Raven, J., & Plowright, P. (2022). Overview of outcome research on compassion focused therapy: A scoping review. In P. Gilbert & G. Simos (Eds.), *Compassion focused therapy: Clinical practice and applications* (pp. 600–616). Routledge.

Beer, R. (2018). Protocol for EMDR therapy in the treatment of eating disorders. In M. Luber (Ed.), *Eye movement desensitization and reprocessing (EMDR) therapy scripted protocols and summary sheets: Treating eating disorders, chronic pain and maladaptive self-care behaviors.* Springer Publishing Company.

Carletto, S., Malandrone, F., Berchialla, P., Oliva, F., Colombi, N., Hase, M., Hofmann, A., & Ostacoli, L. (2021). Eye movement desensitization and reprocessing for depression: A systematic review and meta-analysis. *European Journal of Psychotraumatology, 12*(1), 1894736.

Chen, Y.-R., Hung, K.-W., Tsai, J.-C., Chu, H., Chung, M.-H., Chen, S.-R., Liao, Y.-M., Ou, K.-L., Chang, Y.-C., & Chou, K.-R. (2014). Efficacy of eye-movement desensitization and reprocessing for patients with posttraumatic-stress disorder: A meta-analysis of randomized controlled trials. *PLoS ONE, 9*(8), e103676. https://doi.org/10.1371/journal.pone.0103676

Chen, L., Zhang, G., Hu, M., Liang, X. (2015). Eye movement desensitization and reprocessing versus cognitive-behavioral therapy for adult posttraumatic stress disorder: Systematic review and meta-analysis. *The Journal of Nervous and Mental Disease, 203*(6), 443–451.

Craig, C., Hiskey, S., & Spector, A. (2020). Compassion focused therapy: A systematic review of its effectiveness and acceptability in clinical populations. *Expert Review of Neurotherapeutics, 20*(4), 385–400.

De Jongh, A., Bicanic, I., Matthijissen, S., Amann, B.-L., Hofmann, A., Farrell, D., Lee, C.-L., & Maxfield, L. (2019). The current status of EMDR therapy involving the treatment of complex posttraumatic stress disorder. *Journal of EMDR Practice and Research, 13*(4), 284–290.

Gilbert, P. (2009). Introducing compassion-focused therapy. *Advances in Psychiatric Treatment, 15*(3), 199–208.

Gilbert, P. (2010). *Compassion focused therapy.* Routledge.

Gilbert, P. (2020). Compassion: From its evolution to a psychotherapy. *Frontiers in Psychology,* 3123.

Gilbert, P., & Simos, G. (2022). Compassion focused therapy: An evolution-informed, biopsychosocial approach to psychotherapy: History and challenge. In P. Gilbert & G. Simos (Eds.), *Compassion focused therapy* (pp. 24–89). Routledge.

Gloster, A. T., Walder, N., Levin, M. E., Twohig, M. P.& Karekla, M. (2020). The empirical status of acceptance and commitment therapy: A review of meta-analyses. *Journal of Contextual Behavioral Science, 18*, 181–192.

Griffioen, B. T., Van der Vegt, A. A., De Groot, I. W., & De Jongh, A. (2017). The effect of EMDR and CBT on low self-esteem in a general psychiatric population: A randomized controlled trial. *Frontiers in Psychology, 8*(8), 1910. https://doi.org/10.3389/fpsyg.2017.01910. PMID: 29167649; PMCID: PMC5682328.

Hayes, S. C., Barnes-Holmes, D., & Roche, B. (2001). *Relational frame theory: A post-Skinnerian account of human language and cognition.* Plenum Press.

Hayes, S. C., Barnes-Holmes, D., & Wilson, K. G. (2012). Contextual behavioral science: Creating a science more adequate to the challenge of the human condition. *Journal of Contextual Behavioral Science, 1*, 1–16.

Hayes, S. C., Ciarrochi, J., Hofmann, S. G., Chin, F., & Sahdra, B. (2022). Evolving an idionomic approach to processes of change: Towards a unified, personalised science of human improvement. *Behavior Research and Therapy*, *156*, 104155.

Hayes, S. C., Strosahl, K., & Wilson, K. G. (1999). *Acceptance and commitment therapy: An experiential approach to behavior change*. Guildford Press.

Hofmann, S. (2018). The history and current status of CBT as an evidence-based therapy. In S. C. Hayes & S. G. Hofmann (Eds.), *Process-based CBT: The science and core clinical competencies of cognitive behavioral therapy*. New Harbinger Publications.

Hughes, S. (2018). A brief introduction to the philosophy of science as it applies to clinical psychology. In S. C. Hayes & S. G. Hofmann (Eds.), *Process-based CBT: The science and core clinical competencies of cognitive behavioral therapy*. New Harbinger Publications.

Kashdan, T. B., & Rottenberg, J. (2010). Psychological flexibility as a fundamental aspect of health. *Clinical Psychology Review, 30*(7), 865–878.

Kennedy, F., & Pearson, D. (2020). *Integrating CBT and third wave therapies: Distinctive features*. Routledge.

Kirby, J. N. (2017). Compassion interventions: The programmes, the evidence, and implications for research and practice. *Psychology and Psychotherapy: Theory, Research and Practice*, *90*(3), 432–455.

Korn, D. L. (2009). EMDR and the treatment of complex PTSD: A review. *Journal of EMDR Practice and Research*, *3*(4), 264–278.

Korrelboom, K., Maarsingh, M., & Huijbrechts, I. (2012). Competitive memory training (COMET) for treating low self-esteem in patients with depressive disorders: A randomized clinical trial. *Depression and Anxiety*, *29*(2), 102–110.

Lawrence, V. A., & Lee, D. (2014). An exploration of people's experiences of compassion-focused therapy for trauma, using interpretative phenomenological analysis. *Clinical Psychology & Psychotherapy*, *21*(6), 495–507.

Lucas, J. (2023). *Eight reasons learning acceptance and commitment therapy can make you a better therapist*. www.openforwards.com

Manfield, P., Lovett, J., Engel, L., & Manfield, D. (2017). Use of the flash technique in EMDR therapy: Four case examples. *Journal of EMDR Practice and Research*, *11*(4), 195–205.

Marsden, Z., Lovell, K., Blore, D., Ali, S., & Delgadillo, J. (2018). A randomized controlled trial comparing EMDR and CBT for obsessive-compulsive disorder. *Clinical Psychology and Psychotherapy*, *25*(1), e10–e18.

Marshall, M. B., Zuroff, D. C., McBride, C., & Bagby, R. M. (2008). Self-criticism predicts differential response to treatment for major depression. *Journal of Clinical Psychology*, *64*(3), 231–244.

Millard, L. A., Wan, M. W., Smith, D. M., & Wittkowski, A. (2023). The effectiveness of compassion focused therapy with clinical populations: A systematic review and meta-analysis. *Journal of Affective Disorders*, *326*(1), 168–192.

Mooney, K. A., & Padesky, C. A. (2000). Applying client creativity to recurrent problems: Constructing possibilities and tolerating doubt. *Journal of Cognitive Psychotherapy: An International Quarterly*, *14*, 149–161.

National Institute for Clinical Excellence. (2018). *Post-traumatic stress disorder (PTSD): The management of adults and children in primary and secondary care*. NICE Guidelines.

Neff, K. D., & Vonk, R. (2009). Self-compassion versus global self-esteem: Two different ways of relating to oneself. *Journal of Personality*, *77*(1), 23–50.

Neimeyer, G. J., & Morton, R. J. (1997). Personal epistemologies and preferences for rationalist versus constructivist psychotherapies. *Journal of Constructivist Psychology*, *10*, 109–123.

Ogden, P., Minton, K., & Pain, C. (2006). *Trauma and the body: A sensorimotor approach to psychotherapy*. Norton series on interpersonal neurobiology. W. W. Norton & Company.

Ost, L. G. (2014). The efficacy of acceptance and commitment therapy: An updated systematic review and meta-analysis. *Behavior Research and Therapy, 61*, 105–121.

Parker, Z. J., & Waller, G. (2017). Development and validation of the negative attitudes towards CBT scale. *Behavioural and Cognitive Psychotherapy, 45*(6), 629–646.

Petrocchi, N., Dentale, F., & Gilbert, P. (2019). Self-reassurance, not self-esteem, serves as a buffer between self-criticism and depressive symptoms. *Psychology and Psychotherapy, 92*(3), 394–406.

Salkovskis, P. M. (1991). The importance of behaviour in the maintenance of anxiety and panic: A cognitive account. *Behavioural and Cognitive Psychotherapy, 19*(1), 6–19.

Shapiro, F. (2007). EMDR, adaptive information processing, and case conceptualization. *Journal of EMDR Practice and Research, 1*(2), 68–87.

Shapiro, F. (2018). *Eye movement desensitization and reprocessing (EMDR): Basic principles, protocols and procedures* (3rd ed.). The Guilford Press.

Siegel, D.-J. (2020). *The developing mind: Toward a neurobiology of interpersonal experience* (3rd ed.). The Guilford Press.

Silver, S.-M., Rogers, S., & Russell, M.-C. (2008). Eye movement desensitization and reprocessing (EMDR) in the treatment of war veterans. *Journal of Clinical Psychology: In Session, 64*, 947–957.

Steindl, S., Bell, T., Dixon, A., & Kirby, J. (2023). Therapist perspectives on working with fears, blocks and resistances to compassion in compassion focused therapy. *Counselling and Psychotherapy Research, 23*(3), 850–863.

Stott, R. (2007). When head and heart do not agree: A theoretical and clinical analysis of rational-emotional dissociation (RED) in cognitive therapy. *Journal of Cognitive Psychotherapy, 21*(1), 37–50.

Wakelin, K. E., Perman, G., & Simonds, L. M. (2022). Effectiveness of self-compassion-related interventions for reducing self-criticism: A systematic review and meta-analysis. *Clinical Psychology & Psychotherapy, 29*(1), 1–25.

Walser, R. D. (2019). *The heart of ACT: Developing a flexible, process-based and client-centred practice using acceptance and commitment therapy.* New Harbinger Publications.

Wilson, G., Farrell, D., Barron, I., Hutchins, J., Whybrow, D., & Kiernan, M. D. (2018). The use of eye-movement desensitization reprocessing (EMDR) therapy in treating post-traumatic stress disorder – a systematic narrative review. *Frontiers in Psychology, 9*, 923. https://doi.org/10.3389/fpsyg.2018.00923

Young, J. E., Klosko, J. S., & Weishaar, M. E. (2006). *Schema therapy: A practitioner's guide.* Guilford Press.

Chapter 22

Supervising other CBT practitioners

Jason Roscoe and Natasha Scullane

Introduction

In addition to consolidating knowledge and skills as a therapist, one of the first things qualified CBT therapists do is begin to expand their job role beyond treating clients. Sooner or later, many will find themselves supervising others whether this is through an expressed interest to do so or an organisational expectation (Liness et al., 2017). From our experience as supervisors, and from training others, it is common practice that once you have been qualified for a couple of years, you will start to supervise others. Even if this foray into supervision begins with supervising psychological wellbeing practitioners (PWPs) (as opposed to CBT therapists), this new level of responsibility can be daunting at any stage of one's career. Even more so when one is asked to do this without any specific training as a supervisor.

In this chapter, we consider some of the rewards and challenges of becoming a CBT supervisor. The first section of the chapter provides a theoretical overview of best practices in CBT supervision, building on some of the points made in Chapter 9. There is an emphasis on helping the reader to consider if they have the requisite skills to effectively supervise another practitioner and there is an invitation to reflect on when the supervision they deliver might start to 'drift' from expert recommendations (see Pugh & Margetts, 2020; Roscoe, 2021). Throughout the chapter, we address the 'lived experience' of being a supervisor, providing some examples of the culture of CBT supervision within the UK, particularly England as most of our experience relates to practices within this context. This has undoubtedly shaped our supervisory practice and our supervision schemas. We provide a framework that is born from the lessons we have learned as supervisors. We hope that it helps to ensure that supervision is effective and dynamic, and we have included some reflective exercises to help you to consider aspects where you might identify with our experiences.

Developing knowledge, skills, and confidence as a CBT supervisor

'Are you ready to be a supervisor?' In NHS Talking Therapies settings, it's a question that, in our experience, rarely gets asked. Before you have any time to think

DOI: 10.4324/9781003428527-26

about it you have been designated a supervisee. The pace of an NHS Talking Therapies Service is fast, clinician's caseloads are high; everyone needs supervising, at some point everyone will need to 'muck in'. Ideally, you would go on Supervisor Training before you begin supervising, but depending when the training falls, and how many places your service has on the training, you're likely to be asked to supervise without doing it. This is problematic for several reasons which will be highlighted throughout the chapter. This section focuses on what the research and expert consensus tell us about the skills that make a competent, effective, and dynamic supervisor.

What are the core skills of a CBT supervisor?

You might find yourself experiencing one or more negative automatic thoughts about your level of supervisory skill. The good news is that you don't need to be perfect as a supervisor, in fact, modelling imperfection, especially to trainees who are prone to having 'demanding standards' can be quite useful (Haarhoff, 2006). Also, a healthy level of self-doubt can be a good thing as it prevents us from getting complacent or thinking that we have all the answers.

Personal reflection – Natasha

I've worked as a CBT therapist now for nearly ten years, I'm viewed as an experienced member of the team; however, it doesn't stop those sneaky imposter syndrome thoughts creeping in when it comes to sharing my knowledge in supervision.

- *'What if I don't know the answer to their question?'*
- *'Am I talking too much? Am I being helpful enough?'*
- *'Another supervisor would give much better advice than me!'*

'Remember supervision needs to be normative, formative, restorative – wait, what's formative again?!'

The normative, formative, and restorative functions of supervision

Before you completely fuse with this list of automatic thoughts and write yourself off as unsuitable in the process, it is helpful to consider the core functions of supervision and the specific tasks that a CBT supervisor must undertake (Milne, 2017). These are typically referred to as a range of normative (ethical), formative (educative) and restorative (supportive) duties. The emphasis on each will differ across sessions and will be influenced by the knowledge, skills, and attitudes of the supervisee and what is brought (or not brought) to supervision (Proctor, 1994; Yourman, 2003).

Ideally, these topics are addressed with the supervisee through a range of activities that take them through a cycle of planning, acting, reflecting as described by Kolb (1984). If you provide group supervision there are additional considerations such as managing group dynamics which is beyond the scope of this chapter. In general, 'within' supervision tasks include

- verbal case discussions;
- reviewing videos of therapy sessions and assessing competence using measures such as the Cognitive Therapy Scale-Revised (CTS-R; Blackburn et al., 2001);
- active and experiential methods such as role-play or supervisor modelling, chair work;
- self-practice/self-reflection (SP/SR) of CBT methods such as formulating ruptures, planning behavioural experiments associated with one's own fears (Bennett-Levy, 2019; Pugh, 2019; Pugh & Margetts, 2020).

Personal reflection: Natasha

A challenge for me was learning how to provide quality supervision when I had competing demands on how supervision time should be used. It is common for caseload management to be expected as part of clinical supervision which involves a review of supervisees' caseload, clinical hours, booked sessions, cancellation/DNA rate, as well as addressing their clinical supervision questions, all within one hour. At times it can feel like I am wearing different hats: a 'caseload manager' hat, a 'clinical supervisor' hat, and when I supervisee trainee CBT therapists I wear an extra 'restorative supervisor' hat for providing emotional support, checking they are progressing well on the high-intensity training course, and following the newly learned protocols.

What can we derive from research on standard supervision practices?

There have been relatively few studies that capture what happens routinely in CBT supervision. A study by Townend et al. (2002) which sampled ($n = 170$) the British Association for Behavioural and Cognitive Psychotherapies (BABCP)-accredited therapists found that 36% were supervising despite never having received any supervisor training. This study also found that only 18% reviewed video or audio recordings of therapy sessions in supervision and in comparison, to verbal case discussion, more active methods such as role-play were less common (19%). In addition to this, 53% did not receive supervision of supervision (SoS). My own more recent research with ($n = 38$) supervision workshop attendees also found a similar pattern with 29% never bringing videos, 32% never using role-play, modelling or practising CBT methods on themselves (Roscoe, unpublished). What these findings indicate is that supervisor and supervisee behaviour has altered little in the past few decades.

> **Key Point:** The demands that are placed on how you spend your time within certain working environments can make it more difficult to have adequate preparation time for supervision (e.g. selecting videos for review). With high caseloads, some supervisees might wish to discuss several clients each session or simply 'offload' about their stresses of the job meaning that it is difficult to really 'zoom in' on assessing their skills.

Understanding supervisory drift

There are several potential consequences of supervisors and supervisees (supervision dyads) omitting or underemphasising the more active elements of supervision. Firstly, in failing to review examples of the supervisee's clinical work, misconceptions of CBT theory, poor adherence to protocols and poorly executed interventions may go unnoticed (Murray et al., 2022). Secondly, by failing to utilise role-play or supervisor modelling, novice therapists might struggle to translate the 'declarative' knowledge that they acquire in training into 'procedural' knowledge of how to apply formulations and interventions with real clients (Bennett-Levy, 2006; Roscoe & Wilbraham, 2024). Thirdly, supervision that is not guided by a core set of principles (e.g. Armstrong & Freeston, 2006; Gordon, 2012; Roth & Pilling, 2008) is susceptible to 'drift' because supervision dyads do not have a shared understanding of the tasks of CBT supervision (Milne, 2017; Roscoe, 2021). In these instances, ruptures, where both parties have different (often unexpressed) needs, unfocused supervision or harmful supervision can become the norm (Kennerley & Clohessy, 2010; Milne, 2020; Roscoe et al., 2022; Vekaria et al., 2023). All of this begs the question – if many supervisors are supervising without having had any training or access to effective SoS to reflect on their practice, how do they know how to supervise?

> ### Self-reflection – Natasha
>
> *When I got allocated my first CBT supervisee having not completed the Supervisor Training, I drew on my experience of past supervision to inform my supervisory approach such as:*
>
> - *'What kind of supervision had I experienced?'*
> - *'What kind of supervision methods helped my clinical practice?'*
> - *'What did I like about supervision?'*
> - *'What didn't I like?'*

I aimed to be open, supportive, collaborative, curious, attentive, focused on meeting the supervisee's needs, and ready to answer supervision questions, with clients' treatment and recovery in mind.

Understanding our supervision 'schemas'

Schemas are like filters which help us to organise our experiences both past and present (Segal, 1988). New information (e.g. supervisor behaviour) is screened through the filter of our schema, and behaviour that matches past representations of "what a supervisor is" is assimilated. Information that contradicts the schema may be rejected or 'crushed to fit' the existing one (Butler et al., 2010).

As CBT therapists commence their training, past experiences of being supervised in previous professional roles (e.g. social work, mental health nursing) will in part influence their expectations of what supervision consists of (Robinson et al., 2012). Furthermore, the supervision they receive during training and post-qualification adds to the 'supervision schema' that is in development (e.g. reinforces or challenges; Roscoe & Taylor, 2023).

Like all schemas, supervision schemas are governed by rules ('shoulds' and 'musts' about self and others) and are hypothesised to be resistant to change and self-perpetuating (Young et al., 2006). When supervisor and supervisee have very different expectations of what *should* happen in supervision sessions, a 'schematic mismatch' may ensue. We provide a hypothetical example of this being brought to Supervision of Supervision for exploration.

Schematic mismatch between supervisor and supervisee

Nick (supervisor) brought one of his supervisees Michelle for discussion in Meta-supervision. Michelle struggled with confidence in making decisions around formulation and sequencing of interventions. Despite Nick's best efforts to provide further declarative and procedural knowledge within supervision, Michelle continued to want Nick to provide all the answers about what to do next. Nick felt uncomfortable raising this with Michelle for a fear of upsetting her. There was a clear mismatch between Nick's beliefs about what a supervisor 'should' do and what level of input Michelle believed a supervisor 'should' provide.

Using good 'FORM' in your supervisory practice

Without a means of raising their unspoken schematic clash, Michelle continued to doubt herself as a therapist and rely on Nick to 'spoon feed' her the answers in supervision. Nick continued to feel resentful about doing this but avoided addressing Michelle's helplessness with her. In this section, we provide a framework for ensuring that the issues experienced by Nick and Michelle can be addressed early within the supervisory relationship and effectively. The acronym 'FORM' is used as an easy-to-remember mnemonic and contains details of the four steps to being a dynamic supervisor.

- **Framework** – are you using a recognised framework (e.g. Newcastle 'cake stand' model) to structure supervision sessions, guide content, justify your primary focus; is your supervisee using a recognisable model and treatment plan with their clients?
- **Observation** – are you observing the skills of your supervisee through video feedback, role-play, etc.? Is your supervisee using self-reflective methods to observe their own behaviour within their relationships with clients?
- **Relationships** – is there a sufficient focus on your relationship with your supervisees and of those between your supervisees and their clients?
- **Measurement of processes** – how are you measuring your skills as a supervisor and your supervisees competence? (e.g. SAGE; Milne et al., 2011; CTS-R)

Each part of 'FORM' has a dynamic focus where attention can be directed to the supervisee-client relationship or that of supervisor–supervisee. FORM can also be used as a type of self-audit of supervisory practice or to support discussions within meta-supervision.

Step 1: adhere to a framework

Supervisory drift (SD) is more likely if CBT supervision lacks 'the basics' such as a clear agreement on the goals and tasks (Bordin, 1983). A supervision contract can help to address some of this, but from the outset you should be clear about the model that is underpinning what you do together in supervision. There are several established CBT models of supervision, most notably the tandem (Milne, 2017), the PURE Supervision flower (Corrie & Lane, 2015), and the Newcastle 'cakestand' (Armstrong & Freeston, 2006). The Roth and Pilling (2008) Supervisor competence framework is another useful document that should be kept in sight. Irrespective of the model chosen, a focused and collaborative agenda at the start of each session is essential (see Gordon, 2012, for a useful example).

Top tip: The biggest risk, especially for qualified therapists, is that supervision becomes an informal chat. Your chosen supervision model can act as an anchor if the supervisory focus drifts too far off topic. A supervision model could have helped Nick and Michelle to make sense of their perspectives whilst holding in mind the core aims of their work together.

Tailoring supervision to the needs of the supervisee

How and when you introduce different methods in supervision comes with experience, training, and effective meta-supervision (Newman, 2013). Your first task is tailoring supervision to the needs of the supervisee, followed by maintaining a structure to your sessions and importantly, making supervision an experiential learning experience (Kennerley & Clohessy, 2010; Milne et al., 2011). Tailoring supervision relies on two factors; understanding the *preferences* of the supervisee and gauging where they are at with *skill development*. For example, qualified supervisees who are likely to have greater 'declarative' and 'procedural' knowledge of CBT methods will have different learning needs in comparison to trainees (Bennett-Levy, 2006).

Key Point: The most effective supervisors will adapt the content and structure of their supervision sessions in response to the idiosyncratic needs of their supervisees (Bennett-Levy & Thwaites, 2007; James et al., 2006).

The Socratic approach to supervision

With experienced supervisees, it can be useful to take a more Socratic approach by exploring with them what they hope to gain from supervision (Padesky, 1993). This is because they are likely to have worked with a broader range of clients and understand how to carry out interventions to good effect. Bennett-Levy (2006) refers to this as the acquisition of 'when- then rules'. Trainees and newly qualified therapists are likely to require more educational input from you as a supervisor where information they have acquired/skills they have briefly practised on their training courses, are 'cemented' in supervision through clarification, supervisor modelling or role-play (Roscoe & Wilbraham, 2024). With therapists who have been practising for years, asking the right questions rather than giving them your advice might be more helpful in the long run (Padesky, 1993).

Key Point: Trainees by virtue of their limited clinical experience cannot draw from a 'storehouse' of CBT knowledge and often need to be told how to manage nuanced situations in therapy. As training progresses, supervision can become more Socratic.

Personal reflection: Jason

I have used pre-supervision meetings and a specific questionnaire with both trainees and experienced therapists to highlight strengths, weaknesses, preferences, and intrapersonal or interpersonal factors that might warrant attention on occasions. I find that doing this allows me to get some understanding of how these might play out in supervision before we start working together. For example, if an experienced supervisee does not have many technical questions about CBT Theory, perhaps they might wish to use supervision to reflect on other challenges such as their transference and countertransference reactions with some patients (see Moorey & Byrne, 2019, for useful examples). With a trainee, I would encourage them to reflect on how their previous professional role (e.g. nursing) influences how they use supervision.

Step 2: inject some life into your supervision sessions

Many supervisors can fall into the habit of using verbal case discussion as the mainstay or entirety of their supervision sessions (Townend et al., 2002). Research into why supervisors limit active methods is sparse, however it might be due to a lack of confidence in using more creative or experiential methods (e.g. role-play) or a lack of exposure to this in the supervision that they have experienced as supervisees (Pugh & Margetts, 2020).

Setting up behavioural experiments (BEs) within supervision

Behavioural experiments within supervision can help supervisees to deepen their knowledge of CBT 'from the inside out' (Bennett-Levy et al., 2014). A fictional scenario is provided to show how this can make supervision an active learning experience.

Using CBT Formulation of the supervisee's difficulties

Tracy* brought a client to supervision who would regularly talk at length in an unfocused way. Tracy found it difficult to contain the client due to a fear of upsetting or annoying them. The consequence was that agendas were rarely set, and no progress was being made towards the agreed treatment goals.

Having first checked out if this was a skill deficit (e.g. did Tracy know how to interrupt a client politely?) it was agreed that Tracy held the assumption *'If I interrupt a client then it means that I am rude and they will become upset or angry with me and terminate therapy'*. This was conceptualised as a therapist schema 'rejection-sensitive' (Leahy, 2001) and collaboratively the supervisor agreed to set up a behavioural experiment with Tracy.

Once problematic supervisee behaviour has been formulated, the supervisor can help them to use CBT methods to test out their anxious cognitions. In the example provided, Tracy and her supervisor set up a behavioural experiment to test her prediction. When Tracy interrupted the client in the next session and set the agenda, she was relieved to discover that the client found this helpful and did not react in the ways that she had predicted. This helped to update Tracy's therapist schemas (Leahy, 2001) and generalised to her work with other clients who were prone to rambling.

Utilising other active methods

There are many other 'active' or experiential methods that could be used to achieve a similar effect to a BE. For example, the supervisor could model interrupting Tracy as the client or Tracy could role-play responding in the worst way imagined and they could test out different ways of responding to the client. The supervisor could also ask Tracy to track the activation of various therapist schemas as a homework task. Finally, if Tracy brought a recording of this client to supervision, they would have more accurate information about what Tracy is doing well and where she might change things.

Top tips

- The next time you find yourself about to explain something verbally to your supervisee, ask them *'What would be the best way for me to help you to understand this better?'* (e.g. *I am a visual learner, so I like to see my supervisor demonstrate how to draw out a model or do some role-play on how to deliver an intervention*).
- Try to incorporate CBT methods within supervision sessions (e.g. explore the supervisee's negative automatic thoughts or help them identify 'rules for living' that are getting in the way of therapy).

Get creative – set the supervisee a behavioural experiment to test out some of their predictions. You can also use chairs to help 'embody' their client's perspective or enact different 'parts' of themselves (see Roscoe, 2021).

Step 3: keeping relationships in focus

Dynamic supervisors retain a focus on all of the relationships that are relevant to supervision:

- Supervisor–supervisee
- Supervisee–client

- Supervisor–client
- Meta-supervisor–junior Supervisor

Whilst not originating from the CBT literature, the seven eyed supervision model developed by Hawkins and Shohet (2000) can help to inform our differential focus across sessions.

Self-reflection – Natasha

Setting up solid foundations for supervision is priceless. When supervision goes well, it feels like the most rewarding role in the world. I have witnessed lots of skill development, watched live session clips and discussed cases which have resulted in remarkable recoveries. It's also important to acknowledge the times when issues 'crop up' in supervision. Examples could include

- *lack of preparation;*
- *difficult case discussions;*
- *supervisees not booking in enough clients;*
- *feedback being poorly given/not well received;*
- *interpersonal issues/lack of sensitivity;*
- avoidance (Supervisees not bringing live session clips).

Identifying the preferences of the supervisee

All CBT therapists will have different strengths and weaknesses. For example, some trainees are naturally good at being structured and setting agendas whilst others are better at the relational aspects of therapy. Establishing a baseline of their knowledge, skills, and preferences when contracting for supervision is highly recommended. This process can be aided by a pre-supervision discussion or developing a specific questionnaire. This can be useful for identifying the methods that a supervisee prefers to use (e.g. some trainees love self-practice of CBT methods whilst others detest it). This can also help the supervisor to understand how the supervisee wishes to be addressed (e.g. use of pronouns) and how best to give them feedback on their skills.

Specific challenges associated with supervising experiencing therapists

The dynamics involved in supervising qualified CBT therapists is often a trickier task for several reasons. Firstly, you might find yourself supervising a peer who has a similar level of experience or perhaps more years in the role than you. This can be anxiety provoking as you might think 'what can I tell them that they don't already know?'. This fear exposes a dysfunctional rule and/or assumption about the role of a supervisor (e.g. 'I should have all the answers to my supervisee's questions'). The focus of supervision might be more about enhancing self-reflection, cultural competence and meta-competences than educating the supervisee about CBT models or interventions and (Naz et al., 2019; Whittington & Grey, 2014).

Gauging the alliance

Attending to the supervisory relationship from the outset and at regular intervals (e.g. using the Leeds Alliance in Supervision Scale [LAS] to gauge supervisee satisfaction; Wainwright, 2010) can pay dividends. Whilst there is responsibility on both sides to contribute positively to the development and maintenance of the supervisory relationship, if an issue arises the onus is often on the supervisor to address it. In comparison to other alliance measures, the LAS is brief, measuring three aspects of the alliance each session – the supervisor's approach, how understood the supervisee felt and if the session met their needs.

Formulating difficulties in the relationship

Where supervisor and supervisee experience an impasse or rupture due to their unexpressed assumptions about supervision it could be helpful to formulate this (see Roscoe, 2021, for an illustration of this). Where the relationship is not severely strained, the supervisor could draw this out within a session. Alternatively, the supervisor might need to take this to meta-supervision where the meta-supervisor can help them to construct a formulation without the emotional charge of being in the room with the supervisee.

Natasha: self-reflection – managing 'strains' on the relationship

In my experience, it is 100% possible to address issues in a constructive way. It can be uncomfortable, but it is much better to deal with it than let a problem fester. As you develop your therapy style, you are also likely to develop a supervision style. They may be similar; they may be different.

I received some helpful feedback about my style from a supervisee once. I was made aware at the end of a session that a question I had asked my supervisee had made them feel anxious. I was relieved my supervisee felt able to share this with me, and we had a useful conversation about it. My style can be quite direct as I prefer to cut to the chase when trying to understand something. In treatment with clients, I generally soften my approach to ensure clients feel comfortable and safe. On this occasion, I wanted to understand the reason my supervisee had chosen to use one technique instead of another, and I asked why they had made this choice. I was genuinely curious; however, the way I asked 'why' felt anxiety provoking for the supervisee. They assumed I was being critical about the choice they had made, and it triggered self-critical thoughts. I was quick to acknowledge the impact of my question, and we discussed our perspectives. My overall reflection on this situation was that it's important that I don't forget that supervisees may also benefit from a softened approach at times, especially during training when they experience a lot of self-doubt. This experience helped to evolve my supervision style, to be more mindful of how feedback or questions may be interpreted and remember what it feels like to be a trainee learning on the job.

Step 4: assessing your supervisory competencies

There are various ways that we can 'take stock' of our skills as supervisors. In broad terms, there are formal and informal measures of our supervisory competence. For example, The Supervision Adherence and Guidance Evaluation (SAGE; Milne et al., 2011) and a shorter version (Short SAGE; Reiser et al., 2018) are validated tools, similar in design to the CTS-R (Blackburn et al., 2001). Oxford Cognitive Therapy Centre have also developed a Supervisor Competency Scale (a copy can be obtained from Kennerley & Clohessy, 2010) and either scale can be used to measure specific supervisor competencies. The drawback to their application is that watching full length recordings (e.g. 60 minutes) and undertaking rating scales is time-consuming. Users might also feel like they need training to be confident applying these measures.

Top tips

- On occasions, I (Jason) have used sections of these scales within SoS rather than the full instrument, to rate 10–15 minute clips of supervisions sessions. This allows for some degree of formal rating however, another option is to undertake a brief 'audit' of one's supervision over a specific time period (e.g. six months) by considering if you have had good 'FORM' in your sessions.
- Appendix 2 provides a brief checklist that can either be used to audit your own supervisory practice or can be shared within Supervision of Supervision.

Accessing supervision for your supervisory practice

Many of the challenges discussed in this chapter could potentially be 'nipped in the bud' by taking them to another supervisor often referred to as a 'meta-supervisor'

(Newman, 2013). This is because we can find it difficult to 'see the woods for the trees' when we encounter difficulties in our relationships with supervisees. This last section provides some tips on what to consider when arranging SoS.

Choosing a meta-supervisor

There are many factors that determine the choice that one has over their SoS arrangements. For example, it is recognised that contextual factors such as where one practices (e.g. within a large government health service vs. private practice) can narrow the field of potential meta-supervisors that are available for consultation. In these circumstances, it may be reasonable to consider options such as peer SoS; however, the limitation of this format (e.g. that no one is 'in charge') must be considered. For those with more freedom to select their own meta-supervisor, it is worth cautioning that 'years on the job' does not automatically suggest greater supervisory competence. Continual investment in one's supervisory skills through reading of contemporary literature, attending CPD events and auditing one's own practice are arguably more important facets. It is recommended that you do some 'vetting' when looking for someone who can competently supervise your supervisory practice.

TOP TIP: Don't be afraid to ask a potential meta-supervisor about their experience and commitment to ongoing professional development in this area.

Key points

- Without opportunities to reflect upon habitual ways of delivering supervision, poor supervisory practice might continue into new supervisory relationships and environments.
- The absence of supervisor training means supervisors can end up drawing entirely from their own experiences. Imagine if we delivered therapy based on the therapy, we have received for our personal problems!
- Being an effective supervisor does not mean that you need to have all the answers. Whilst some 'teaching' forms a part of supervision, most other methods such as role-play, SP/SR, and video feedback are collaborative ventures.

Top tips

1. Always use a supervision contract which includes goals for supervision and set clear expectations of what supervisees need to do to prepare for supervision.

2. The same principles that help CBT treatment stay on track also help supervision stay on track.
3. Seek feedback from the supervisee about how they are finding your supervision sessions and encourage open discussions about their preferences and expectations of supervision.

Conclusion

Many CBT therapists become supervisors yet are often asked to do so without prior training. Consequently, novice supervisors are likely to draw upon their own experiences of supervision which has several inherent problems associated with this. The research indicates that many supervisory relationships lack 'active' components. Years 'on the job' as a supervisor do not necessarily lead to a change in supervisory habits therefore committing to ongoing supervision training and SoS are recommended. This chapter has only been able to offer a whistlestop tour of some of the main challenges to providing effective supervision. It is hoped that it generates a reflective space for 'budding' or experienced supervisors to change the culture of supervision, one supervisor at a time.

*(supervisee name changed to protect anonymity)

Further reading

Gordon, P. K. (2012). Ten steps to cognitive behavioural supervision. *The Cognitive Behaviour Therapist, 5*(4), 71–82.
Roscoe, J. (2021). Conceptualising and managing supervisory drift. *The Cognitive Behaviour Therapist, 14*, E37. https://doi.org/10.1017/S1754470X21000350
Roth, A. D., & Pilling, S. (2008). *A competence framework for the supervision of psychological therapies.* https://www.ucl.ac.uk/pals/sites/pals/files/background _document_supervision_competences_july_2015.pdf

References

Armstrong, P. V., & Freeston, M. H. (2006). Conceptualising and formulating cognitive therapy supervision. In N. Tarrier (Ed.), *Case formulation in cognitive behaviour therapy* (pp. 349–371). Routledge/Taylor & Francis Group.
Bennett-Levy, J. (2006). Therapist skills: A cognitive model of their acquisition and refinement. *Behavioural and Cognitive Psychotherapy, 34*, 57–78.
Bennett-Levy, J. (2019). Why therapists should walk the talk: The theoretical and empirical case for personal practice in therapist training and professional development. *Journal of Behavior Therapy and Experimental Psychiatry, 62*, 133–145. https://doi.org/10.1016/j.jbtep.2018. 08.004
Bennett-Levy, J., & Thwaites, R. (2007). Self and self-reflection in the therapeutic relationship: A conceptual map and practical strategies for the training, supervision and self-supervision of interpersonal skills. In P. Gilbert & R. L. Leahy (Eds.), *The therapeutic relationship in the cognitive behavioral psychotherapies.* Routledge.
Bennett-Levy, J., Thwaites, R., Haarhoff, B., & Perry, H. (2014). *Experiencing CBT from the inside out: A self-practice/self-reflection workbook for therapists.* Guilford Publications.

Blackburn, I. M., James, I. A., Milne, D. L., Baker, C., Standart, S., Garland, A., & Reichelt, F. K. (2001). The revised cognitive therapy scale (CTS-R): Psychometric properties. *Behavioural and Cognitive Psychotherapy, 29*, 431.

Bordin, E. S. (1983). A working alliance based model of supervision. *The Counseling Psychologist, 11*(1), 35–42. https://doi.org/10.1177/0011000083111007

Butler, G., Fennell, M., & Hackmann, A. (2010). *Cognitive-behavioral therapy for anxiety disorders: Mastering clinical challenges.* Guilford Press.

Corrie, S., & Lane, D. A. (2015). *CBT supervision.* Sage.

Gordon, P. K. (2012). Ten steps to cognitive behavioural supervision. *The Cognitive Behaviour Therapist, 5*(4), 71–82.

Haarhoff, B. A. (2006). The importance of identifying and understanding therapist schema in cognitive therapy training and supervision. *New Zealand Journal of Psychology, 35*, 126–131.

Hawkins, P., & Shohet, R. (2000). *Supervision in the helping professions.* Open University Press.

James, I., Milne, D., Marie-Blackburn, I., & Armstrong, P. (2006). Conducting successful supervision: Novel elements towards an integrative approach. *Behavioural and Cognitive Psychotherapy, 35*, 191–200.

Kennerley, H., & Clohessy, S. (2010). Becoming a supervisor. In M. Mueller, H. Kennerley, F. McManus, & D. Westbrook (Eds.), *Oxford guide to surviving as a CBT therapist.* Oxford University Press.

Kolb, D. A. (1984). *Experiential learning: Experience as the source of learning and development.* Prentice Hall.

Leahy, R. (2001). *Overcoming resistance in cognitive therapy.* Guilford Press.

Liness, S., Lea, S., Nestler, S., Parker, H., & Clark, D. M. (2017). What IAPT CBT high-intensity trainees do after training. *Behavioural and Cognitive Psychotherapy, 45*(1), 16–30.

Milne, D. L. (2017). *Evidence-based CBT supervision: Principles and practice.* John Wiley & Sons.

Milne, D. (2020). Preventing harm related to CBT supervision: A theoretical review and preliminary framework. *The Cognitive Behaviour Therapist, 13*, E54. https://doi.org/10.1017/S1754470X20000550

Milne, D. L., Reiser, R. P., Cliffe, T., & Raine, R. (2011). SAGE: Preliminary evaluation of an instrument for observing competence in CBT supervision. *The Cognitive Behaviour Therapist, 4.*

Moorey, S., & Byrne, S. (2019). Supervision and the therapeutic relationship. In S. Moorey & A. Lavender (Eds.), *The therapeutic relationship in cognitive behavioural therapy.* Sage.

Murray, H., Grey, N., Warnock-Parkes, E., Kerr, A., Wild, J., Clark, D., & Ehlers, A. (2022). Ten misconceptions about trauma-focused CBT for PTSD. *The Cognitive Behaviour Therapist, 15*, e33. https://doi.org/10.1017/S1754470X22000307

Naz, S., Gregory, R., & Bahu, M. (2019). Addressing issues of race, ethnicity and culture in CBT to support therapists and service managers to deliver culturally competent therapy and reduce inequalities in mental health provision for BAME service users. *The Cognitive Behaviour Therapist, 12*, e22.

Newman, C. F. (2013). Training cognitive behavioral therapy supervisors: Didactics, simulated practice, and 'metasupervision'. *Journal of Cognitive Psychotherapy, 27*, 5–18.

Padesky, C. A. (1993). *Socratic questioning: Changing minds or guiding discovery?* Invited keynote address presented at the 1993 European Congress of Behaviour and Cognitive Therapies, London. www.padesky.com/clinicalcorner/publications

Proctor, B. (1994). Supervision – competence, confidence, accountability. *British Journal of Guidance & Counselling, 22*, 309–318.

Pugh, M. (2019). Working with maladaptive therapist modes: An action-experiential approach to supervision. *Schema Therapy Bulletin, 3*, 10–14.

Pugh, M., & Margetts, A. (2020). Are you sitting (un) comfortably? Action based supervision and supervisory drift. *The Cognitive Behaviour Therapist, 13,* e17. https://doi.org/10.1017/S1754470X20000185

Reiser, R. P., Cliffe, T., & Milne, D. L. (2018). An improved competence rating scale for CBT supervision: Short-SAGE. *The Cognitive Behaviour Therapist, 11,* e7.

Robinson, S., Kellett, S., King, I., & Keating, V. (2012). Role transition from mental health nurse to IAPT high intensity psychological therapist. *Behavioural and Cognitive Psychotherapy, 40,* 351–366. https://doi.org/10.1017/S1352465811000683

Roscoe, J. (2021). Conceptualising and managing supervisory drift. *The Cognitive Behaviour Therapist, 14,* E37. https://doi.org/10.1017/S1754470X21000350

Roscoe, J., & Taylor, J. (2023). Maladaptive therapist schemas in CBT practice, training and supervision: A scoping review. *Clinical Psychology & Psychotherapy,* 1–18. https://doi.org/10.1002/cpp.2802

Roscoe, J., Taylor, J., Harrington, R., & Wilbraham, S. (2022). CBT supervision behind closed doors: Supervisor and supervisee reflections on their expectations and use of clinical supervision. *Counselling and Psychotherapy Research, 22*(4), 1056–1067. https://doi.org/10.1002/capr.12572

Roscoe, J., & Wilbraham, S. (2024). 'When it goes well, it works fantastically': Motivations to train and their impact on the practice of CBT. *The Cognitive Behaviour Therapist, 17,* e6.

Roth, A. D., & Pilling, S. (2008). *A competence framework for the supervision of psychological therapies.* https://www.ucl.ac.uk/pals/sites/pals/files/background_document_supervision_competences_july_2015.pdf

Segal, Z. V. (1988). Appraisal of the self-schema construct in cognitive models of depression. *Psychological Bulletin, 103*(2), 147–162. https://doi.org/10.1037/0033–2909.103.2.147

Townend, M., Iannetta, L., & Freeston, M. H. (2002). Clinical supervision in practice: A survey of UK cognitive behavioural psychotherapists accredited by the BABCP. *Behavioural and Cognitive Psychotherapy, 30,* 485.

Vekaria, B., Thomas, T., Phiri, P., & Ononaiye, M. (2023). Exploring the supervisory relationship in the context of culturally responsive supervision: A supervisee's perspective. *The Cognitive Behaviour Therapist, 16,* E22. https://doi.org/10.1017/S1754470X23000168

Wainwright, N. A. (2010). *The development of the Leeds Alliance in supervision scale (LASS): A brief sessional measure of the supervisory alliance.* University of Leeds.

Whittington, A., & Grey, N. (Eds.). (2014). *How to become a more effective CBT therapist: Mastering metacompetence in clinical practice.* John Wiley & Sons.

Young, J. E., Klosko, J. S., & Weishaar, M. E. (2006). *Schema therapy: A practitioner's guide.* Guilford Press.

Yourman, D. B. (2003). Trainee disclosure in psychotherapy supervision: The impact of shame. *Journal of Clinical Psychology, 59*(5), 601–609.

Chapter 23

Venturing into private practice

Sarah D. Rees

Introduction

One minute, you're buried nose-deep in textbooks and training, soaking up all that knowledge. Next, you are a qualified therapist about to put all the theory into practice and make a genuine difference in people's lives. It's an exhilarating time, you're standing at the starting line of an incredible career!

The allure of private practice has grown in recent years, with many organisations in crisis, long waiting lists, small budgets and unrealistic targets all placing enormous strain on services and staff. Alongside this, there's a growing demand for therapy as the stigma around seeking treatment reduces and mental health is generally more widely discussed.

Thousands of people struggle to access the treatment and support they need from traditional services, so they begin to turn to and explore other options. Private practice will be a valuable part of bridging the treatment-need gap.

Whilst there may have been little talk about private practice during training, your qualification has provided you with many exciting choices. One of those choices is to set up your own private practice.

In this chapter, I will walk you through an overview of opportunities and obstacles to help you decide if private practice is right and lay down some of the initial foundations you need to consider; by the end of the chapter, you will know.

- If you are ready to venture into private practice?
- What the common opportunities and obstacles are.
- Have an overview of what it takes to start a private practice.

I have the privilege each day to work alongside many therapists setting up and building their private practice inside my online community, 'Therapists Corner. co.uk'. Common themes regularly arise for therapists when considering this path, for example, uncertainty about whether it will work, anxiety around where referrals will come from, a desire for increased autonomy and flexibility, hoping for more financial security and the ability to work more creativity with less organisational boundaries.

DOI: 10.4324/9781003428527-27

This chapter aims to provide you with a starting point and a balanced view of what awaits you in private practice, but every journey is unique and shaped by personal aspirations, values, and individual goals; your individuality will add that special touch and steer you forward.

My journey

My career started as a mental health nurse at the time I believed I'd be in that role for life; however, as the healthcare landscape evolved, I was drawn to a more holistic and creative approach, supporting people to be their best and recover from mental health challenges. This curiosity steered me towards psychology, and I eventually trained as a cognitive behavioural therapist (CBT). The idea of private practice flickered in my mind and seemed foreign initially. I began watching entrepreneurs on social media reading business books, and the idea gradually grew.

When I first qualified as a CBT therapist, I joined an Improving Access to Psychological Therapies (IAPT) in the National Health Service (NHS) and soon realised CBT didn't have all the answers for the clients I was working with because they had more complex needs and high levels of self-criticism that required more than a single model approach, this led me to discover compassion-focused therapy (CFT). At that time, CFT wasn't as popular as it is now, and the NHS couldn't finance the training. Eager to continue learning and developing my therapist skills, private practice became the only option to fund this training and my burgeoning book collection.

Although traditional employment offers the comforts of paid holidays, sick leave, a consistent salary, and structured retirement plans, the appeal of private practice and its choice, flexibility, and potential were compelling. I could always return to a conventional job if private practice didn't pan out as expected.

Is private practice right for you?

Private practice certainly is a more challenging option. It demands self-motivation, commitment, and dedication, but if personal and professional goals compel you and a clear vision anchors you, the journey is worth every challenge. For me, private practice made sense financially and professionally; it promised and delivered the finances I needed for further training and the autonomy to balance my work and personal life. Plus, when I was a relatively new therapist, it gave me far more reflection time and supervision than would have been possible in an employed role.

Determining if private practice aligns with your aspirations is a weighty choice. It necessitates thoroughly evaluating potential benefits and obstacles, considering your personal and professional objectives, comfort with autonomy, adaptability, and willingness to handle various business responsibilities. Moreover, consider your current life situation, available support, and the additional time investment required.

Getting the balance right for you

It doesn't have to be an all-or-nothing choice. Many therapists successfully balance private practice with part-time employed roles, reaping the benefits of both worlds.

In my book 'The Therapist Guide to Private Practice: Building a Values-Based Business' (2023), I don't start with the practical steps you need to take. Instead, I encourage people to consider why they choose this route and to begin with the end in mind.

Exercise

Picture your future private practice. What do you hope it will look like? What will you have achieved? Is it the ability to have more flexibility, the potential to earn more, or the freedom to work with specific client groups? Will you be working part-time, online or delivering workshops? Visualise your end game and let this vision guide your every step. See the space you've created, whether modern or cosy, filled with satisfied clients you're passionate about serving. What are the values you want to infuse your work? Recall your reasons for this journey. Then, write out your vision in as much detail as possible.

Reflective exercise: my future private practice – the vision

Top tips

- **Start with the End in Mind:** Your first year in private practice will demand more hours and may yield minimal rewards. Having a long-term vision can help you stay motivated.
- **Patience is Key:** Building a thriving private practice requires time and persistence. Whilst setting things up is one aspect, it takes time to establish your business, gain a solid caseload, build a strong reputation, and achieve a sustainable income. Be prepared for the journey.
- **Values:** are the bedrock of a business. They differentiate us from others, sharpen our message, and guide our every decision. Think of them as a sieve – ensuring our choices align with our goals, especially during challenging times.
- **Financial Uncertainty and Long Hours:** Starting your own practice often means facing financial uncertainty and working longer hours initially. Consider whether you're ready for these challenges and who in your support network is willing to join you on this journey.

The opportunities and obstacles

Opportunities

Imagine the freedom and potential private practice could offer you; at its core, it is about carving out your unique space in the vast therapeutic landscape. Picture this: You're not just a therapist but an entrepreneur. You set the rhythm of your days, decide when it's time for that well-deserved holiday, you choose the training courses that resonate with you and determine your own salary (you might throw in a bonus or two when you've outdone yourself!). The direction of your career? That's all up to you.

The beauty of private practice lies in its customisation. It's a canvas awaiting your unique touch. No more generic sessions, organisational constraints, or frustrating politics; instead, you can offer flexible, tailored therapeutic experiences that cater to your client's needs. When you face a challenging client or a tricky case, you can reach out to an expert in that area for guidance, just as I've done several times.

Instead of a one-size-fits-all approach, you can tailor your services for your clients with your clients, ensuring they align with what sets your heart on fire and it's not limited to traditional therapy. Have you ever thought of running a workshop? How about supervising other therapists or crafting online resources? The world is your oyster, opening doors to diverse revenue streams and passive income streams, which means you can earn even when you're not actually working. The possibilities are endless! It's an expedition of discovery, growth, and endless possibilities.

Obstacles

With great freedom comes its fair share of responsibilities. Stepping into private practice isn't just about enriching therapy sessions; it's also about diving head first into the intricacies of running a business. You're not just a therapist anymore; you are also a business owner. Your role pivots from being solely a service provider to a strategic thinker, ensuring the heartbeat of your practice is sustained by both impactful client outcomes and viable business strategies.

Setting up that inviting, comforting therapy space, gathering all the essential tools, and letting the world know about your unique practice on websites with professional branding and photographs and getting the word out about your practice don't come cheap; it's an investment, both in your time and money. Imagine juggling tasks from branding to billing, from drafting that perfect marketing message to ensuring your website echoes your unique voice. Those out-of-hour crises? They now land on your plate. And yes, those pesky administrative duties, legal checks, and ethical considerations? They're part of the package, too.

Whilst private practice can pave the way to financial independence, it doesn't happen overnight. It's a journey. Unlike the steady paycheck of employed roles, the financial landscape here is full of highs and lows. You're in the driver's seat, setting your rates, handling invoices, crunching taxes, and planning for those quieter times when client appointments might be sparse.

A realistic and warranted concern for therapists considering private practice is feeling isolated, especially if you enjoy the camaraderie of a team and the benefits of small talk during a coffee break. Yes, networking events and professional supervision can bridge this gap, but it's a facet to consider and plan for so you can sidestep it. My reality is that I've never felt more connected in my career.

The foundations of a private practice

Setting up in private practice is an exhilarating shift that demands preparation, planning, and the right support system. Picture it as standing at the shore of a vast sea; the enormity of the decision merges with the anticipation of the unknown. Yet, with planning and guidance, this journey becomes manageable.

If there is one thing that I wish I had prioritised at the start of my private practice, it would have been planning and developing a business plan. It's not essential to meticulously detail every aspect, but a considered, structured approach to setting up lays a robust groundwork for your private practice. A business plan is a live and evolving document and even in its simplest form, it trumps having no plan at all, leading to unnecessary setbacks and misdirection.

If you spent some time on the previous exercise, you should have a clear vision of your business in your mind's eye. Now it's time to get more details and explore the mission of your private practice.

- **The Strategy:** why will your private practice exist in the world? What is your vision, the mission you are on, the values you will uphold, and the goals you will be driving your private practice forward? The more clarity you have in this area, the more it will shine through in your messaging and attract your ideal clients. We often look at what others are doing in private practice and follow this but the more you can embrace your individuality, diversity, and uniqueness, the better because when people are choosing a therapist, they are choosing a person they connect with; if you try to appeal to everyone, you will appeal to no-one. This is called developing a business strategy and is what will set you apart in the therapeutic landscape.
- **Crafting Your Ideal Working Week:** The beauty of private practice is that you're at the helm of designing your week; ask yourself:

  - What will my ideal week resemble?
  - How many clients will I see?
  - Which days are strictly for work and which will be reserved for admin tasks or rest?

It's not merely about maximising client sessions; it's about ensuring you have the space for self-care, professional growth and the other myriad aspects of running your business. After all, a balanced therapist is a more effective one.

- **The first practical step in your plan:** Decide on the name of your private practice. Even if you don't decide to have a website straight away, I'd recommend you buy the domain name for your private practice – this is the online address where you would host a website; you can purchase a domain name for about £10 a year from platforms like 34SP or Namecheap.

- **Marketing and Sales Strategies:** How will clients find out about you? Will you register with referral companies, become an associate or focus on attracting self-funding clients? If it's the latter, you will need to set up a website and other visibility tools, such as social media platforms and online directories.
- **Websites:** Act as your digital storefront, the first glimpse potential clients get of your practice. It must reflect who you are, your services and how a potential client can contact you. However, a striking website is useless if it's buried in the vastness of the internet. This is where Search Engine Optimisation (SEO) steps in. SEO is about optimising a website to improve its visibility in search engine results, making it easier for people to find and access the site. This involves techniques like using relevant keywords, improving site speed and ensuring that it contains up-to-date, original, high-quality content, elevating your website's visibility and ensuring clients find you precisely when they seek your expertise.
- **Referrals and Collaborations:** Referrals are the heartbeat of any thriving private practice. Setting up a website can take three to six months to start working for you and bringing in regular referrals. Consider also forging relationships with other healthcare professionals, local schools, services, or community organisations. Will you be a sole practitioner, work in a group practice, or be an associate for a company? Collaborating with referral companies, working as an associate or aligning with insurance companies can help create a steady stream of clients.

> **Top tip:** Weigh the administrative demands and potential constraints such collaborations might present. For example, report writing can add on unpaid hours. Ensure each partnership aligns with your values and vision.

Conclusion

Running a private therapy practice is hard work. It's certainly not an easy option, so clarity on why you chose this path is important and will give you regular injections of motivation. With careful planning, hard work, and a commitment to your vision and goals, building a successful and fulfilling practice as a therapist is possible. By focusing on the key considerations outlined above and balancing all the opportunities and obstacles, you can take important steps towards achieving your dream of running your own private practice.

Running a private practice is not just about enhancing your income; it's a testament to your motivation, resilience, commitment to your work and business and ability to maintain this balance. Private practice demands more than therapeutic expertise. You need an entrepreneurial spirit, creativity, consistency, business acumen, and a genuine desire to make a difference.

Reflecting on my decade in private practice, the hours poured in and the obligations met were unparalleled. Yet the rewards went beyond the financial. It's brought exciting opportunities my way, given me full autonomy and facilitated deeper client relationships. Each time a new client walks into your office, it isn't a business win; it's an endorsement of all your hard work, expertise, professional standing and personal brand.

Private practice is as much about self-discovery as it is about professional growth. As you navigate this journey, remember to continually reassess, ensuring your path aligns with your vision and values. If you're ready for this challenge, surround yourself with people already in private practice for support and guidance and anticipate a transformative journey, both personally and professionally. The road might be challenging and feel long at times, but with determination, resilience, and belief, success is within reach. People choosing a therapist are choosing a person they can connect with and trust, so embrace your individuality and diversity and then your ideal clients who need your support can find you. Are you prepared to embrace all challenges and the possibilities of private practice? If so, exciting times await!

Key points

- **Financial considerations**: Draft a clear budget. Account for initial start-up costs, recurring expenses, expected income and projections for growth. Remember to factor in peaks and troughs in client appointments, which can fluctuate. Decide on the structure of your business:
- Will you be a sole trader or a limited company?
- Plan to inform the tax office, set up a business bank account and establish financial systems like invoicing and taking payments. Decide what you need to earn and the hourly rate you will charge clients.
- **Operational Plan:** Detail the day-to-day operations. Set up your insurance for seeing clients and the necessary policies and paperwork – for example, a 'therapy agreement', data protection policies, and cancellation policies.
- Where will your office be located?
- Will you employ anyone or work with an accountant?
- What's your plan for appointments, cancellations, data protection and emergencies?
- **Regulatory and Ethical Considerations**: Outline your strategy for ensuring all interactions comply with your professional code of conduct, local regulations, and the highest ethical standards of the therapy profession. This includes client confidentiality, data protection, and registering with the Information Commissioner's Office (ICO) if you are in the UK, risk management protocols, health and safety requirements, and a plan for continued professional development.
- **Getting Support and Mentorship:** A crucial step, yet often overlooked, is finding support and mentorship. Embarking on a private practice journey can feel

overwhelming. But remember, many have walked this path before you and their insights and experience will give you a real advantage. Join communities like 'Therapist Corner.co.uk', where fellow therapists share their experiences and lessons learned. Through this support, you gain invaluable insights and create a network of colleagues who understand your journey.

- **Review:** Set regular intervals, quarterly and annually, to review and tweak your business plan and strategy; this ensures you stay agile, adapting to changing circumstances and seizing new opportunities.

A flexible, values-based business plan, clear marketing, sound financial strategies, adherence to regulatory standards, and the value of mentorship are key to establishing a private practice. Regular reflection and adaptation will also ensure you navigate successfully.

Further reading

Data protection – https://ico.org.uk
Register your business – www.gov.uk/set-up-business
Therapists Register – https://babcp.com/CBTRegister/Search#/
Websites for therapists – https://pocketsite.co.uk/
Community Support – www.therapistscorner.co.uk/
DBS check -www.gov.uk/request-copy-criminal-record
Therapists Share their private practice journey www.therapistscorner.co.uk/s/
    therapist-spotlight
Referral sources – https://sarahdrees.co.uk/referral-sources-in-private-practice/
Setting up in private practice – https://sarahdrees.co.uk/setting-up-in-private-practice/
Work hour your hourly fee – https://pocketsite.co.uk/therapist-fee-calculator/

Reference

Rees, S. (2023). The therapist guide to private practice: Building a values-based business. Routledge.

Chapter 24

From surviving to thriving

Going the distance as a CBT therapist

Jason Roscoe

Introduction

The word 'thrive' is defined as growing, developing, or being successful, and each chapter within this book has sought to offer advice and guidance on how the trainee and newly qualified CBT therapist can continue to thrive in each step of their journey. Thriving therefore, will mean different things at different stages of the journey.

It is worth stating that thriving is not simply the product of an individual's efforts. Just as a flower needs water, sunlight, and soil to grow, we all require the correct conditions to survive the training course (reasonable service targets, helpful supervision, and high-quality teaching) and to thrive throughout our career once qualified. Figure 24.1 illustrates this interplay in the form of a 'thriving matrix'. The inner circle represents the *stages* that novices pass through when developing skills as a CBT therapist whilst the outer boxes represent the *processes* that are hypothesised to be key in supporting this. This final chapter summarises how this book can be used to assist trainees in moving through the stages by instigating and supporting the different processes.

Thriving from day one

Arguably, thriving as a CBT therapist begins before we submit the training application. We can use our initiative to download some journal papers that can help us with our interview preparation. We can request to meet with qualified CBT therapists or email course tutors to find out what it is really like to do this job. Chapters 1–4 contain a range of tips for getting off to the best possible start. Beyond this, the pathway to thriving or struggling, can be influenced by the first place that we practice our skills and meet with our clients. Limited access to rooms, poor technology, unsuitable venues, inadequate or infrequent supervision, limited opportunities to shadow qualified peers, insufficient reflection our own troublesome schemas, all impact on our capacity to thrive. Negative experiences at the start of our journey can dampen the enjoyment of learning new ideas and skills. Being able to see CBT 'work' is also crucial for our engagement with the models we routinely use. Chapters 8–10 are particularly relevant to combating these stressors.

DOI: 10.4324/9781003428527-28

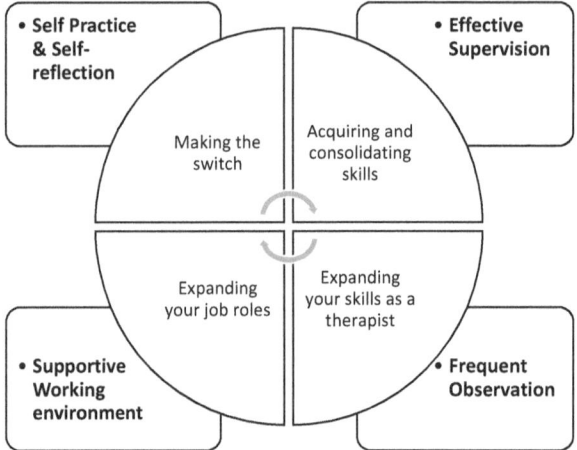

Figure 24.1 Thriving matrix

Thriving through self-reflection

Being reflective of our practice can be taken as a 'given', yet we are all prone to experiencing blind spots in our work as therapists. Effective use of supervision and continually applying CBT to our own personal and professional lives deepen our reflective capacity, paving the way towards engaging in behaviours that will help us in continuing to thrive (Bennett-Levy, 2019). This is particularly important given that the literature frequently highlights how therapists are especially vulnerable to burnout (e.g. Kaeding et al., 2017). The degree to which initiatives such as self-practice/self-reflection (SP/SR) are embedded within training courses varies considerably; therefore, Chapters 5–7 and 17–19 will help to 'kickstart' your reflective practice.

Thriving through inclusivity

We also thrive by learning to use CBT more flexibly whilst retaining its core features. This is especially important when we look to make CBT more inclusive to minoritised groups (Faheem, 2023). Thankfully, CBT training courses are making advances in this respect, embedding Equality and Diversity within teaching and assessment and involving experts by experience on interview panels and co-producing workshops. There is also a greater focus on adapting formulations and treatment plans to take account of individual differences. Chapters 11 and 12 provide excellent examples of ensuring that we practice CBT in an inclusive way.

Thriving as a profession

One way that we can help CBT 'as a whole' to thrive is by continuing to ask questions rather than passively accepting the status quo (e.g. being 'scientist-practitioners').

We need more clinicians contributing to research and sharing their clinical experiences through teaching the next generation of trainees. The 'shopfloor' experience that many CBT therapists possess is vital to help personalise teaching, strengthen supervision and target key areas for further research. The lived experience of CBT therapists is also important when it comes to designing new and more effective protocols.

Creating your own development plan to thrive

The final section of this chapter invites you to complete a personal development plan. Have a read through the notes you have made across the other chapters in the book to help you complete this. This will help you to 'zoom in' on aspects of your skill development that require specific attention now and in the future.

Reflective exercise

My 'surviving to thriving' development plan

Congratulations on making it through your training! Once you have had some time to adjust to life as a qualified therapist (e.g. bigger caseload, more contacts, more variety of presentations), have a go at answering the questions below to help you consider what the next 6–12 months will involve in terms of consolidating, fine-tuning, or expanding your skills and knowledge.

What are your current strengths and weaknesses as a CBT therapist? (e.g. perhaps you are good at implementing change methods in session but don't spend enough time on eliciting client feedback on homework tasks)

What are your priorities in terms of consolidating your understanding of CBT theories and interventions over the next six months? (e.g. which formulations can you draw out easily and which do you struggle with? Which techniques come easy to you and which do you struggle to understand/implement or try to avoid or delay using?)

What do you like and dislike about CBT? (your answers to this might help you to consider if it is the correct career path for you or it might help to identify topics that require further attention in supervision, attending CPD events or reading relevant research/book chapters)

How will you improve specific skills? (e.g. role-play in supervision and attend CPD events to plug gaps in knowledge and skills)

Conclusion

Thriving is not about being invincible – being a psychological therapist of any modality is hard work. Regardless of how long we have been qualified, it is the case for most of us that sometimes we feel that we make a real difference to another person's life, other times we can feel completely useless. That said, there are common problems that arise during CBT training (see Appendix 3), some of which persist beyond training if they are not addressed within supervision or through CPD. This is especially true when delivering CBT in contexts where our perceived worth is dependent on changes in arbitrary outcome measures (Roscoe, 2021). The frequently mooted 'Love yourself as a person, doubt yourself as a therapist' is very apt and having the capacity to treat ourselves with compassion is vital for trainees and experienced therapists alike (Nissen-Lie et al., 2017). The final point to make is that it is crucial that we never become complacent as we never reach a point as therapists where there is no more to learn. My advice is to stay humble, stay curious and stay in touch with your values, if you hold this in mind, you will not stray too far from the path towards thriving (see Skovholt & Starkey, 2010).

References

Bennett-Levy, J. (2019). Why therapists should walk the talk: The theoretical and empirical case for personal practice in therapist training and professional development. *Journal of Behavior Therapy and Experimental Psychiatry*, *62*, 133–145. https://doi.org/10.1016/j.jbtep.2018. 08.004

Faheem, A. (2023). 'It's been quite a poor show' – exploring whether practitioners working for improving access to psychological therapies (IAPT) services are culturally competent to deal with the needs of Black, Asian and Minority Ethnic (BAME) communities. *The Cognitive Behaviour Therapist*, *16*, E6. https://doi.org/10.1017/S1754470X22000642

Kaeding, A., Sougleris, C., Reid, C., van Vreeswijk, M. F., Hayes, C., Dorrian, J., & Simpson, S. (2017). Professional burnout, early maladaptive schemas, and physical health in clinical and counselling psychology trainees. *Journal of Clinical Psychology*, *73*(12), 1782–1796.

Nissen-Lie, H. A., Rønnestad, M. H., Høglend, P. A., Havik, O. E., Solbakken, O. A., Stiles, T. C., & Monsen, J. T. (2017). Love yourself as a person, doubt yourself as a therapist?. *Clinical Psychology & Psychotherapy*, *24*(1), 48–60.

Roscoe, J. (2021). Your worth is not your recovery rate. *CBT Today*, *49*(4), 7–9.

Skovholt, T. M., & Starkey, M. T. (2010). The three legs of the practitioner's learning stool: Practice, research/theory, and personal life. *Journal of Contemporary Psychotherapy*, *40*, 125–130.

Afterword

Lucy Hale

Background

The UK has a complex and diverse group of professions contributing to delivering cognitive behavioural therapy (CBT), including multiple psychological professions. NHS workforce planning policies (e.g. The Long-Term Plan, 2019; Psychological Professions Workforce Plan for England, 2021) call for evidence-based psychological therapies to expand faster than ever in several areas, including services for people with severe mental health problems, specialist eating disorder services, perinatal mental health services, and children and young people (see Lack et al., 2024). Given the Standards of Proficiency for Practitioner Psychologists stipulate that qualified clinical psychologists must be able to implement therapeutic interventions from a range of evidence-based models, including CBT (Health and Care Professions Council; HCPC, 2023), gaining recognised accreditation from the British Association of Behavioural and Cognitive Psychotherapies (BABCP) is one way to demonstrate that a recognised multi-professional marker of CBT competence is met.

This book has focused on one of the routes to accreditation in CBT (training as a CBT therapist). Recently, there has been an expansion of routes to accreditation in CBT through clinical psychology doctoral training programmes. It is hoped that this will increase the number of qualified clinical psychologists who can demonstrate that they have met recognised markers of specific competences in evidence-based psychological therapy nationally, to support recent NHS workforce planning policies.

Progress so far

The growth of clinical psychology doctoral programmes accredited to Level 2 with the BABCP has been progressing. Since 2022, the number of courses committed to delivering Level 2-BABCP-accredited pathways (between 2021 and 2026) has expanded from 5 to 22 (Lack et al., 2024).

There have been numerous strengths in relation to expanding routes to recognition in CBT competence through BABCP accreditation. Early work evaluating

DOI: 10.4324/9781003428527-29

trainee experiences ($n = 7$) of being on a CBT pathway as part of the Doctorate of Clinical Psychology at the University of Surrey used a focus group design to collect qualitative data. Results highlighted benefits such as the added value of audio recording routinely, in addition to detailed CBT-specific feedback and dedicated CBT supervision (Daley et al., 2022). The initial evaluation of the pathway highlighted the importance of integrating a trainee perspective to further develop this route to Level 2 accreditation. Further research is underway at the University of Surrey exploring the experiences of trainees, supervisors, and trainers involved in development and delivery of such pathways, as well as investigating the extent to which pathway graduates pursue and maintain their accreditation.

In addition to expanding pathways to accreditation in the trainee population, there have been drivers to increase the number of qualified clinical psychologists in the UK who meet the BABCP minimum training standards (MTS; BABCP, 2022) to become accredited cognitive behavioural psychotherapists. This directly supports the expansion agenda as these psychologists can then provide clinical supervision and teaching and assess academic work that facilitates the routes to trainee accreditation. In 2021, NHS England (NHS-E – formerly Health Education England) funded the development of a comprehensive, online CBT 'top-up' training and supervision programme for qualified clinical psychologists wishing to gain their BABCP accreditation across England and Wales. This has been led by clinical psychology programmes at the University of Oxford and the University of Exeter. The initial cohort of this training ran from 2022 to 2023 with 231 qualified applied psychologists taking part (see Lack et al., 2024).

Challenges

Lack et al. (2024) provide an overview of some of the key challenges facing the expansion work around routes to BABCP accreditation. Key issues include differences in access to BABCP-accredited practitioners needed to support pathways to accreditation. At the course level, there are various challenges in meeting the MTS requirements to gain accreditation. This requires time and knowledge to map existing programmes on to these specific requirements.

Two initial qualitative evaluations of a pathway to CBT accreditation on one clinical psychology programme ($n = 7$ in each) suggested that trainees noticed significant additional workload when they compared themselves to other trainees not on the pathway and highlighted that trainee beliefs about CBT, in addition to supporting trainees to apply CBT in complex settings relatively early on in training, were important (see Rodwell et al., 2023; Daley et al., 2022). Working closely with training providers to include trainers and supervisors is key when thinking about supporting trainees to develop sound CBT competence and be able to apply CBT to a range of difficulties in a way that is meta-competently adherent.

Opportunities

Expanding routes to accreditation has led to several opportunities to work collaboratively with professionals at local, regional, and national levels. Collaboration has helped to navigate some of the challenges through sharing information and proactive problem-solving together. At local level, collaboration across training clinical psychology doctoral programmes and postgraduate diploma programmes in CBT has enabled curricula to be delivered in line with the MTS (e.g. at the University of Surrey, see Daley et al., 2022). At regional and national levels, the expansion agenda has created opportunities for collaboration across networks both within the clinical psychology community and also more widely with the BABCP. An example of this is the development of a national working group within the Group of Trainers in Clinical Psychology (GTiCP). The group comprises people from different professional backgrounds (such as clinical and counselling psychologists and CBT therapists) with a shared passion for expanding routes to CBT accreditation in clinical psychology. NHS-E has also ring-fenced funding for courses developing routes to CBT accreditation to facilitate this process and support courses fund dedicated roles to set up and maintain the pathways to accreditation. This will support the feasibility and viability of developing such routes to CBT accreditation.

Initial evaluation work in this area highlights a wealth of opportunity that some of the expansion work has brought. Continuing to explore experiences of those involved in the development of pathways to accreditation could continue to be beneficial (e.g. Daley et al., 2022). This will not only support further development of pathways to accreditation but also refinement of processes around this for pathways already established.

Threats

Whilst the rapid growth in developing additional routes to accreditation with the BABCP shows promise, there are undoubtedly some limitations related to this expansion. Firstly, the capacity to accredit the numbers needed (both in terms of individual applications but also at course level) given current infrastructure within the BABCP has been a challenge. Diverse perspectives as to the value of CBT (both generally but also within clinical psychology) may also pose a threat to expanding routes to CBT accreditation (see Lack et al., 2024). In a recent exploratory study using a focus group design with trainee clinical psychologists, a theme that emerged was reluctance to apply CBT and how one's own beliefs about CBT might impact fidelity to the model and perceived value across healthcare settings (Rodwell et al., 2023). Such beliefs towards the model may impact how the model is viewed and valued more generally which could influence whether people support current expansion plans. Further research and understanding of this would be beneficial. Finally, the national divers for the expansion to routes to accreditation may also raise questions or even be a threat to professional identity. Whilst some research has highlighted the challenges of transitioning roles when in CBT training

(Wilcockson, 2020), developing research specifically exploring relationship to professional identity for clinical psychologists who also hold practitioner accreditation with the BABCP as a CBT therapist could be a fruitful line of enquiry.

Conclusion

The current expansion programmes to increase routes to CBT accreditation are ambitious and have been largely successful in their initial stages. The challenges moving forward will be to ensure that courses secure routes to Level 2 accreditation through pathways and whole cohort course accreditation. Continuing to monitor progress of this and exploration of potential threats to the expansion work will remain important. Research into the effect of the expansion of routes to accreditation will be crucial moving forward. This could be both impact in terms of the effect of CBT accreditation on practitioners' CBT practice and also the benefits to those accessing services.

References

BABCP. (2022). *Minimum training standards*. Retrieved March 3, 2024, from www.babcp.com/Portals/0/Files/About/BABCP%20Minimum%20Training%20Standards%200823.pdf?ver=2023-08-01-143802-047

Daley, J., Hale, L., & Patton, B. (2022). Clinical psychology trainees' experiences of following a specialised cognitive behavioural therapy (CBT) pathway accredited by the British Association of Behavioural and Cognitive Psychotherapies (BABCP): A pilot evaluation. *Clinical Psychology Forum, 349*, 28–34.

Health and Care Professions Council. (2023). *Standards of Proficiency for Practitioner Psychologists*. Retrieved February 6, 2024, from www.hcpc-uk.org/globalassets/resources/standards/standards-of-proficiency – practitioner-psychologists.pdf

Lack, S., Handley, R., Barr, L., Rivers, M., Patel, A., Coe, M., & Hale, L. (2024). CBT accreditation for clinical psychologists: A limitation or an opportunity to apply and maintain our organisational and systemic influence and leadership? *Clinical Psychology Forum, 375*. https://doi.org/10.53841/bpscpf.2023.1.371.4

NHS Long Term Plan. (2019). Retrieved December 19, 2023, from www.longtermplan.nhs.uk/wp-content/uploads/2019/01/nhs-long-term-plan-june-2019.pdf

Psychological professions workforce plan for England 2020/21–2023/24. (2021). Retrieved December 19, 2023, from www.hee.nhs.uk/sites/default/files/documents/Psychological%20Professions%20Workforce%20Plan%20for%20England%20-%20Final.pdf

Rodwell, D., Kent, T., & Hale, L. (2023). Trainee clinical psychologists' views on the facilitators and barriers to cognitive behavioural practice: A thematic exploration. *Clinical Psychology Forum, 362*, 64–70. https://doi.org/10.53841/bpscpf.2023.1.362.64

Wilcockson, M. D. (2020). Transition to cognitive behavioural therapy from different core professional backgrounds: three grounded theory studies. *The Cognitive Behaviour Therapist, 13*, E35. https://doi.org/10.1017/S1754470X20000331

Alignment to CBT scale

The scale has not been subject to a research trial and is based largely on observations of trainees across multiple cohorts in a single CBT training site. The scale is intended to aid self-reflection rather than to determine a 'cut-off score' for suitability.

The scale has five sections:

(1) *Receptiveness to structure*
(2) *Attitudes towards measurement*
(3) *Responsibility for change*
(4) *Use of sessions*
(5) *Capacity for tolerating distress*

Whilst there is no 'cut-off' score, the more that you identify with the questions, the more suited you might be to CBT as a career. Score each item based on the following:

0 – Not at all like me
1 – A little like me
2 – Quite like me
3 – Moderately like me
4 – Mostly like me
5 – Very much like me

Personal characteristic	*Score 0–5*

Receptiveness to structure

1. I like sessions to be focused on specific problems rather than talking about whatever is on the clients mind that day
2. I think it is important for clients to be set homework tasks between sessions
3. It is important that sessions do not overrun, even if this means interrupting a client

Attitudes towards measurement

4. It is important to have an objective measure of the effectiveness of therapy and questionnaires are helpful in achieving this
5. Diagnostic classification helps to pinpoint formulation and treatment plans
6. I like to follow evidence-based treatment plans rather than using my intuition about what the client needs from me

Responsibility for change

7. I do not have to have all the answers to my clients' problems to be of help to them
8. I can refrain from sharing my own personal experiences with clients
9. I do not try to persuade clients of the need to change

Use of sessions

10. I like to be active during therapy sessions rather than simply talking about a client's difficulties
11. I would enjoy going out into the community and helping clients to face their fears
12. I like being creative in how I help clients to make sense of their difficulties and to change their thinking and behaviour

Capacity for tolerating distress

13. I recognise that helping clients to change involves them facing difficult thoughts, emotions, memories, and bodily sensations
14. I am willing to encourage clients to talk about aversive life experiences such as rape, sexual abuse, or torture to help them process the memories
15. I can tolerate my own anxiety about the outcome of various interventions
16. I can help to contain the client if they become distressed or dissociated during therapy sessions

Supervision audit

Supervisory task	Every time	Every other time	Twice a year	Once a year	Never
Outcome monitoring: We review patient outcome measures to track progress and effectiveness of interventions used in therapy					
Direct observation of supervisee skills: Watching/listening to recordings of therapy sessions/sitting in on live sessions					
Use of active methods: Supervisor modelling, role-play, self-practice of CBT methods					
Mutual feedback: Formal review of goals, progress, supervisory alliance					

FAQ's during training and supervision

Problem	Question	Solutions
Delayed or absent agenda	'How do I contain them as *I can't get a word in edgeways?!*'	Ask yourself 'Is it me or is it them?' Is it due to the client talking at length in an unfocused way or it is your own resistance towards agenda setting?
Timekeeping	'Why do my sessions *always overrun*'	Set an agenda with no more than two to three items. Set an alarm to go off ten minutes before the session ends Learn to respectfully but assertively interrupt and focus the client.
Keeping sessions active	'*What is a change method?*'	A good CBT session has a beginning, middle, and an end. After undertaking a mood check and homework review the agenda should be set, with a plan on how to build on the previous session. The middle part should be the longest part of the session and is either spent formulating, teaching the client a new skill or testing out predictions.
Incomplete homework	'*What if they keep forgetting/avoiding?*'	Allow sufficient time to collaboratively set a homework task. Check they understand and agree with it. Consider barriers. Don't minimise the importance of it.
Client resistance	'*They keep saying "yes but, how do I manage this?"*'	Have you developed a shared understanding of their problems rather than offered your 'expert' opinion? Formulate and be curious about any resistance (e.g. what is the function of the behaviour?); Consider chair work to interview that 'part' of the client.

(Continued)

(Continued)

Problem	Question	Solutions
Lack of affect in the room	'How do I help them to access their emotions?'	Have you elicited the hottest cognition? Can you get them to close their eyes and relive a recent experience to allow greater access to their feelings? Can you do an experiment in the session to generate affect? Are you doing things to protect the client from experiencing strong emotions?
Client wants you to tell them what to do	'I've given the suggestions but they don't think any will work, what now?'	Resist the urge to always 'educate' or explain. Practice Socratic Dialogue. Formulate their helpless behaviour.
Collusion	'But their life really is terrible?'	Many reactions to adversity are understandable but not inevitable. Two people can experience the same type of trauma and react very differently. Always pick out the meaning of the event to the individual and explore the workability of their responses to it.

Index